DATE DUE

Neuroimmunoendocrinology

Chemical Immunology

Vol. 69

Series Editors

Luciano Adorini, Milan
Ken-ichi Arai, Tokyo
Claudia Berek, Berlin
J. Donald Capra, Oklahoma City, Okla.
Anne-Marie Schmitt-Verhulst, Marseille
Byron H. Waksman, New York, N.Y.

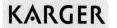

Basel · Freiburg · Paris · London · New York ·
New Delhi · Bangkok · Singapore · Tokyo · Sydney

....

Neuroimmunoendocrinology

3rd, revised and enlarged edition

Volume Editor   *J. Edwin Blalock,* Birmingham, Ala.

45 figures, 20 in color, and 17 tables, 1997

KARGER   Basel · Freiburg · Paris · London · New York ·
New Delhi · Bangkok · Singapore · Tokyo · Sydney

Chemical Immunology

Formerly published as 'Progress in Allergy'
Founded in 1939 by Paul Kallòs

Vol. 43 (1st edition)
Neuroimmunoendocrinology
Editors: J. Edwin Blalock; Kenneth L. Bost, Birmingham, Ala.
X + 166 p., 17 fig., 1 cpl., 13 tab., hard cover, 1988. ISBN 3–8055–4774–9

Vol. 52 (2nd edition)
Neuroimmunoendocrinology
Editor: J.E. Blalock, Birmingham, Ala.
XII + 196 p., 22 fig., 3 cpl., 14 tab., hard cover, 1992. ISBN 3–8055–5488–5

Cover illustration: Molecular structure of the interferon-γ receptor complex. Reproduced with permission from M.R. Walter et al., Nature 1995;376:230–235.

Bibliographic Indices. This publication is listed in bibliographic services, including Current Contents® and Index Medicus.

....
Contents

Structural Biology of Cytokines, Their Receptors, and Signaling Complexes: Implications for the Immune and Neuroendocrine Circuit

M.R. Walter, Birmingham, Ala.

Noradrenergic and Peptidergic Innervation of Lymphoid Organs

S. Y. Stevens-Felten, D. L. Bellinger, Rochester, N.Y.

Neuroendocrine Peptide Receptors on Cells of the Immune System

H. H. Garza, Jr., D. J. J. Carr, New Orleans, La.

Contents

Neuroendocrine Peptide Hormone Regulation of Immunity
B.A. Torres, H.M. Johnson, Gainesville, Fla.

Hormonal Activities of Cytokines
E.M. Smith, Galveston, Tex.

Interactive Signaling Pathways of the Neuroendocrine-Immune Network
T.L. Roszman, W.H. Brooks, Lexington, Ky.

Introduction to the 1st Edition

The study of interactions between the immune and neuroendocrine systems is a currently popular and rapidly advancing field which had its foundation in anecdotal observations of the association between 'personality' and disease. A measure of scientific credence was afforded to the area by the observation that, like many other physiologic responses, immune reactions could be conditioned in a classical Pavlovian fashion [1]. A possible mechanism was then found in Selye's [2] observation of thymic involution during 'stress'. The concept of the effects of stress on immunity turned out to be a two-edged sword. On the one hand, it provided a molecular basis, in the form of adrenal glucocorticoids, for neuroendocrine control of immunity. On the other hand, it led to the general and often currently held notion that steroid hormones are the sole players in neuroendocrine modulation of the immune system. Of course, recent studies have shown that this is clearly not the case since stressed adrenalectomized animals are functionally immunosuppressed [3]. Another impediment to the development of the area was the ability to have immunologic responses proceed in vitro. This inadvertently led to the idea that the immune system is a totally autonomous and self-regulating unit. If this were the case, then the immune system would be unlike all other organ systems. Furthermore, this view overlooks the rich hormonal milieu in which many in vitro immune responses occur. The end result of this series of events is the thought that if immune neuroendocrine interactions occur, they are mediated by steroid hormones. The picture has been further clouded by the predominance of studies of the psychological aspects of immune neuroendocrine interactions. Though it is not necessarily our view, such studies have given the field an aura of being a 'soft' science, thus the intent of *Neuroimmunoendocrinology* is to highlight the cellular and molecular aspects of this field.

References

1   Ader R: A historical account of conditioned immunobiologic responses; in Ader (ed): Psychoneuro-
    immunology. New York, Academic Press, 1981, pp 321–349.
2   Selye H: Thymus and adrenals in the response of the organism to injuries and intoxications. Br J
    Exp Pathol 1936;17:234–248.
3   Keller SE, Weiss JM, Schleifer SJ, Miller NE, Stein M: Stress-induced suppression of immunity in
    adrenalectomized rats. Science 1983;221:1301–1304.

J. Edwin Blalock, PhD, Department of Physiology and Biophysics, Center for Neuroimmunology,
The University of Alabama at Birmingham, 896 Basic Health Sciences Building,
1918 University Boulevard, Birmingham, AL 35294-0005 (USA)
Tel. (205) 934 6439, Fax (205) 934 1446, E-Mail: blalock@phybio.bhs.uab.edu

Introduction to the 2nd Edition

In the 3 years since the first publication of this volume, we have witnessed an explosion of information on immune neuroendocrine interactions. This has been evidenced by numerous international congresses, the inclusion of many symposia at the annual meetings of immunology, endocrinology, and neuroscience societies and the initiation of at least two new journals on the subject (i.e., *Progress in NeuroEndocrinImmunology* and *Advances in Neuroimmunology*). Among the highlights which have fueled the scientific growth of this discipline are: the tremendous increase in the number of neuroendocrine hormones and peptide neurotransmitters as well as their receptors which are endogenous to the immune system; the finding of cytokines such as IL-1 and IL-6 as well as their receptors in neural and endocrine tissues; and the profound effects of bidirectional communication between the immune and neuroendocrine systems on an animal's physiology. As an example, it is interesting to note that IL-1 is probably a more potent activator of the hypothalamic pituitary adrenal axis than is corticotropin releasing factor (CRF). Thus the paradox that without knowing it immunologists discovered a most potent 'hypothalamic releasing factor'. Contrariwise, CRF is a very effective inducer of IL-1. Thus, endocrinologists without knowing it discovered a cytokine. Such are the strange but exciting ironies of the development of a new discipline.

As a result of the great accumulation of new knowledge and the overwhelming success of the first edition, myself, and the coauthors have written the present revised edition of *Neuroimmunoendocrinology*. Once again, the emphasis is on the molecular, cellular, and physiologic aspects of immune neuroendocrine interactions. Because of the expansion of the literature in this area, most chapters and bibliographies are longer. It is our fondest hope that this volume will be a valuable resource to the evolution of this exciting new discipline.

J. Edwin Blalock, PhD, Department of Physiology and Biophysics, Center for Neuroimmunology,
The University of Alabama at Birmingham, 896 Basic Health Sciences Building,
1918 University Boulevard, Birmingham, AL 35294-0005 (USA)
Tel. (205) 934 6439, Fax (205) 934 1446, E-Mail: blalock@phybio.bhs.uab.edu

....

Introduction to the 3rd Edition

Interest in the area of immune neuroendocrine interactions has experienced unabated growth since the publication of the first edition of *Neuroimmunoendocrinology* in 1988. This interest, coupled with a continued expansion of information in this research discipline, made the first and second editions of this volume the most successful in the *Chemical Immunology* series with virtually every copy of the book being sold. As a result of this level of reader interest and a wealth of new data in the field, myself and the coauthors have written the present revised edition of *Neuroimmunoendocrinology*.

The third edition of this volume continues to emphasize the molecular, cellular and physiologic aspects of bidirectional communication between the immune and neuroendocrine systems. Most chapters have been extensively revised and expanded with up-to-date bibliographies which reflect the latest findings in the area. In addition, our present level of knowledge has allowed for the inclusion of a new chapter by Mark R. Walter on the structural biology of certain cytokines, hormones, and receptors which form the basis for part of the immune neuroendocrine circuitry. In this regard, it is particularly gratifying to now witness our first fascinating glimpses of the three-dimensional structures of signaling molecules and receptors which are shared by the nervous, immune, and endocrine systems.

In addition to the structural biology, there are numerous other highlights which should continue to fuel the growth of neuroimmunoendocrinology as a new discipline. Among these are a new and detailed understanding of the molecular regulation of cytokine genes in the central nervous system and molecular definition of hormone and neurotransmitter receptors that reside on immune cells. While the existence of peptide hormones and neurotransmitters in immunocytes has been known for some time, the last year has witnessed the first demonstration of nonpeptide neurotransmitters, catecholamines, being produced by T lymphocytes. New immunoregulatory functions have been assigned to hormones and neurotransmitters and novel hormonal activities have been associated with even more cytokines. Studies of the interactions of cytokines and neuroendocrine peptides are beginning. In particular, cortico-trophin-releasing factor was found to sensitize the pituitary gland to the direct action of IL-1 in terms of ACTH release. Perhaps most profoundly, in intact animals, lymphocytes have been shown to cause analgesia via corticotropin-releasing factor-induced production of β-endorphin which acts locally on sensory nerves. Thus, the immune system does seem to serve a sensory function and the neuroendocrine system has an immunoregulatory role. These are but a few of the exciting new developments which form the basis for the 3rd edition of *Neuroimmunoendocrinology* and portend an exciting future for this area of research.

J. Edwin Blalock, PhD, Department of Physiology and Biophysics, Center for Neuroimmunology,
The University of Alabama at Birmingham, 896 Basic Health Sciences Building,
1918 University Boulevard, Birmingham, AL 35294-0005 (USA)
Tel. (205) 934 6439, Fax (205) 934 1446, E-Mail: blalock@phybio.bhs.uab.edu

Blalock JE (ed): Neuroimmunoendocrinology, 3rd rev ed.
Chem Immunol. Basel, Karger, 1997, vol 69, pp 1–30

....
Production of Peptide Hormones and Neurotransmitters by the Immune System

Douglas A. Weigent, J. Edwin Blalock

Department of Physiology and Biophysics, University of Alabama at
Birmingham, Ala., USA

Introduction

Among the newly recognized similarities between the immune and neuroendocrine systems is the observation in both systems of an increasing number
of peptides and proteins that are used as intercellular messengers. The number
of neuroendocrine peptide hormones and peptide neurotransmitters found in
the immune system to date is listed in table 1. These molecules were largely
deemed to be endogenous informational substances for the system from which
they were originally isolated. Recent evidence, however, strongly supports the
notion that neuroendocrine peptides are endogenous to the immune system and
are used for both intraimmune system regulation, as well as for bidirectional
communication between the immune and neuroendocrine systems. The focus of
more recent studies has been to identify the factors involved in the lymphocyte
production of these substances as well as determine their role in immunity.
The findings suggest that there are both similarities and differences in the
lymphocyte production of these peptides compared to the neuroendocrine
system and that they may play pivotal roles in immunity.

Production and Structure of Leukocyte-Derived Peptide Hormones

Pituitary Hormones
Corticotropin (ACTH) was one of the first neuroendocrine peptide hormones to be described and was the first de novo synthesized hormone to be

Table 1. Stimuli for immunologically derived peptide hormones and neurotransmitters

Hormone or neurotransmitter	Stimuli	References
Corticotropin	Newcastle disease virus	2, 3, 10, 11
	lymphotropic viruses	13
	bacterial lipopolysaccharide	4, 15, 123, 140, 141
	corticotropin-releasing factor	66, 99, 100
	arginine vasopressin	66
	interleukin-1	100
	thymopentin	105
	cellular stress factors	59
	unknown	6
Endorphins	Newcastle disease virus	2, 3, 11
	bacterial lipopolysaccharide	4,16, 120, 147
	corticotropin-releasing factor	66, 99, 100
	arginine vasopressin	66
	interleukin-1	100
	psychoactive drugs	98
	cold water stress	148
Thyrotropin	staphylococcal enterotoxin A	22
	thyrotropin-releasing hormone	23, 24
Chorionic gondadotropin	mixed lymphocyte reaction	36
Luteinizing hormone	luteinizing hormone-releasing hormone	38–40
Follicle-stimulating hormone	concanavalin A	45, 46
Growth hormone	unknown	47
	growth hormone-releasing hormone	48
	thyrotropin	112
	growth hormone	49
	mitogens	54
Prolactin	concanavalin A	25–27
	retinoic acid	109
	unknown	28–30
Corticotropin releasing factor	unknown	56
	cellular stress factors	59
Growth hormone-releasing hormone	unknown	64, 65

Table 1 (continued)

Hormone or neurotransmitter	Stimuli	References
Luteinizing hormone-releasing hormone	unknown PHA PRL, TPA	60–62 115 63
[Met]enkephalin	concanavalin A	19
Arginine vasopressin	unknown	77, 78
Oxytocin	unknwon	77, 79
Neuropeptide Y	unknown	75
Vasoactive intestinal peptide	histamine liberators hypersensitivity unknown	67 69 70, 71
Somatostatin	hypersensitivity unknown	69 68, 70
Substance P	unknown	76
Parathyroid hormone-related protein	human T cell lymphotropic virus I	82
Calcitonin gene-related peptide	hypersensitivity	69
Insulin-like growth factor	growth hormone	85
Suppressin	concanavalin A	92
Neuroimmune protein	developmental concanavalin A bacterial lipopolysaccharide	96 95 95

found in the immune system [1, 2]. ACTH is a 39 amino acid peptide whose production is primarily associated with the pituitary gland and whose classical action is to elicit a glucocorticoid response from the adrenal glands during times of stress. In the immune system, human peripheral blood lymphocytes and mouse spleen cells were initially observed to express an ACTH-like peptide following virus infection or interaction with transformed cells or bacterial lipopolysaccharide (LPS) [2–4]. In contrast to the inducible synthesis of ACTH and endorphins by most lymphocytes, a subpopulation of mouse splenic macrophages, as well as some rat lymphocytes in the tunica propia, produced these peptides in a constitutive fashion [4–6]. More recently, the presence of proopiomelanocortin (POMC)-like mRNA and the ACTH peptide have also been identified in murine Thy1+ dendritic cells by Northern blot analysis and immunostaining, respectively [7]. Pituitary ACTH is derived from a large precursor protein, POMC, which contains the endogenous opioid peptides, endorphins [8]. Likewise, leukocyte-derived endorphins are coordinately expressed along with ACTH, and this is most likely due to their derivation from POMC. In fact, there would seem to be no other source for these peptides, since all ACTH and endorphins are derived from a single POMC gene. Among the many shared characteristics between immune system and pituitary-derived ACTH and endorphins are: shared antigenicity as determined with monospecific antibodies against synthetic peptides hormones; identical retention times on reverse-phase, high-performance liquid chromatography (HPLC) columns; identical molecular weights; and shared biological activities [9, 10] and the presence of POMC-related mRNA in lymphocytes and macrophages [6, 11–17]. The identity between pituitary and leukocyte ACTH has been unequivocally established by demonstrating that the amino acid and nucleotide sequences of mouse splenic and pituitary ACTH were identical [15, 16]. Although previous reports have identified truncated forms of POMC mRNA, a more recent analysis has demonstrated that mononuclear cells also produce full-length POMC transcripts [18]. Primer extension analysis identified a band which migrated with a size equivalent to a full-length POMC transcript in mitogen-stimulated mononuclear cells. The presence of all three POMC exons was confirmed by the sequence analysis of 5'-RACE-tailed PCR products. Cells of the immune system also seem to synthesize another family of endogenous opiates, the enkephalins, that are related to the endorphins. Abundant levels of preproenkephalin mRNA have been found in mitogen- or antigen-activated but not resting T helper (h) cells. This mRNA represented from 0.1 to 0.5% of the total mRNA depending on the particular T_h line which was induced. The mRNA was apparently translated and the product was secreted since immunoreactive (ir) [Met] enkephalin was detected in T_h cell culture supernates [19]. The results with human peripheral blood mononuclear cells show that primary cells also express preproenkephalin mRNA and that monocytes, but not T cells, process the propeptide to met enkephalin [20]. By RT-PCR it has reently been demonstrated that T helper 2 cytokines IL-4 and IL-10 are more potent in upregulating preproenkephalin mRNA expression in human PBL than the T helper 1 cytokines IL-2 and IFNγ [21]. Therefore, at the site of inflammation, it appears that local immune networks of opioid peptides and cytokines may influence inflammation and pain.

Thyrotropin (TSH) was the first de novo synthesized glycoprotein hormone to be found in the immune system. Its induction was initially observed in response to activation of human peripheral blood cells by a particular T-cell mitogen, staphylococcal enterotoxin A (SEA) [22]. More recently, TSH has been shown to be constitutively produced by human T-cell leukemia lines [23]. In these studies, the lymphocyte-derived TSH was recognized by a monospecific antibody to TSH-β and was shown to have the same molecular weight as pituitary TSH. Further, the intact molecule was shown to be composed of two polypeptide chains of the molecular weight of TSH-α and TSH-β. Whether the immune system-derived hormone is biologically active and will stimulate thyroid cells remains to be established. With regard to identity with the pituitary hormone, TSH-β-related mRNA has been observed in human and mouse lymphocytes [23, 24].

The idea that lymphocytes could serve as a source of PRL was first suggested when it was reported that concanavalin A (ConA) could induce lymphocyte production of a prolactin-related mRNA [25] and prolactin-like molecules [26]. The mRNA (10 kb) was larger than that in the pituitary gland [25] and the lymphocyte associated prolactin-like molecule had a molecular weight of 48 kD compared to pituitary prolactin of 23–24 kD [27]. Friesen and co-workers [28–30] have conclusively demonstsrated the presence of prolactin and its mRNA in an IM9 human B lymphoblastoid cell line. The IM9 mRNA was 150 nucleotides longer than the pituitary transcript due to an elongation of the 5′ untranslated region. This extension resulted from the use of a new 5′ noncoding exon that was 5–7 kb upstream of the human pituitary prolactin gene exon 1. In contrast to de novo synthesis, Clevenger et al. [31] reported that IL-2-stimulated T lymphocytes accumulated prolactin by internalization from the culture medium. Thus, at present it would appear that there are at least three mechanisms for prolactin association with cells of the immune system: (1) active uptake from extracellular fluids; (2) constitutive production by lymphoid cells, and (3) antigen- or mitogen-induced synthesis from lymphocytes. Since these early observations, several groups have reported the presence of a PRL RNA in lymphocytes that is similar to pituitary RNA by restriction [32] and sequence analysis [33, 34]. There appears, however, to be considerable size heterogeneity with protein products ranging from 11 to 36 kD and 46 to 60 kD [34, 35]. The size variations observed in these proteins may be due to posttranslational modification, including proteolysis, glycosylation, and aggregation.

Interestingly, mixed lymphocyte reactions (MLR) result in T-cell mitogenesis but unlike SEA or ConA do not evoke the production of TSH or prolactin. Rather, this allogeneic stimulus results in the production of an ir chorionic gonadotropin (CG) [36]. CG production, as monitored by immunofluorescence with antibody to CGβ, paralleled the blastogenic response of the MLR. Gel filtration of the de novo synthesized lymphocyte-derived CG showed that this material comigrated with the human (h)CG standard at a molecular weight of approximately 58 kD. This molecule was apparently glycosylated since it bound to a ConA affinity column. The lymphocyte-derived CG was also dissociable into two subunits of the molecular weight of CGα and β, 32 and 18 kD, respectively. The material from the MLR was biologically active since it elicited testosterone production from Leydig cells and this activity was neutralized by antiserum to CG. The finding that mouse, as well as human, lymphocytes produce CG is important since controversy lingers as to whether mouse placentas produce the molecule. The results with the murine MLR would seem to support the notion that rodents have the equivalent of hCG. The presence of lymphocyte CG has also been studied by two-color immuno-histochemistry in sections of human thymus [37]. Immunolabeling of lympho-cytes for hCG was found especially in the medulla of the thymus as well as in peripheral lymphoid organs.

Besides CG, two other gonadotropins have been found in the immune system. In response to luteinizing hormone (LH)-releasing hormone (RH), human [38, 39], mouse [40, 41] and porcine [42–44] lymphocytes were shown to synthesize and release irLH. The lymphocyte-derived LH-shared antigenicity, molecular mass, subunit structure, glycosylation and reverse-phase HPLC profile with the pituitary hormone [38]. Most recently, the amino-terminal sequence of the lymphocyte LHβ chain was shown to be identical to LHβ [Smith, pers. commun.]. An ir follicle-stimulating hormone (FSH) was also detected in cultured rat lymphocytes [45]. The levels of this hormone were markedly elevated by a T-cell mitogen (ConA) and the biologically active irFSH existed in two molecular weight forms. One form was quite similar to pituitary FSH (30 kD) while the other (54 kD) was not [46]. Collectively, these data show that a number of different animal species' leukocytes can produce the three principal gonadotropins (i.e. CG, LH, and FSH).

All of the aforementioned peptide hormones have required an inductive event for their synthesis by lymphocytes. In contrast, splenic lymphocytes spontaneously produce growth hormone (GH) mRNA after about 4–6 h of in vitro culture [47]. Thus, in vivo the lymphocyte GH gene must be under tonic suppression. In spite of this spontaneous production, GHRH [48] as well as GH [49] marginally augmented lymphocyte GH synthesis. GH-related RNA has been detected in cells from spleen, thymus, bone marrow, and peripheral blood [50]. The production of GH by rodent and human lympho-cytes as well as cell lines has been reported in a number of studies [25, 49, 51–54]. The mRNA has the same molecular weight as GH mRNA and is translated into a 22-kD biologically active irGH [47]. In addition, we have cloned and sequenced a cDNA from rat lymphocytes corresponding in se-quence to that obtained for the four exons of pituitary GH cDNA [55]. Similar findings have been obtained in the human Burkitt lymphoma Ramos cell lines [52].

Hypothalamic Releasing Factors

In general, each pituitary hormone is positively regulated by a given releasing hormone from the hypothalamus. Evidence has recently accumulated suggesting that a similar situation may exist in the immune system. Stephanou et al. [56] were the first to demonstrate a hypothalamic releasing factor-like peptide in leukocytes. They found an ir corticotropin-releasing factor (CRF), also referred to synonymously as corticotropin-releasing hormone (CRH), in human lymphocytes and neutrophils which eluted earlier than standard CRF on HPLC. The lymphocyte CRF-like mRNA was 1.7 kb in comparison with the 1.5 kb mRNA for hypothalamic CRF. More recent work suggests that the molecule produced in the rat thymus and spleen and human T lymphocytes is structurally similar to hypothalamic CRF but that the regulation of the synthesis of lymphocyte CRF is different [57, 58]. The ability of human lymphocytes and mouse splenocytes to secrete CRF in vitro in response to hyperthermia, hyperosmolarity and hypoxia has also been shown [59]. Although originally identified as the central regulator of the hypothalamic-pituitary-gonadal axis, Emanuele et al. [60] demonstrated a biologically active irLHRH from lymphocytes that was indistinguishable from hypothalamic LHRH. Furthermore, the irLHRH was apprently encoded by LHRH mRNA [61], and we have found that the sequences of hypothalamic and lymphocyte LHRH are identical [62]. The level of irLHRH, approximately 500 pg/20 × 10^6 lymphocytes, represented about 15% of the entire spleen content since 100–120 × 10^6 lymphocytes were obtained per splenic preparation. As such, the amount of irLHRH in spleen is quite comparable to that of single whole rat hypothalami. In other studies using the rat Nb2 T cell line, Wilson et al. [63], in addition to full-length LHRH messenger RNA, identified an alternatively spliced LHRH messenger RNA in cells stimulated with PRL. The smaller LHRH transcript could produce a truncated GnRH-associated peptide that may serve as a negative regulator for the pituitary and/or the local production of PRL. The LHRH messenger RNA has a very short half-life and uses the same transcription start site as the hypothalamus [63].

Rat lymphocytes also synthesized and released relatively large amounts (200 pg/mg protein) of irGHRH as compared to hypothalamic cells (1,000 pg/mg protein) [64]. Once again, when we consider the greater protein content of the spleen relative to the hypothalamus, the potential RH output of these two organs is of the same order of magnitude. Northern gel analysis showed that lymphocyte GHRH-related RNA was polyadenylated and of the same molecular mass (0.8 kD) as GHRH mRNA [65]. The 5-kD irGHRH bound the GHRH receptor and increased GH mRNA synthesis in pituitary cells. Collectively, these studies demonstrate the production of hypothalamic RHs by immunocytes. Since immunocytes also contain the pituitary hormones that are regulated by these hypothalamic releasing factors, the data suggest that the immune system may regulate itself by using peptides that are analogous to those of the hypothalamic-pituitary axis. This idea is made particularly attractive by the observation that CRF can elicit lymphocyte ACTH production [66] and GHRH can elevate levels of lymphocyte GH [48].

Neuropeptides

In addition to the pituitary hormones and their releasing factors, a number of neuropeptides have been isolated from cells of the immune system. Vasoactive intestinal peptide (VIP) and somatostatin (SOM) have been immunologically detected in platelets, mononuclear leukocytes, mast cells and polymorphonuclear (PMN) leukocytes [67–71]. Although the amino acid sequences have not been completed, the immune-derived SOM_{28}, appears to be larger than the authentic neuropeptide [69] and to have a similar but not identical amino acid composition [68]. The presence of SOM-specific mRNA in spleen and thymus has been documented by the S1 nuclease protection assay whereas the protein has been identifed by immunocytochemistry [72]. The presence of this hormone has been confirmed recently by showing that cell proliferation is increased by eliminating the expression of lymphocyte SOM with antisense oligodeoxynucleotides [73]. VIPs from rat basophilic leukemia cells consist of VIP_{10-28} free acid and a mixture of amino terminally extended 'big' VIPs, which are apparently obtained from a novel prepro-VIP encoded by an alternately spliced mRNA [69].

High levels of neuropeptide tyrosine (NPY) and its RNA have been found in rat peripheral blood cells, bone marrow, and spleen. A combination of in situ hybridization and immunocytochemistry was used to show that the NPY-like material was present in megakaryocytes (i.e. platelet precursors) [74]. Neuropeptide Y mRNA expression has been reported in human peripheral blood mononuclear cells and lymphoid tissues by RT-PCR [75]. The PCR products had the expected size and Northern blotting demonstrated the presence of the 0.8 kb NPY mRNA. Another cell type, macrophages, were recently shown to synthesize ir substance P and its mRNA [76]. Arginine vasopressin (AVP), oxytocin, and neurophysin are detectable in a lymphoid-associated organ, the thymus, although they are apparently not localized to lymphocytes [77, 78]. The apparent source of these ir peptides are thymic 'nurse' cells [79]. Using immunocytochemical staining with antiserum to AVP, both plasma cells and IgG-negative smaller cells in rat spleen were found to be positive [80]. Thymus extracted oxytocin and neurophysin eluted in the same position as reference standards on Sephadex G-75. The authenticity of oxytocin was also confirmed by biological assay and HPLC analysis. irAVP coeluted with the authentic peptide on reverse-phase HPLC [78].

A number of other neuroendocrine peptides, including parathyroid hormone-related protein [81, 82], calcitonin gene-related peptide [69], and insulin-like growth factor I (IGF-I) [83–87], have also been shown to be synthesized by or associated with cells of the immune system. Another report has appeared showing that endotoxin induces parathyroid hormone-related protein gene expression in splenic stromal and smooth muscle cells but not in lymphocytes [88]. The continuing studies with IGF have confirmed the expression of lymphocyte insulin-like growth factors and identified their binding proteins in human PBL using RT-PCR and Western ligand binding [89]. Kelley and co-workers have shown that developing macrophage express IGF-1 receptors and transcribe class I IGF-1 mRNA transcripts [86]. Macrophages can also be a source of IGF-1 binding proteins [87]. These data are consistent with an important role for the IGF system during development and/or inflammation. Thus, when one considers the number of molecules so far identified, it seems likely that virtually all known neuroendocrine peptides or proteins will be found in the immune system.

New Substances

In addition to known neuroendocrine peptides and proteins, a move is afoot to identify novel molecules that are associated with the neuroendocrine and immune systems. Two different approaches have been successfully employed. First, a neuroendocrine tissue, the pituitary gland, was evaluated for the presence of new immunoregulatory substances. This led to the discovery of a novel (63 kD) protein, suppressin, which inhibited the growth of transformed and normal lymphoid and neuroendocrine cells, enhanced natural killer cell activity, and induced interferon [90–92]. The suppressin-producing population in the pituitary was composed of somatotrophs, lactotrophs, corticotrophs, thyrotrophs, and mammosomatotrophs, while gonadotrophs did not produce suppressin. In studies specifically with lactrotrophs, suppressin production was observed primarily in non-PRL-secreting lactotrophs or in lactotrophs secreting a high amount of PRL, suggesting a potential regulatory relationship between the synthesis and secretion of suppressin and PRL [93]. Suppressin was subsequently shown also to be synthesized by lymphocytes. Suppressin is found intracellularly in all unstimulated lymphocyte subsets, monocytes, and in phytohemagglutinin-activated T lymphocytes immunopositive for the low-affinity IL-2 receptor. The biological actions of suppressin in vitro include the inhibition of mitogen-induced proliferation and immunoglobulin synthesis of lymphocytes and the suppression of IL-2-dependent CTLL-2 cell proliferation. These results suggest that suppressin may be a major negative regulator of cell proliferation in the immune system [94].

The second approach involved the use of selective hybridization and molecular cloning to isolate cDNA derived from genes expressed predominantly in the neuroendocrine and immune systems. Two such rat genes, named neuro-immune 1 and 2, were identified [95, 96]. Sequence analysis showed that the gene products were unique and hybridization studies suggest that neuroimmune 1 protein may play a role during early postnatal neural development. It is anticipated that these two approaches and others will eventually lead to the discovery of a number of new peptides and proteins that are involved in immune neuroendocrine interactions. Interestingly, there are now data showing that lymphocytes can synthesize catecholamines [97]. Lymphocytes appear to utilize the classical pathway of catecholamine synthesis and T lymphocytes appear to be the major producers. The biological significance of this finding and its mechanism of action or role in immunity requires further study [97].

Regulation of Leukocyte-Derived Peptide Hormones

With regard to those peptide hormones that have been shown to be inducibly synthesized by lymphocytes in response to immunostimulants, a possibly interesting pattern seems to emerge. That is, in many instances, a given stimulus results in a particular hormone (table 1). For instance, LPS, SEA, and MLR induce ACTH, TSH and CG, respectively. If this pattern continues to be followed and expanded then in the future we may be able to assign certain aspects of the pathophysiology of infectious diseases and tumors to a particular hormone or group of hormones that are produced by the immune system. Thus, changes in adrenal function during bacterial and viral infections might in part be associated with leukocyte ACTH while changes in thyroid function might occur during cell-mediated immune responses and involve T-cell production of TSH.

In addition to immunoregulation of leukocyte-derived hormones, there are also control elements that are similar to those in the hypothalamic pituitary axis. For instance, β-endorphin follows a circadian rhythm though it differs from the pituitary [98]. In the central axis, the anterior pituitary gland contains at least five different types of secretory cells with each cell type containing a minimum of one hormone formed in this gland. Production and secretion of a particular hormone by anterior pituitary cells is controlled by a specific hormone from the hypothalamus. These are termed hypothalamic releasing factors or hormones and are usually controlled in a negative fashion by end products of the particular neuroendocrine cascade. Thus, glucocorticoid hormones, for example, suppress pituitary ACTH production and release. Cells of the immune system, in addition to responding to immunostimulants, also respond with fidelity to the classical hypothalamic regulators of anterior pituitary hormones (table 2). For instance, CRF was observed to cause the de

Table 2. Pituitary hormones and their hypothalamic releasing factors

Hypothalamic releasing factor	Hormone	Pituitary cell type	Lymphocyte response to releasing factor
Corticotropion releasing factor	corticotropin	corticotroph	marked elevation of corticotropin
Growth hormone-releasing hormone	growth hormone	somatotroph	marginal elevation of growth hormone
Thyrotropin-releasing hormone	thyrotropin	thyrotroph	marked elevation of thyrotropin
Luteinizing hormone-releasing hormone	luteinizing hormone	gonadotroph	marked elevation of luteinizing hormone
Vasoactive intestinal peptide[1]	prolactin	lactotroph	not tested

[1] Derived from lactotroph rather than hypothalamus.

novo synthesis and release of leukocyte-derived ACTH and β-endorphin in vitro [66] and in vivo [99]. While it occurred at about 10-fold higher concentrations, AVP (a less potent regulator of pituitary ACTH) alone was also observed to have intrinsic CRF activity on leukocytes. At concentrations that are frequently used on cultured pituitary cells, CRF and AVP together acted in an additive fashion to induce POMC-derived peptides and such induction was blocked by the synthetic glucocorticoid hormone, dexamethasone. Thus, on the surface, leukocytes seem quite similar to corticotrophs with respect to control of the POMC gene by CRF and AVP and feedback inhibition by a synthetic glucocorticoid hormone. Upon closer exmination, however, it was found that both the actions of CRF as well as dexamethasone were indirect (fig. 1). Heijnen and co-workers [100] have shown that CRF actually causes IL-1 production by macrophages and that the IL-1, rather than CRF, then elicits POMC production by B lymphocytes. The production of IL-1 in response to CRF is particularly interesting since the converse occurs in hypothalamic neurons. That is, IL-1 causes CRF release [101]. This observation was soon extended to CRF release in vivo, and a controversy ensued [102]. In vivo, the IL-1-mediated release of pituitary ACTH appeared to be indirectly mediated through the ability of IL-1 to cause hypothalamic CRH release, rather than through a direct effect on the pituitary gland. This, of course, was in marked contrast to the numerous reports of the ability of IL-1 to directly

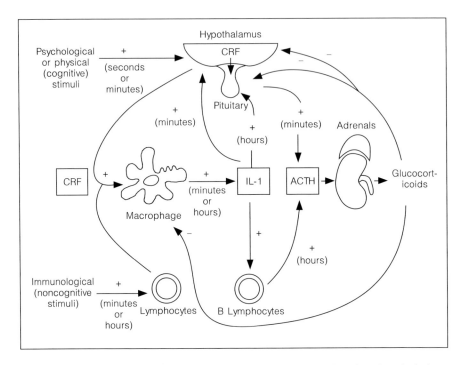

Fig. 1. Potential interplay of IL-1 and CRF in the lymphoid adrenal and pituitary adrenal axes. Cognitive or noncognitive stimuli are recognized by the nervous or immune systems, respectively, and hypothalamic or lymphoid CRF is released. CRF can in turn cause IL-1 release from macrophages or ACTH release from the pituitary gland. IL-1 can then elicit CRF from the hypothalamus and ACTH from the pituitary or B lymphocytes. ACTH then evokes a glucocorticoid response which can feedback inhibit IL-1 production from macrophages, CRF from the hypothalamus or ACTH from the pituitary. + = Positive response; − = inhibitory response; ( ) = the time required for the response. Reproduced with permission from Blalock [102].

cause ACTH production from pituitary cells [see Smith, this vol., for details]. This controversy has recently been resolved by the observation that hypothalamic CRH, released in response to IL-1, causes both the direct release of pituitary ACTH and sensitizes the pituitary gland to the direct ACTH-releasing activity of IL-1 [103].

Like CRH, glucocorticoids were shown to act indirectly by blocking macrophage production of IL-1 instead of B-cell POMC itself [104]. These findings collectively suggest that the POMC gene in B lymphocytes is regulated differently from that in pituitary cells. In fact, we have shown that lymphocytes basally transcribe at least two POMC transcripts that are upregulated by CRF

Table 3. Effect of hormones on lymphocyte and pituitary PRL synthesis

Hormone	Lymphocyte PRL	Pituitary PRL
Dexamethasone	–	–
Dopamine	0	–
Triiodothyronine	0	+
TRH	0	+
VIP	0	+
EGF	0	+
Estrogen	–	+
Progesterone	–	0
Retinoic acid	+	ND
PRL	–	ND

+ = Enhancement; – = suppression; 0 = no effect; ND = not determined.

presumably via IL-1 [17]. Of the 3 exons of POMC, the two lymphocyte mRNAs lacked exons 1 and 2 but contained either most or all of exon 3 which encodes most POMC-derived peptides (including ACTH) [16]. Since lymphocytes do not directly respond to CRF we initially considered that this transcriptional difference resulted from the B lymphocyte use of an IL-1, rather than CRF, control element for the POMC gene. If this were the case, one would expect IL-1 to cause alternate transcription initiation in pituitary cells. However, pituitary cells upregulate only the expected 1-kb (3 exon) mRNA in response to either CRF or IL-1 indicating some other cause for the truncated mRNAs in lymphocytes [Galin, LeBoeuf, Blalock, unpubl. obs.]. Mononuclear cells can produce full-length POMC mRNA after ConA treatment [18], suggesting that the nature of the POMC product produced in the immune system is dependent on the cell type, the microenvironment as well as the nature of the stimulus [105, 106]. Based on these findings, it is tempting to speculate on the alternative explanation that some genetic rearrangement in proximity to the lymphocyte POMC gene leads to altered transcription initiation. Concomitant with this postulated rearrangement there is the apparent loss of the glucocorticoid regulatory element. Such rearrangement could easily be envisioned in the mouse B lymphocyte since the immunoglobulin heavy chain locus as well as the POMC gene are both located on chromosome 12.

It appears the mechanisms controlling lymphocyte PRL and pituitary PRL differ markedly (table 3). Early studies showed that mitogen stimulation increases the expression of lymphocyte PRL [25]. It has been shown that the synthesis of lymphocyte PRL mRNA is inhibited by phorbol ester whereas the expression of pituitary PRL is enhanced [107]. Most of the hormones that modulate PRL secretion by the pituitary gland, e.g. estradiol, TRH, prostaglandin, VIP, EGF, dopamine and insulin have no effect on PRL expression by IM-9-P3 [108]. Dexamethasone inhibits both pituitary and lymphocyte PRL production by producing a four-fold reduction in the half-life of PRL mRNA. On the other hand, retinoic acid increases the stability of the PRL transcript in lymphoid cells [109]. Alternative promoter usage appears to be the basis of the tissue specificity of hormonally regulated PRL expression [110]. For the expression of lymphocyte GH, however, lymphocytes appear to use the same first exon and promoter as the pituitary. In studies with GH promoter constructs coupled to luciferase, we have data in lymphocytes to suggest that overexpression of GHRH is able to increase luciferase expression [Weigent, unpubl. obs.]. Despite this, there are also differences along with similarities between the expression of lymphocyte and pituitary GH. Thus, in both tissues, GHRH stimulates, whereas SOM inhibits, GH synthesis [48]. IGF-1 also suppresses lymphocyte GH synthesis [85], although another group [111] found it ineffective in this regard. The in vitro culture of rat splenocytes and thymocytes results in spontaneous lymphocyte GH gene transcription, with maximal levels of GH mRNA being attained within only 8 h. Furthermore, exogenous GHRH augments endogenous GH secretion by nonstimulated and phytohemagglutinin (PHA)-stimulated peripheral blood mononuclear cells [111]. Thyrotropin also stimulates the release of GH from lymphocytes, whereas dexamethasone is inhibitory in this regard [112]. Both T- and B-cell mitogens enhance lymphocyte GH expression [113]. Pit-1 is expressed in human and rat lymphoid tissues and cell lines, and our findings that the expression of GH in lymphocytes from dwarf animals is near normal [114] thus raise the possibility that another protein may substitute for Pit-1 in immune cells. It has also been strongly suggested that Pit-1 has no role in the regulation of nonpituitary PRL gene expression [110].

With regard to other hormones, the following is known about regulation. Thyrotropin-releasing hormone (TRH) has been found to induce the synthesis of TSH in mouse leukocytes and the human T-cell leukemia cell line (MOLT-4) and such induction was blocked by T3 [23]. LHRH induction of lymphocyte LH is another example of hypothalamic RF control of an immune system hormone [38–40, 44]. LHRH increases in cells activated by PHA [115], PRL, TPA or pokeweed mitogen [63]. Another current study suggests that LHRH production by T cells is dependent on the activation of protein kinase C, protein tyrosine phosphorylation and calcium [116]. Thus, although there can be novel intermediates such as IL-1 involved, cells of the immune system seem quite similar to circulating pituitary cells with respect to their ability to positively respond to hypothalamic releasing factors and to have such responses blunted by the appropriate neuroendocrine end products of the particular hypothalamic pituitary axis (table 2).

Processing of Leukocyte-Derived Peptide Hormones

Many peptide hormones and peptide neurotransmitters are synthesized as large prohormones that must be cleaved to release the active fragments. In the ACTH and endorphin system, this seems to result from cleavage of the precursor POMC at pairs of basic amino acids by a unique set of proteases. The site of POMC production can determine the final set of active peptides. For instance, in the anterior lobe of the pituitary gland, POMC is ultimately cleaved into an N-terminal fragment, ACTH(1-39) and β-lipotropin while the intermediate lobe ultimately yields γ-melanocyte-stimulating hormone (MSH), α-MSH, corticotropin-like intermediate lobe peptide (CLIP), γ-lipotropin and β-endorphin [117]. To date, pituitary proteases have been described which yield POMC-processing patterns which are similar, if not identical, to those seen in the anterior and intermediate lobes of the pituitary [118, 119]. The discovery of POMC production by cells of the immune system has led to the observation of processing pathways that are unique to leukocytes as well as composites of those observed in the anterior and intermediate lobe of the pituitary gland. With regard to previously described pituitary pathways, we have found that Newcastle disease virus (NDV) or CRF elicits the production of ACTH(1-39) and β-endorphin from cultured leukocytes [2, 66]. By Western blot analysis with specific antibody to ACTH, we have observed an increase in nonglycosylated ACTH, a biosynthetic intermediate as well as full-length POMC (31 kD) after mitogen treatment [18]. Others have shown that a subpopulation of mouse splenic macrophages spontaneously produce POMC which is processed into ACTH and β-endorphin [5]. In contrast, bacterial endotoxin or LPS treatment of leukocytes results in a novel processing pattern. It elicits the production of ACTH(1-25) [15] and endorphins which correspond to the molecular weight of α- or γ-endorphin from B lymphocytes [4, 120].

These findings point to some proteolytic cleavages of POMC as have been previously observed in the anterior and intermediate lobe of the pituitary as well as the hypothalamus. Of course, the results also suggest that cells of the immune system differ from virtually all other extrapituitary tissues where the major proteolytic cleavages are similar to those in the intermediate lobe of the pituitary gland [117]. The production of α-melanocyte-stimulating hormone (α-MSH) has been demonstrated in murine [121] and human [122] monocytic cell lines. The results suggest that the proinflammatory cytokine, tumor necrosis factor, can induce macrophages to increase the production of α-MSH which can modulate inflammation by inhibiting the production of nitric oxide. In another example, bacterial LPS induction of ACTH(1-25) suggests a quite novel processing pathway. In fact, we have demonstrated a B-cell-derived enzyme which may be responsible for this alternate processing. This protease is induced or activated by LPS and at pH 5 cleaves ACTH(1-39) to a form that comigrates with ACTH(1-24) on polyacrylamide gels [123]. Such differential processing points to cells of the immune system having processing pathways which are both unique and in some instances composites of those seen in the anterior and intermediate lobe of the pituitary gland. A further interesting implication of this work is the suggestion of a possible stimulus-specific B lymphocyte-processing mechanism for POMC. This could be quite different from previously described pathways which are largely determined by the cell type (i.e. intermediate vs. anterior lobe pituitary cells) in which the POMC is processed. Perhaps this is related to the level of maturity of the B cell. Within the immune system, such differential processing could have important immunoregulatory consequences. For instance, α- but not β-endorphin suppresses in vitro antibody responses while β- but not α-endorphin enhances T-cell mitogenesis [124, 125]. Also, ACTH(1-39) but not ACTH(1-24) suppresses in vitro antibody production [124]. Thus, the type of POMC stimulus may determine the processing pathway and ultimately the specific peptides which result. The specific peptide, in turn, then determines which immunologic cell type and function will be affected. Of course, the end result would be that different stimuli would elicit different responses via the same prohormone. Similarly, the isolation of distinct fragments of VIP(1-28) from lymphocytes, mast cells, and other leukocytes is another example of posttranslational peptidolysis [69]. In this system, the peptide variants bind differently to lymphocyte than to neural receptors, suggesting that each member of the VIP family may have a distinct immunoregulatory role [126].

In addition to having proteolytic processing enzymes, macrophages, at least, must also contain acetylating enzymes. This is based on the finding that while the major endorphin species in mouse spleen macrophages is endorphin (β-EP$_{1-31}$), there are smaller amounts of N-acetylated β-EP$_{1-16}$ (endorphin), β-EP$_{1-27}$ (γ-endorphin), β-EP$_{1-27}$ and β-EP$_{1-31}$ [12]. While the study of regulatory factors which control leukocyte-derived hormone genes and enzymes which posttranslationally modify their products are in their infancy, it is clear that this will be an important and exciting area of future investigation.

Immunologic Cell Types that Produce Peptide Hormones

Several reports have recently appeared on the production of peptide hormones by particular cell types within the immune system (table 4). Essentially, the cellular origin of the peptide depends on the particular hormone and the stimulus for production. For instance, when human peripheral blood cells are infected with NDV and all cells harbor the virus, then all cells produce POMC-derived peptides. Thus, in response to this stimulus, every major cell type (T and B lymphocytes, NK cells, and macrophages) has the potential to produce POMC-derived peptides [127]. On the other hand, when these cells are treated with bacterial LPS only, B cells produce the peptides [120]. Since all of the cells have the potential to produce this group of hormones, this is apparently an instance where the stimulus is only recognized by B lymphocytes and hence only these cells produce ACTH and endorphins. More recent work has identified a truncated form of POMC mRNA and ACTH and the parent POMC molecule with specific antibody immunostaining of Thy-1+ dendritic cells of the mouse [7]. The kinetics of ACTH expression has been evaluated in both ConA and LPS treated rat splenic leukocyte populations [128]. The results indicate that rat splenic macrophages, B, CD8 +, and CD4 + lymphocytes can all be stimulated to express the ACTH peptide. In contrast, the production of TSH seems to be limited to T lymphocytes regardless of the stimulus [129]. Thus, in this instance, only T cells seem to have the potential to make this hormone [22, 23]. In contrast to TSH, T and B cells as well as macrophages produce GH [50]. Interestingly, GH is primarily an enhancer of immune response and within the T-cell compartment, T-helper cells produce more GH than T cytotoxic/suppressor cells. The location and type of cells involved in lymphocyte PRL synthesis in humans provides evidence that PRL mRNA is expressed in normal human thymus, spleen, tonsil, and lymph node as well as in tumorous lymphoid tissues [130]. Studies in isolated lymphocytes suggest PRL expression is mainly associated with the T-lymphocyte population [33]. Although the findings with other lymphocyte-derived neuroendocrine hormones is just beginning to be investigated, a few observations are worthy of mention (table 4). In general, the peptides are found in numerous cell types of the immune system and the levels increase after immunostimulation. Both T and B lymphocytes can be stimulated by ConA and LPS, respectively, to secrete CRF which can be inhibited by hydrocortisone [59]. Neuropeptide Y [75] and VIP gene [131] expression has been found in both T and B cells in central and peripheral lymphoid organs. Immunohistochemistry with anti-CD3 antibodies revealed a strong CD3 expression on hCG-immunoreactive cells, whereas CD3-negative cells were hCG-negative [37]. An important role for LHRH in the immune response was suggested by the finding that rat

Table 4. Cellular source of immunologically derived neuropeptides

Hormone	Cell types or tissue	References
Corticotrophin and endorphins	T, B, NK, Mac, dendritic cells	1, 120, 128
Thyrotropin	T cells	22, 129
CG	thymus, T cells	36, 37
GH	T, B, NK, Mac	50, 137
PRL	spleen, thymus, T cells	33, 130
LH	T cells, thymus	45, 150
CRF	thymus, spleen, T and B cells	57–59
LHRH	spleen, T cells	61, 63, 115
Neuropeptide Y	T and B cells	75
VIP	T and B cells	131
Catecholamines	T cells	97

splenic and thymic cells and human CD4 and CD8 T cells contain LHRH peptide and express mRNA for LHRH [61, 115]. Both subsets of T cells produce comparable amounts of LHRH which could be significantly increased when cells were activated by either PHA or anti-CD3 antibody [115]. Obviously, a great deal of work remains to be done in this area. However, the preliminary results indicate there may be some immune cell specificity to certain hormonal responses.

Functions of Leukocyte-Derived Peptide Hormones

At least two possibilities exist relative to the function of peptide hormones and neurotransmitters that are produced by the immune system. First they act on their classic neuroendocrine target tissues. Second, they may serve as endogenous regulators of the immune system. With regard to the latter possibility, it is clear that neuroendocrine peptide hormones can directly modulate immune functions, and this is discussed in detail in another chapter of this book [Torres and Johnson]. These studies, however, do not address endogenous as opposed to exogenous regulation by neuroendocrine peptides. A number of investigators have now been able to demonstrate that such regulation is endogenous to the immune system (fig. 2). Specifically, TSH is a pituitary hormone that can be produced by lymphocytes in response to TRH and, like TSH, TRH enhanced the in vitro antibody response [132]. This TRH enhancement was not observed with GHRH, AVP, or LHRH and was blocked by antibodies to the β-subunit of TSH [24]. Thus, it appears that TRH specifi-

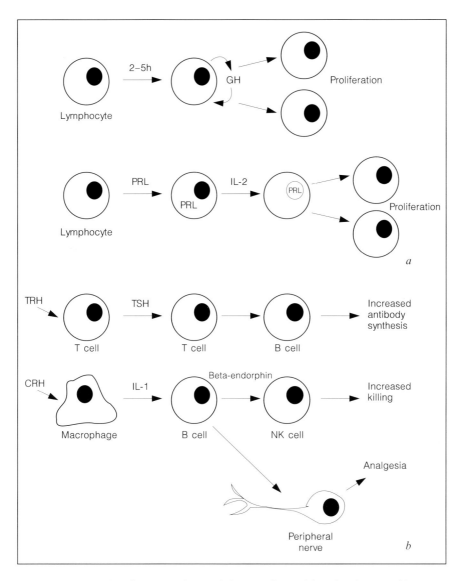

Fig. 2. Examples of (*a*) autocrime and (*b*) paracrine activity of various peptide neuro-transmitters and hormones synthesized by lymphocytes and macrophages. See text for details. CRH = Corticotropin-releasing hormone; GH = growth hormone; IL-2 = interleukin 2; NK = natural killer; PRL − prolactin; TRH = thyrotropin-releasing hormone; TSH = thyroid-stimulating hormone; β-end = β-endorphin.

cally enhances the in vitro antibody response via production of TSH. This was apparently the first demonstration that a neuroendocrine hormone (TSH) can function as an endogenous regulator within the immune system. In a similar study, antibody to prolactin was shown to inhibit mitogenesis through neutralization of the lymphocyte-associated prolactin [133]. An elegant example of paracrine activity of hormones synthesized by lymphocytes and macrophages can be found in the production of POMC (fig. 2). As discussed earlier, glucocorticoids inhibit, whereas CRH induces, lymphocyte-derived POMC peptides. However, closer examination reveals that the action of both substances is indirect; CRH causes macrophages production of IL-1, which then induces B-cell production of POMC [100, 101, 104]; and glucocorticoids block macrophage production of IL-1, rather than directly blocking B-cell synthesis of POMC. The ability of human T and B lymphocytes and mouse splenocytes to secrete CRF and ACTH in response to hyperthermia, hyperosmolarity and hypoxia has also been demonstrated and this secretion could be inhibited by anti-CRF antibodies and by hydrocortisone [59]. These findings support the idea that CRF could provide a link between external stimuli such as cellular stress factors and ACTH secretion by immunocytes leading to corticosteroid production and, subsequently, to nonspecific defense reaction of the organism.

Two new and different approaches have provided further convincing evidence that endogenous neuroendocrine peptides have autocrine or paracrine immunoregulatory functions. First, an opiate antagonist was shown to indirectly block CRF enhancement of NK cell activity by inhibiting the action of immunocyte-derived opioid peptides [134]. Second, Weigent et al. [135] have used an antisense oligodeoxynucleotide (ODN) to the translation start site of GH mRNA to specifically inhibit leukocyte production of GH. The ensuing lack of GH resulted in a marked diminution in basal rates of DNA synthesis in such antisense ODN-treated leukocytes which was overcome by exogenously added GH. Another group, in a similar kind of study, examining SOM found that antisense oligodeoxynucleotides to SOM dramatically increased lymphocyte proliferation in culture [73].

A second major function of GH produced by cells of the immune system is the induction of the synthesis of IGF-1 [85], which, in turn, may inhibit the synthesis of both lymphocyte GH mRNA and protein. Our previous studies show that both exogenous [48] and endogenous [136] GHRH can stimulate the synthesis of lymphocyte GH. Taken together, these findings support the existence of a complete regulatory loop within cells of the immune system, and they provide a molecular basis whereby GHRH, GH, IGF-1 and its binding protein may be intimately involved in regulating each other's synthesis. Furthermore, data obtained by immunofluorescence techniques suggest the cells producing GH also produce IGF-1, which suggests that an intracrine regulatory circuit may be important in the synthesis of these hormones by cells of the immune system [137].

Certain experimental models and clinical observations would also seem to support the view that leukocyte-derived hormones can sometimes also act on their classic neuroendocrine targets. The finding that cells of the immune system are a source of secreted ACTH suggested that stimuli which elicit the leukocyte-derived hormone should not require a pituitary gland for an ACTH-mediated increase in corticosteroid. This seemed to be the case since NDV (an in vitro inducer of leukocyte ACTH) infection of hypophysectomized mice caused a time-dependent increase in corticosterone production which was inhibitable by dexamethasone. Unless such mice were pretreated with dexamethasone, their spleens were positive for ACTH by immunofluorescence [10]. However, two other groups have failed to reproduce these findings in mice [138] and rats [139], and have concluded that the positive results stemmed from incomplete removal of the pituitary gland, such that pituitary remnants release ACTH. Although this may be the case in rodent models, a more recent study in the chicken has strongly suggested that B lymphocytes can be responsible for extrapituitary ACTH and glucocorticoid production. In this report, hypophysectomized chickens were shown to produce ACTH and corticosterone in response to *Brucella abortus*. This ACTH and corticosterone response was ablated if B lymphocytes were deleted by bursectomy prior to hypophysectomy [140]. Similar results have been observed in humans. For example, when children who were pituitary ACTH-deficient were pyrogen tested (typhoid vaccine, another in vitro inducer of leukocyte ACTH), they showed an increase in the percentage of ACTH-positive mononuclear leukocytes [141]. Both the response in hypophysectomized mice and hypopituitary children peaked at approximately 6–8 h after administration of virus and typhoid vaccine, respectively. These findings might explain the earlier observation of bacterial polysaccharide (Piromen)-induced cortisol responses in 7 of 8 patients who underwent pituitary stalk sectioning [142]. Such studies have been furthered by the report of Fehm et al. [143] that CRF administration to pituitary ACTH-deficient individuals results in both an ACTH and a cortisol response.

Gram-negative bacterial infections and endotoxin shock may represent yet another situation in which leukocyte hormones act on the neuroendocrine system. For instance, endorphins have been implicated in the pathophysiology associated with these maladies since the opiate antagonist, naloxone, improved survival rates and blocked a number of cardiopulmonary changes associated with these conditions [144]. Further, two separate pools of endorphins have been observed following endotoxin, bacterial LPS, administration and it was suggested that one pool might originate in the immune system [145]. Considering the potent immunological effects of endotoxin, as well as its ability to induce in vitro leukocyte production of endorphins, cells of the immune system seem the most likely source of endogenous opiates that are observed during gram-negative sepsis and endotoxin shock. Consistent with this idea is the observation that lymphocyte depletion, like naloxone treatment, blocked a number of endotoxin-induced cardiopulmonary changes [146]. Our interpretation of these results is that lymphocyte depletion removes the source of the endorphins while naloxone blocks their effector function. In a different approach, LPS-resistant inbred mice which have essentially no pathophysiologic response to LPS were shown to have a defect in leukocyte processing of POMC to endorphins. If leukocyte-derived endorphins were administered to such LPS-resistant mice, they then showed much of the pathophysiology associated with LPS administration to sensitive mice [147]. A final and exciting new development in the opioid field has come with the demonstration that activation of endogenous opioids in rats by a cold water swim results in a local antinociceptive effect in inflamed peripheral tissue. This local antinociception in the inflamed tissue apparently results from production by immune cells of endogenous opioids which interact with opioid receptors on peripheral sensory nerves [148]. A more recent study strongly suggests that the immune system plays an essential role in pain control [149]. The findings identify locally expressed CRF as the main agent to induce opioid release within inflamed tissue. The opioid receptor-specific antinociception in inflamed paws of rats could be blocked by intraplantar α-helical CRF or antiserum to CRF or CRF-antisense oligodeoxynucleotide. This later treatment reduced the amount of CRF extracted from inflamed paws, as well as the number of CRF-immuno-stained cells [149]. These observations seem to offer new potential insights into pain occurring in normal and immunosuppressed conditions. Perhaps with a greater understanding of this paradigm, it will be possible to alleviate pain by manipulation of the immune system.

In conclusion, cells of the immune system can now be considered a source of neuroendocrine peptides. In many respects, the production and regulation of these peptides in leukocytes is remarkably like that observed in neuroendo-crine cells. There are, however, a number of noteworthy differences which suggest that rules which apply to pituitary hormone production are not necessarily applicable to the immune system. First, there may not be an immediate response of the immune system since, unlike the pituitary gland, the hormones are usually not stored but are synthesized de novo and this requires a number of hours. Second, plasma hormone concentrations do not have to reach the levels required when the pituitary gland is the source because immune cells are not fixed but are mobile and can locally deposit the hormone at the target site. Third, on a per cell basis, leukocytes produce considerably less hormone than pituitary cells. This difference, however, is more than compensated for by the greater number of cells in the immune system as compared with the pituitary gland. Once produced, these peptide hormones seem to function in at least two capacities. They are endogenous regulators of the immune system as well as conveyors of information from the immune to the neuroendocrine system. It is our bias that the transmission of such information to the neuroendocrine system represents a sensory function for the immune system wherein leukocytes recognize stimuli that are not recognizable by the central and peripheral nervous systems [127]. These stimuli have been termed noncognitive and include bacteria, tumors, viruses, and antigens. The recognition of such noncognitive stimuli by immunocytes is then converted into information, in the form of peptide hormones and neurotransmitters, lymphokines and monokines, which is conveyed to the neuroendocrine system and a physiologic change occurs.

Acknowledgments

We thank faculty colleagues, students and postdoctoral fellows who were pivotal to the studies reported herein. I am also grateful to Diane Weigent for expert editorial assistance. These studies were supported in part by NIH grants AI41651 (D.A.W.), AI37670 (J.E.B.), MH52527 (J.E.B.), and NS29719 (J.E.B.).

References

1   Blalock JE, Smith EM: Human leukocyte interferon: Structural and biological relatedness to adreno-corticotropic hormone and endorphins. Proc Natl Acad Sci USA 1980;77:5972–5974.
2   Smith EM, Blalock JE: Human lymphocyte production of corticotropin and endorphin-like substances: Association with leukocyte interferon. Proc Natl Acad Sci USA 1981;78:7530–7534.
3   Blalock JE, Smith EM: Human leukocyte interferon (HuIFN-alpha): Potent endorphin-like opioid activity. Biochem Biophys Res Commun 1981;101:472–478.
4   Harbour-McMenamin D, Smith EM, Blalock JE: Bacterial lipopolysaccharide induction of leukocyte-derived corticotropin and endorphins. Infect Immun 1985;48:813–817.
5   Lolait SJ, Lim ATW, Toh BH, Funder JW: Immunoreactive β-endorphin in a subpopulation of mouse spleen macrophages. J Clin Invest 1984;73:277–280.
6   Endo Y, Sakata T, Watanabe S: Identification of proopiomelanocortin-producing cells in the rat pyloric antrum and duodenum by in situ mRNA-cDNA hybridization. Biomed Res 1985;6:253–256.
7   Farooqui JZ, Medrano EE, Boissy RE, Tigelaar RE, Nordlund JJ: Thy-1 + dendritic cells express truncated form of POMC mRNA. Exp Dermatol 1995;4:297–301.
8   Herbert E: Discovery of pro-opiomelanocortin: A cellular polyprotein. Trends Biochem Sci 1981; 6:184–186.
9   Blalock JE, Smith EM: A complete regulatory loop between the immune and neuroendocrine systems. Fed Proc 1985;44:108–111.
10   Smith EM, Meyer WJ, Blalock JE: Virus-induced corticosterone in hypophysectomized mice: A possible lymphoid adrenal axis. Science 1982;218:1311–1312.

11   Westly HJ, Kleiss AJ, Kelley KW, Wong PKY, Yuen PH: Newcastle disease virus-infected splenocytes express the pro-opiomelanocortin gene. J Exp Med 1986;163:1589–1594.

12   Lolait SJ, Clements JA, Markwick AJ, Cheng C, McNally M, Smith AI, Funder JW: Pro-opiomelano-cortin messenger ribonucleic acid and posttranslational processing of beta endorphin in spleen macrophages. J Clin Invest 1986;77:1776–1779.

13   Oates EL, Allaway GP, Armstrong GR, Boyajian RA, Kehr JH, Probhakar BS: Human lymphocytes produce pro-opiomelanocortin gene-related transcripts: Effects of lymphotropic viruses. J Biol Chem 1988;263:10041–10044.

14   Buzzetti R, McLoughlin L, Lavender PM, Clark AJ, Rees LH: Expression of pro-opiomelanocortin gene and quantification of adrenocorticotropic hormone-like immunoreactivity in human normal peripheral mononuclear cells and lymphoid and myeloid malignancies. J Clin Invest 1989;83:733–737.

15   Smith EM, Galin FS, LeBoueuf RD, Coppenhaver DH, Harbour DV, Blalock JE: Nucleotide and amino acid sequence of lymphocyte-derived corticotropin: Endotoxin induction of a truncated peptide. Proc Natl Acad Sci USA 1990;87:1057–1060.

16   Galin FS, LeBoueuf RD, Blalock JE: A lymphocyte mRNA encodes the adrenocorticotropin/β-lipotropin region of the pro-opiomelanocortin gene. Prog NeuroEndocrinImmunol 1990;3:205.

17   Galin FS, LeBoueuf RD, Blalock JE: Corticotropin-releasing factor upregulates expression of two truncated pro-opiomelanocortin transcripts in murine lymphocytes. J Neuroimmunol 1991;31:51–58.

18   Lyons PD, Blalock JE: Pro-opiomelanocortin gene expression and protein processing in rat mononu-clear leukocytes. J Neuroimmunol 1997, in press.

19   Zurawski G, Benedik M, Kamb BJ, Abrams JS, Zurawski SM, Lee FD: Activation of mouse T-helper cells induces abundant preproenkephalin mRNA synthesis. Science 1986;232:772–775.

20   Kuis W, Villiger PM, Leser HG, Lotz M: Differential processing of proenkephalin-A by human peripheral blood monocytes and T lymphocytes. J Clin Invest 1991;88:817–824.

21   Kamphuis S, Kavelaars A, Brooimans R, Kuis W, Zegers BJM, Heijnen CJ: T helper 2 cytokines induce preproenkephalin mRNA expression and proenkephalin A in human peripheral blood mononuclear cells. J Neuroimmunol 1997;in press.

22   Smith EM, Phan M, Kruger TE, Coppenhaver DH, Blalock JE: Human lymphocyte production of immunoreactive thyrotropin. Proc Natl Acad Sci USA 1983;80:6010–6013.

23   Harbour DV, Kruger TE, Coppenhaver D, Smith EM, Meyer WJ 3d: Differential expression and regulation of thyrotropin (TSH) in T cell lines. Mol Cell Endocrinol 1989;64:229–241.

24   Kruger TE, Smith LR, Harbour DV, Blalock JE: Thyrotropin: An endogenous regulator of the in vitro immune response. J Immunol 1989;142:744–747.

25   Hiestand PC, Mekler P, Nordmann R, Grieder A, Permmongkol C: Prolactin as a modulator of lymphocyte responsiveness provides a possible mechanism of action for cyclosporine. Proc Natl Acad Sci USA 1986;83:2599–2603.

26   Montgomery DW, Zukowski CF, Shah NG, Buckley AR, Pacholczyk T, Russell DH: Concanavalin A-stimulated murine leukocytes produce a factor with prolactin-like bioactivity and immunoreactiv-ity. Biochem Biophys Res Commun 1987;145:692–698.

27   Kenner JR, Holaday JW, Bernton EW, Smith PF: Prolactin-like protein in murine lymphocytes: Morphological and biochemical evidence. Prog NeuroEndocrinImmunol 1990;3:188–199.

28   DiMattia GE, Gellersen B, Bohnet HG, Friesen HG: A human β-lymphoblastoid cell line produces prolactin. Endocrinology 1988;122:2508–2517.

29   DiMattia GE, Gellersen B, Duckworth ML, Friesen HG: Human prolactin gene expression: The use of an alternative noncoding exon in decidua and the IM-9-P3 lymphoblast cell line. J Biol Chem 1990;2165:16412.

30   Friesen HG, DiMattia GE, Too CKL: Lymphoid tumor cells as models for studies of prolactin gene regulation and action. Prog NeuroEndocrinImmunol 1991;4:1–9.

31   Clevenger CV, Russell DH, Appasamy PM, Prystowsky MB: Regulation of interleukin 2-driven T-lymphocyte proliferation by prolactin. Proc Natl Acad Sci USA 1990;87:6460–6464.

32   Jurcovicova J, Day RN, MacLeod RM: Expression of prolactin in rat lymphocytes. Prog NeuroEn-docrinImmunol 1992;2:256–263.

33   Pellegrini I, Lebrun J-I, Ali S, Kelly PA: Expression of prolactin and its receptor in human lymphoid cells. Mol Endocrinol 1992;6:1023–1031.

34   O'Neal KD, Montgomery DW, Truong TM, Yu-Lee L-Y: Prolactin gene expression in human thymocytes. Mol Cell Endocrinol 1992;87:R19–R23.

35   Montgomery DW, Shen GK, Ulrich ED, Steiner LL, Parrish PR, Zukoski CF: Human thymocytes express a prolactin-like messenger ribonucleic acid and synthesize bioactive prolactin-like protein. Endocrinology 1992;131:3019–3026.

36   Harbour-McMenamin D, Smith EM, Blalock JE: Production of immunoreactive chorionic gonadotropin during mixed lymphocyte reactions: A possible selective mechanism for genetic diversity. Proc Natl Acad Sci USA 1986;83:6834–6838.

37   Batanero E, deLeeuw FE, Jansen GH, vanWichen DF, Huber J, Schuurman HJ: The neural and neuro-endocrine component of the human thymus. II. Hormone immunoreactivity. Brain Behav Immun 1992;6:249–264.

38   Ebaugh MJ, Smith EM: Human lymphocyte production of immunoreactive luteinizing hormone (abstract). FASEB J 1988;2:7811.

39   Smith EM, Ebaugh MJ: Luteogenic activity from human leukocytes. Ann NY Acad Sci 1990;594:492–493.

40   Blalock JE, Costa O: Immune neuroendocrine interactions: Implications for reproductive physiology. Ann NY Acad Sci 1989;564:261–266.

41   Costa O, Mulchahey JJ, Blalock JE: Structure and function of luteinizing hormone releasing hormone (LHRH) receptors on lymphocytes. Prog NeuroEndocrinImmunol 1990;3:55–60.

42   Maier RM, Chew BP: Stimulation of progesterone secretion by blood monocytes and lymphocytes in the porcine. Theriogenology 1989;33:1045–1056.

43   Standaert FE, Chew BP, Wong TS: Influence of blood monocytes and lymphocytes on progesterone production by granulosa cells from smalll and large follicles in the pig. Am J Reprod Immunol 1990;22:49–55.

44   Standaert FE, Chew BP, Wong TS, Michal JJ: Porcine lymphocytes secrete factors in response to LHRH to stimulate progesterone production by granulosa cells in vitro (abstract). Biol Reprod 1990;42:75.

45   Gorospe WC, Kasson BG: Lymphokines from concanavalin-A-stimulated lymphocytes regulate rat granulosa cell steroidogenesis in vitro. Endocrinology 1989;123:2462–2471.

46   Kasson BG, Tuchel TL: Identification and characterization of a lymphocyte-produced substance with gonadotropin-like activity (abstract). Endocrinology 1989;75.

47   Weigent DA, Baxter JB, Wear WE, Smith LR, Bost KL, Blalock JE: Production of immunoreactive growth hormone by mononuclear leukocytes. FASEB J 1988;2:2812–2818.

48   Guarcello V, Weigent DA, Blalock JE: Growth hormone releasing hormone receptors on thymocytes and splenocytes from rats. Cell Immunol 1991;136:291–302.

49   Hattori N, Shimatsu A, Sugita M, Kumagai S, Imura H: Immunoreactive growth hormone (GH) secretion by human lymphocytes: Augmented release by exogenous GH. Biochem Biophys Res Commun 1990;168:396–401.

50   Weigent DA, Blalock JE: The production of growth hormone by subpopulations of rat mononuclear leukocytes. Cell Immunol 1991;135:55–65.

51   Kao TL, Harbour DV, Meyer WJ 3d: Immunoreactive growth hormone production by cultured lymphocytes. Ann NY Acad Sci 1992;650:179–181.

52   Lytras A, Quan N, Vrontakis ME, Shaw JE, Cattini PA, Friesen HG: Growth hormone expression in human Burkitt lymphoma serum-free Ramos cell line. Endocrinology 1993;132:620–628.

53   Varma S, Sabharwal P, Sheridan JF, Malarkey WB: Growth hormone secretion by human peripheral blood mononuclear cells detected by an enzyme-linked immunoplaque assay. J Clin Endocrinol Metab 1993;76:49–53.

54   Weigent DA, Blalock JE: Associations between the neuroendocrine and immune systems. J Leukocyte Biol 1995;58:137–150.

55   Rohn WA, Weigent DA: Cloning and nucleotide sequencing of rat lymphocyte growth hormone cDNA. Neuroimmunomodulation 1995;2:108–114.

56   Stephanou A, Jessop DS, Knight RA, Lightman SL: Corticotrophin-releasing factor-like immunoreactivity and mRNA in human leukocytes. Brain Behav Immun 1990;4:67–73.

57   Aird F, Clevenger CV, Prystowsky MB, Redei E: Corticotropin-releasing factor mRNA in rat thymus and spleen. Proc Natl Acad Sci USA 1993;90:7104–7108.

58   Ekman R, Servenius B, Castro MG, Lowry PJ, Cederlund AS, Bergman O, Sjogren HO: Biosynthesis of corticotropin-releasing hormone in human T-lymphocytes. J Neuroimmunol 1993;44:7–13.

59   Kravchenco IV, Furalev VA: Secretion of immunoreactive CRF and ACTH by T- and B-lymphocytes in response to cellular stress factors. Biochem Biophys Res Commun 1994.204:828–834.

60   Emanuele NV, Emanuele MA, Tentler J, Kirsteins L, Azad N, Lawrence AM: Rat spleen lymphocytes contain an immunoactive and bioactive luteinizing hormone-releasing hormone. Endocrinology 1990;126:2482–2486.

61   Azad N, Emanuelle NV, Halloran MM, Tentler J, Kelley MR: Presence of luteinizing hormone-releasing hormone (LHRH) mRNA in spleen lymphocytes. Endocrinology 1992;128:1679–1681.

62   Maier CC, Marchetti B, LeBoeuf RD, Blalock JE: Thymocytes express a mRNA that is identical to hypothalamic luteinizing hormone-releasing hormone mRNA. Cell Mol Neurobiol 1992;12: 447–454.

63   Wilson TM, Yu-Lee L, Kelley MR: Coordinate gene expression of luteinizing hormone-releasing hormone (LHRH) and the LHRH-receptor after prolactin stimulation in the rat Nb2 T-cell line: Implications for a role in immunomodulation and cell cycle gene expression. Mol Endocrinol 1995; 9:44–53.

64   Weigent DA, Blalock JE: Immunoreactive growth hormone-releasing hormone in rat leukocytes. J Neuroimmunol 1990;29:1–13.

65   Weigent DA, Riley JE, Galin FS, LeBoeuf RD, Blalock JE: Detection of growth hormone and growth hormone-releasing hormone-related messenger RNA in rat leukocytes by the polymerase chain reaction. Proc Soc Exp Biol Med 1991;198:643–648.

66   Smith EM, Morrill AC, Meyer WJ 3d, Blalock JE: Corticotropin releasing factor induction of leukocyte-derived immunoreactive ACTH and endorphins. Nature 1986;321:881–882.

67   Cutz E, Chan W, Track N, Goth A, Said S: Release of vasoactive intestinal peptide in mast cells by histamine liberators. Nature 1978;275:661–662.

68   Giachetti A, Goth A, Said SI: Vasoactive intestinal polypeptide (VIP) in rabbit platelets, and rat mast cells. Fed Proc 1978;37:657.

69   Goetzl EJ, Grotmol T, Van Dyke RW, Turck CW, Wershil B, Galli SJ, Sreedharan SP: Generation and recognition of vasoactive intestinal peptide by cells of the immune system. Ann NY Acad Sci 1990;594:34–44.

70   Lygren I, Revhaug A, Burhol PG, Giercksky E, Jenssen TG: Vasoactive intestinal peptide and somatostatin in leukocytes. Scand J Clin Lab Invest 1984;44:347–351.

71   O'Dorisio MS, O'Dorisio TM, Cataland S, Balcerzak SP: Vasoactive intestinal peptide as a biochemical marker for polymorphonuclear leukocytes. J Lab Clin Med 1980;96:666–670.

72   Aguila MC, Dees WL, Haensly WE, McCann SM: Evidence that somatostatin is localized and synthesized in lymphoid organs. Proc Natl Acad Sci USA 1991;88:11485–11489.

73   Aguila MC, Rodriguez AM, Aguila-Mansila HN, Lee WT: Somatostatin antisense oligodeoxynucleotide-mediated stimulation of lymphocyte proliferation in culture. Endocrinology 1996;137:1585–1590.

74   Ericsson A, Larhammar D, McIntyre KR, Persson H: A molecular genetic approach to the identification of genes expressed predominantly in the neuroendocrine and immune systems. Immunol Rev 1987;100:261–277.

75   Schwarz H, Villiger PM, von Kempis J, Lotz M: Neuropeptide Y is an inducible gene in the human immune system. J Neuroimmunol 1994;51:53–61.

76   Pascual DW, Bost KL: Substance P production by P388D1 macrophages: A possible autocrine function for this neuropeptide. Immunology 1990;71:52–56.

77   Kelly PA, Blalock JE, Chrousos GP, Yu-Lee L-Y, Geenen V: Neuroendocrine hormones and the immune system; in Cuello AC, Collier B (eds): Pharmacological Sciences: Perspectives for Research and Therapy in the Late 1990s. Basel, Birkhauser, 1995, pp 365–372.

78   Markwick AJ, Lolait SJ, Funder JW: Immunoreactive arginine vasopressin in the rat thymus. Endocrinology 1986;119:1690–1696.

79   Geenen V, Robert F, Martens H, Benhida A, De Giovanni G, Defresne MP, Boniver J, Legros JJ, Martial J, Franchimont P: Biosynthesis and paracrine/cryptocrine actions of 'self' neurohypophysial-related peptides in the thymus. Mol Cell Endocrin 1991;76:C27–31.

80 Jessop DS, Chowdrey HS, Lightman SL, Larsen PJ: Vasopressin is located within lymphocytes in the rat spleen. J Neuroimmunol 1995;56:219–223.

81 Adachi N, Yamaguchi K, Miyake Y, Honda S, Nagasaki K, Akiyama Y, Adachi I, Abe K: Parathyroid hormone-related protein is a possible autocrine growth inhibitor for lymphocytes. Biochem Biophys Res Commun 1990;166:1088–1094.

82 Fukumoto S, Matsumoto T, Watanabe T, Takhashi H, Miyoshi I, Ogata E: Secretion of parathyroid hormone-like activity from human T-cell lymphotropic virus type I-infected lymphocytes. Cancer Res 1989;49:3849–3852.

83 Rom WN, Basset P, Fells GA, Nukiwa T, Trapnell BC, Crystal RG: Alveolar macrophages release an insulin-like growth factor I-type molecule. J Clin Invest 1988;82:1685–1693.

84 Merimee TJ, Grant MB, Broder CM, Cavalli-Sforza LL: Insulin-like growth factor secretion by human B-lymphocytes: A comparison of cells from normal and pygmy subjects. J Clin Endocrinol Metab 1989;69:978–984.

85 Baxter JB, Blalock JE, Weigent DA: Characterization of immunoreactive insulin-like growth factor-I from leukocytes and its regulation by growth hormone. Endocrinology 1991;129:1727–1734.

86 Arkins S, Rebeiz N, Biragyn A, Reese DL, Kelley KW: Murine macrophages express abundant IGF-I class I, Ea and Eb transcripts. Endocrinology 1993;133:2334–2343.

87 Li YM, Arkins S, McCusker RH Jr, Donovan SM, Liu Q, Jayaraman S, Dantzer R, Kelley KW: Macrophages synthesize and secrete a 25 KDa protein that binds insulin-like growth factor-I. J Immunol 1996;156:64–72.

88 Funk JL, Lausier J, Moser AH, Shigenaga JK, Huling S, Nissenson RA, Strewler GJ, Grunfeld C, Feingold KR: Endotoxin induces parathyroid hormone-related protein gene expression in splenic stromal and smooth muscle cells, not in splenic lymphocytes. Endocrinology 1995;136:3412–3422.

89 Nyman T, Pekonen F: The expression of insulin-like growth factors and their binding proteins in normal human lymphocytes. Acta Endocrinol 1993;128:168–172.

90 LeBoeuf RD, Burns JN, Bost KL, Blalock JE: Isolation, purification, and partial characterization of suppressin, a novel inhibitor of cell proliferation. J Biol Chem 1990;265:158–165.

91 LeBoeuf RD, Carr DJJ, Green MM, Blalock JE: Cellular effects of suppressin: A biological response modifier of cells of the immune system. Proc NeuroEndocrinImmunol 1990;3:176–187.

92 Carr DJ, Blalock JE, Green MM, LeBoeuf RD: Immunomodulatory characteristics of a novel antiproliferative protein, suppressin. J Neuroimmunol 1990;30:179–187.

93 Ban EM, Propst SM, Blalock JE, LeBoeuf RD: Identification of suppressin-producing cells in the rat pituitary. Endocrinology 1993;133:241–247.

94 Ban EMH, LeBoeuf RD: Suppressin: An endogenous negative regulator of immune cell activation. Immunol Res 1995;13:1–9.

95 Ericsson A, Barbany G, Friedman WJ, Persson H: Molecular cloning and characterization of genes predominantly expressed in the neuroendocrine and immune systems. Prog NeuroEndocrinImmunol 1991;4:26–41.

96 Ericsson A, Barbany G, Persson H: Regional and temporal distribution of the neuroimmune mRNA NI-1 in the rat central nervous system. Prog NeuroEndocrinImmunol 1991;4:42–55.

97 Musso NR, Brenci S, Setti M, Indiveri F, Lotti G: Catecholamie content and in vitro catecholamine synthesis in peripheral human lymphocytes. J Clin Endocrinol Metab 1996;81:1–5.

98 Sacerdote P, Ciciliato IA, Rubboli F, Panerai AE: Effects of psychoactive drugs on lymphocyte neuropeptides. Ann NY Acad Sci 1990;594:270–279.

99 Kavelaars A, Berkenbosch F, Croiset G, Ballieux RE, Heijnen CJ: Induction of beta-endorphin secretion by lymphocytes after subcutaneous administration of corticotropin-releasing factor. Endocrinology 1990;126:759–764.

100 Kavelaars A, Ballieux RE, Heijnen CJ: The role of IL-1 in the corticotropin-releasing factor and arginine-vasopressin-induced secretion of immunoreactive beta-endorphin by human peripheral blood mononuclear cells. J Immunol 1989;142:2338–2342.

101 Schettini G: Interleukin-1 in the neuroendocrine system: From gene to function. Prog NeuroEndocrinImmunol 1990;3:157–166.

102 Blalock JE: The syntax of immune-neuroendocrine communication. Immunol Today 1994;15:504–511.

103 Payne LC, Weigent DA, Blalock JE: Induction of pituitary sensitivity to interleukin-1: A new function for corticotropin-releasing hormone. Biochem Biophys Res Commun 1994;198:480–484.

104 Kavelaars A, Ballieux RE, Heijnen CJ: Beta-endorphin secretionby human peripheral blood mononuclear cells: Regulation by glucocorticoids. Life Sci 1990;46:1233–1240.

105 Buzzetti R, Valente L, Barietta C, Scavo D, Pozzilli P: Thymopentin induces release of ACTH-like immunoreactivity by human lymphocytes. J Clin Lab Immunol 1989;29:157–159.

106 Clarke BL, Gebhardt BM, Blalock JE: Mitogen-stimulated lymphocytes release biologically active corticotropin. Endocrinology 1993;132:983–988.

107 Gellersen B, DiMattia GE, Friesen HG, Bohnet HG: Phorbol ester stimulates prolactin release but reduces prolactin mRNA in the human β-lymphoblastoid cell line IM-9-P. Mol Cell Endocrinol 1989;66:153–161.

108 Gellersen B, DiMattia GE, Friesen HG, Bohnet HG: Regulation of prolactin secretion in the human B-lymphoblastoid cell line IM-9-P3 by dexamethasone but not other regulators of pituitary prolactin secretion. Enddocrinology 1989;125:2853–2861.

109 Gellersen B, Kempf R, Hartung S, Bonhoff A, DiMattia GE: Posttranscriptional regulation of the human prolactin gene in IM-9-P3 cells by retinoic acid. Endocrinology 1992;131:1017–1025.

110 Gellersen B, Kempf R, Telgmann R, DiMattia GE: Nonpituitary human prolactin gene transcription is independent of Pit-1 and differentially controlled in lymphocytes and in endometrial stroma. Mol Endocrinol 1994;8:356–373.

111 Hattori N, Shimormura K, Ishihara T, Moridera K, Hino M, Ikekubo K, Kurahachi H: Growth hormone (GH) secretion from human lymphocytes is up-regulated by GH, but not affected by insulin-like growth factor-1. J Clin Endocinol Metab 1993;76:937–939.

112 Kao TL, Meyer WJ: Inhibition of immunoreactive growth hormone secretion from lymphoid cell lines by dexamethasone. Life Sci 1992;51:1033–1039.

113 Weigent DA, Blalock JE: Growth hormone and the immune system. Prog NeuroEndocrinImmunol 1990;3:231–241.

114 Weigent DA, Blalock JE: Effect of the administration of growth hormone-producing lymphocytes on weight gain and immune function in dwarf mice. Neuroimmunomodulation 1994;1:50–58.

115 Azad N, LaPaglia N, Jurgens KAJ, Kirsteins L, Emanuele NV, Kelley MR, Lawrence AM, Mohagheghpour N: Immunoactivation enhances the concentration of luteinizing hormone-releasing hormone peptide and its gene expression in human peripheral T-lymphocytes. Endocrinology 1996;133:215–223.

116 Mohagheghpour N, Abel K, LaPaglia N, Emanuele NV, Azad N: Signal requirements for production of luteinizing hormone releasing-hormone by human T cells. Cell Immunol 1995;163:280–283.

117 Krieger DT: Brain peptides. Science 1983;222:975–985.

118 Loh YP, Parish DC, Tuteja R: Purification and characterization of a paired basic residue-specific pro-opiomelanocortin converting enzyme from bovine pituitary intermediate lobe secretory vesicles. J Biol Chem 1985;260:7194–7205.

119 Cromlish JA, Seidah NG, Chretein M: Selective cleavage of human ACTH beta-lipotropin, and the N-terminal glycopeptide at pairs of basic residues by IRCM-serine protease. I. Subcellular localization in small and large vesicles. J Biol Chem 1986;261:10857–10859.

120 Harbour-McMenamin D, Smith EM, Blalock JE: B lymphocyte-enriched populations produce immunoreactive endorphin that binds to delta opiate receptors and may play a role in endotoxic shock. ICSU short reports. Adv Gene Technol 1986;4:378–379.

121 Star RA, Rajora N, Huang J, Stock RC, Cattania A, Lipton JM: Evidence of autocrine modulation of macrophage nitric oxide synthase by alpha-melanocyte-stimulating hormone. Proc Natl Acad Sci USA 1995;92:8016–8020.

122 Rajora N, Ceriani G, Catania A, Star RA, Murphy MT, Lipton JM: Alpha-MSH production, receptors, and influence on neopterin in a human monocyte/macrophage cell line. J Leuk Biol 1996;59:248–253.

123 Harbour DV, Smith EM, Blalock JE: Novel processing pathway for proopiomelanocortin in lymphocytes: Endotoxin induction of a new prohormone-cleaving enzyme. J Neurosci Res 1987;18:95–101.

124 Johnson HM, Smith EM, Torres BA, Blalock JE: Neuroendocrine hormone regulation of in vitro antibody formation. Proc Natl Acad Sci USA 1982;79:4171–4174.

125 Gilman SC, Schwartz JM, Milnher RJ, Bloom FE, Feldman JD: β-Endorphin enhances lymphocyte proliferative responses. Proc Natl Acad Sci USA 1982;79:4226–4230.

126 Wenger GD, O'Dorisio MS, Goetzl EJ: Vasoactive intestinal peptide: Messenger in a neuroimmune axis. Ann NY Acad Sci 1990;594:104–119.

127 Blalock JE: The immune system as a sensory organ. J Immunol 1984;132:1067–1070.

128 Lyons PD, Blalock JE: The kinetics of ACTH expression in rat leukocyte subpopulations. J Neuroimmunol 1995;63:103–112.

129 Kruger TE, Blalock JE: Cellular requirements for thyrotropin enhancement of in vitro antibody production. J Immunol 1986;137:197–200.

130 Wu H, Devi R, Malarkey WB: Expression and localization of prolactin messenger ribonucleic acid in the human immune system. Endocrinology 1996;137:349–353.

131 Gomariz RP, Leceta J, Garrido E, Garrido T, Delgado M: Vasoactive intestinal peptide (VIP) mRNA expression in rat T and B lymphocytes. Regul Pept 1994;50:177–184.

132 Blalock JE, Johnson HM, Smith EM, Torres BA: Enhancement of the in vitro antibody response by thyrotropin. Biochem Biophys Res Commun 1984;125:30–34.

133 Hartmann DP, Holaday JW, Bernton EW: Inhibition of lymphocyte proliferation by antibodies to prolactin. FASEB J 1989;3:2194–2202.

134 Carr DJ, DeCosta BR, Jacobson AE, Rice KC, Blalock JE: Corticotropin-releasing hormone augments natural killer cell activity through a naloxone-sensitive pathway. J Neuroimmunol 1990;28:53–61.

135 Weigent DA, Blalock JE, LeBoeuf RD: An antisense oligodeoxynucleotide to growth hormone messenger ribonucleic acid inhibits lymphocyte proliferation. Endocrinology 1991;128:2053–2057.

136 Payne LC, Rohn W, Weigent DA: Lymphocyte-derived growth hormone releasing hormone is an autocrine modulator of lymphocyte-derived growth hormone (abstract). Endocrinology 1994;A1255:514.

137 Weigent DA, Baxter JB, Blalock JE: The production of growth hormone and insulin-like growth factor-I by the same subpopulation of rat mononuclear leukocytes. Brain Behav Immun 1992;6:365–376.

138 Dunn AJ, Powell ML, Gaskin JM: Virus-induced increases in plasma corticosterone. Science 1987;238:1423–1425.

139 Olsen NJ, Nicholson WE, DeBold CR, Orth DN: Lymphocyte-derived adrenocorticotropin is insufficient to stimulate adrenal steroidogenesis in hypophysectomized rats. Endocrinology 1992;130:2113–2119.

140 Bayle JE, Guellati M, Ibos F, Roux J: Brucella abortus antigen stimulates the pituitary-adrenal axis through the extra-pituitary B-lymphoid system. Prog NeuroEndocrinImmunol 1991;4:99–105.

141 Meyer WJ, Smith EM, Richards GE, Cavallo A, Morrill AC, Blalock JE: In vivo immunoreactive adrenocorticotropin (ACTH) production by human mononuclear leukocytes from normal and ACTH-deficient individuals. J Clin Endocrinol Metab 1987;64:98–105.

142 Van Wyk JJ, Dugger GS, Newsome JF, Thomas PZ: The effect of pituitary stalk section in the adrenal function of women with cancer of the breast. J Clin Endocrinol Metab 1960;20:157–172.

143 Fehm HL, Holl R, Spath-Schwalbe E, Voigt KH, Born J: Ability of human corticotropin releasing factor (hCRF) to stimulate cortisol secretion independent from pituitary ACTH. Life Sci 1988;42:679–686.

144 Reynolds DG, Gurll NJ, Vargish T, Lechner RB, Faden AI, Holaday JW: Blockade of opiate receptors with naloxone improves survival and cardiac performance in canine endotoxic shock. Circul Shock 1980;7:39–48.

145 Carr DB, Bergland R, Hamilton A, Blume H, Kasting N, Arnold M, Martin MB, Rosenblatt M: Endotoxin-stimulated opioid peptide secretion: Two secretory pools and feedback control in vivo. Science 1982;217:845–848.

146 Bohs CT, Fish JC, Miller TH, Traber DL: Pulmonary vascular response to endotoxin in normal and lymphocyte depleted sheep. Circ Shock 1979;6:13–21.

147 Harbour DV, Smith EM, Blalock JE: Splenic lymphocyte production of an endorphin during endotoxic shock. Brain Behav Immun 1987;1:123–133.

148 Stein C, Hassan AHS, Przewlocki R, Gramsch C, Peter K, Herz A: Opioids from immunocytes interact with receptors on sensory nerves to inhibit nociception in inflammation. Proc Natl Acad Sci USA 1990;87:5935–5939.

149 Schafer M, Mousa SA, Zhang Q, Carter L, Stein C: Expression of corticotropin-releasing factor in inflamed tissue is required for intrinsic peripheral opioid analgesia. Proc Natl Acad Sci USA 1996;93:6096–6100.

150 Sabharwal P, Varma S, Malarkey WB: Human thymocytes secrete luteinizing hormone: An autocrine regulator of T-cell proliferation. Biochem Biophys Res Commun 1992;187:1187–1192.

J. Edwin Blalock, PhD, Department of Physiology and Biophysics,
Center for Neuroimmunology, The University of Alabama at Birmingham,
896 Basic Health Sciences Building, 1918 University Boulevard,
Birmingham, AL 35294–0005 (USA)
Tel. (205) 934 6439, Fax (205) 934 1446, E-Mail: blalock@phybio.bhs.uab.edu

Blalock JE (ed): Neuroimmunoendocrinology, 3rd rev ed.
Chem Immunol. Basel, Karger, 1997, vol 69, pp 31–75

....

Cytokines: Influence on Glial Cell Gene Expression and Function

Etty N. Benveniste

Department of Cell Biology, The University of Alabama at Birmingham,
UAB Station, Birmingham, Ala., USA

Introduction

The central nervous system (CNS) has traditionally been considered as an 'immunologically privileged' site for several reasons: (1) a poor alloreactive response to tissue engraftment within the CNS [1]; (2) lack of a lymphatic system that drains the tissues and captures potential antigens; and (3) protection from the blood by a unique blood-brain barrier (BBB) composed of specialized endothelial cells that restricts the passage of cellular elements and many soluble substances (immunoglobulins, cytokines, growth factors) from the circulation into the CNS [2]. Additionally, cells of the CNS (neurons, macroglia, microglia) express very low levels of proteins with immunological properties (class I and II major histocompatibility complex (MHC) antigens, adhesion molecules, costimulatory molecules), which all play a fundamental role in the induction and regulation of immune responses [3]. However, recent studies have demonstrated that the separation of the brain from the immune system is not absolute even under normal conditions, i.e. an intact BBB. Activated T cells in very low numbers can traffic through the CNS for purposes of immune surveillance [4], and the presence of lymphatic-like capillaries in the brain provides a possible natural, untraumatized, entryway for lymphoid cells into the CNS [5]. Thus, there may exist a low level immune response in the CNS as a mechanism to eliminate potential antigens. In addition, endogenous glial cells can be activated to participate in CNS immune reactivity [3].

During human diseases such as viral encephalitis [6], multiple sclerosis (MS) [7–9], and AIDS dementia complex (ADC) [10], and animal models of CNS disease such as experimental allergic encephalomyelitis (EAE) [11], inflammatory infiltrates composed of activated T cells, B cells, and macrophages are found in the brain. The presence of leukocytes in the CNS results from recruitment of cells from the circulating compartment and the disruption of the BBB, which are crucial steps in the development of these diseases.

There is a growing body of literature which demonstrates that communication exists between cells of the immune system and the CNS. This communication can occur by cell-cell contact or by the production of soluble factors from lymphoid/mononuclear cells that are able to modulate the growth and function of cells found within the CNS; specifically, macroglia and microglial cells. Furthermore, glial cells can be activated to secrete immunoregulatory products that influence immune cells, as well as the glial cells themselves. Thus, the potential exists for bidirectional communication between lymphoid cells and glial cells, which is mediated via soluble factors such as cytokines and chemokines.

In this chapter, the 'traditional' functions of various glial cells and their antigenic determinants will be described. Following this will be a focus on various neurological disease states in which glial cells themselves are involved in inflammation and immunological events occurring in the brain. The topics to be discussed include the ability of glial cells to both respond to, and synthesize, a variety of cytokines/chemokines within the CNS. The capacity of glial cells to acquire MHC antigens and costimulatory molecules and function as antigen-presenting cells (APC) within the CNS will also be covered. The implications of these functions, cytokine secretion and antigen presentation, by glial cells will be discussed with respect to intracerebral immune responses, demyelination, and inflammation in neurological diseases that have an immunological component.

Glial Cells: Classification and Function

The first account of neuroglia was cited by Dutrochet in 1824, who noticed the existence in the CNS of non-neuronal components made up of spindle-shaped cells which were morphologically distinct from neurons. These cells were considered as a form of connective tissue within the CNS, and were called 'neuroglia', which means nerve glue [12]. There are two broad subgroups of glial cells; the *macroglia*, which consists of astrocytes, oligodendrocytes and ependymal cells, and *microglia*. The cells to be described and discussed in this chapter are astrocytes, oligodendrocytes and microglia.

Astrocytes

Astrocytes are the most numerous of the glial cells, and in the mammalian brain, outnumber neurons 10:1. Astrocytes have been implicated as the cell type most involved in the development and maintenance of the CNS, particularly with respect to keeping the interstitial milieu compatible for neuronal functioning. The astrocyte has critical roles in the development and support of neurons, repair of injured neurons, formation and maintenance of the BBB, neurotransmitter uptake, and maintenance of ion and metabolite homeostasis within the brain [13].

Origins and Characterization

Astrocytes are derived from the neuroectoderm of the neural tube. There are two morphological types of astrocytes; protoplasmic astrocytes found predominantly in gray matter and in relation to capillaries, which appear as 'bushy' cells with numerous radiating short processes, and fibrous astrocytes, localized primarily in the white matter, having long, thin ramified processes. Astrocytes can be distinguished from other CNS cell types by their expression of glial fibrillary acidic protein (GFAP), an astrocyte-specific intermediate filament [14]. The function of GFAP intermediate filaments has been obscure; however, the recent generation of mice deficient in GFAP has shed some light regarding its function. GFAP-deficient mice have normal development and fertility, and show no gross alterations in CNS morphology or behavior [15, 16]. However, the GFAP-deficient mice do have subtle changes in astrocyte morphology and show enhanced long-term potentiation in hippocampal neurons [15], suggesting that GFAP is important for astrocyte-neuronal interactions and modulating synaptic efficacy in the CNS. Glutamine synthetase (GS) is an enzyme that has been localized to astrocytes [17, 18], and is often used as a marker of astrocytes in vitro and in vivo. GS helps to regulate the levels of the neurotransmitter glutamate (see below), and also participates in ammonia detoxification in the CNS [19]. S100β is a calcium-binding protein localized primarily in astrocytes, and increases in expression as the astrocyte matures [20, 21]. Antisense inhibition of astrocyte S100β production causes alterations in cell morphology and cytoskeletal organization, and inhibits astrocyte proliferation [22], providing direct evidence for a role of S100β in glial cell structure and function. Astrocytes also secrete a biologically active form of S100β that functions as a trophic factor for certain neuronal populations and acts in an autocrine manner as a mitogenic factor for astrocytes [23]. In addition, S100β can initiate a pathogenic autoimmune T-cell response, implicating S100β as an astrocyte-derived autoantigen [24].

Astrocyte Functions

The Blood-Brain Barrier. As mentioned previously, the BBB, interposed between the circulatory system and the CNS, is relatively impermeable to ions, small peptides, proteins, and cells, and prevents access of the majority of circulating substances in the blood to the brain. The BBB is a layered structure of endothelial cells of cerebral vessels, basement membrane, and the perivascular glia limitans. Endothelial cells of the BBB differ from those in most peripheral capillaries in a fundamental manner; tight junctions with high electrical resistance are present between the brain capillary endothelial cells, and thus serve to limit entry of blood-borne elements in the CNS [25–27]. Astrocytes are the main element of the perivascular glia limitans. It has been shown that astrocytes influence the formation and maintenance of the BBB in vitro, both by elaboration of soluble mediators and by cell-cell contact [28–31]. In vivo, astrocyte foot processes are in close apposition to the abluminal surface of the microvascular endothelium of the BBB; thus, astrocytes contribute to both the structural and functional integrity of the BBB [27]. These findings indicate that astrocyte-endothelial cell interactions are crucial for the maintenance of an intact BBB, and for other brain endothelial cell properties necessary for both passive and active regulation at the blood-brain interface.

Guidance of Neurons during Development. Radial glia are cells of astrocytic lineage that appear transiently during a short developmental period, and then transform, presumably into GFAP-positive astrocytes [32–34]. These cells are elongated, often bipolar, and have two or more principal cell processes extending long distances throughout the neural tissue. Radial glia play a crucial role in the construction of the nervous system by providing scaffolding for migrating neurons and by participating in the formation of diverse glial cell lineages. In the developing nervous system, contact between radial glia and migrating neurons plays a crucial role in the selection of the migration pathways taken by neurons [35, 36]. In addition, radial glia generate signals for the displacement of neurons. This process of migration and displacement is mediated by a variety of adhesion molecules present on neuronal, glial or on both neuronal and glial cell surfaces [37, 38].

Regulation of K^+ Levels. Neurons in the CNS are maintained in a highly regulated environment. Neuronal activity results in the release of neurotransmitters and in extracellular pH changes, which can modify neuronal function. In addition, depolarization of neurons results in the opening of voltage-gated K^+ channels, release of K^+ because of membrane depolarization with subsequent accumulation of K^+ within the extracellular space ($[K^+]_0$). Appropriate synaptic transmission is particularly sensitive to $[K^+]_0$ variations, thus, the increase in $[K^+]_0$ needs to be buffered. Astrocytes play a major role in this regulatory process by employing several homeostatic mechanisms to regulate $[K^+]_0$ levels, including K^+ channel-mediated influx, K^+ cotransporters, and (Na^+, K^+) ATPase-mediated transport [39]. Astrocytes accumulate K^+ at a far higher rate than do neurons, indicating the importance of these cells in K^+ regulation.

Levels of $[K^+]_0$ can also be regulated by K^+ transport via current flow through glial cells by a process called 'K$^+$ spatial buffering' [39]. K^+ spatial buffering leads to the transfer of extracellular K^+ from regions where it is highest to regions where K^+ is low. Astrocytes, due to their distribution within the CNS and their electrical coupling, are believed to be the glial cell principally involved in spatial buffering.

Neurotransmitter Uptake. Astrocytes envelope synapses in a manner that allows them to intercept neurotransmitter molecules that overflow from the synaptic cleft; furthermore, they are equipped with transport systems and enzymes that are necessary to degrade most known neurotransmitters. One of the best-studied systems involves the metabolism of glutamate, the major excitatory neurotransmitter in the CNS [40]. Glutamate interaction with specific membrane receptors is responsible for many neurologic functions including cognition, memory, movement and sensation. Excessive extracellular glutamate levels can lead to activation of NMDA receptor channels present within neuronal synaptic membranes, leading to an increase in Ca^{2+} influx, and, eventually, neurotoxicity and cell death, which is termed 'excitotoxicity' [41]. Glutamate transport is the primary mechanism for the inactivation of synaptically released glutamate [42, 43]. The astrocyte glutamate transporters GLAST and GLT–1 provide the majority of functional glutamate transport, and are essential for maintaining low extracellular glutamate levels and for preventing chronic glutamate excitotoxicity [44, 45]. Glutamate that is taken up by astrocytes can be converted into glutamine via the enzyme GS that is present in astrocyte processes closely surrounding glutamatergic synapses [17, 18]. The glutamine is then released in the extracellular space to be taken up by neurons where it serves as a precursor of glutamate synthesis [40, 46].

Astrogliosis. Trauma, ischemia and many neurodegenerative diseases including Alzheimer's, Huntington's, MS, and ADC produce a glial reaction characterized by astrocyte proliferation, morphological changes, and enhancement of GFAP expression, that is termed astrogliosis [47]. The function of reactive astrocytes in the pathology of or recovery from neurological insult is not well understood. Depending on the circumstances, astrogliosis can be viewed as beneficial by aiding neuronal survival through the production of growth factors, neurotrophins, and extracellular matrix components that support neurite growth. However, astrogliosis may be of detriment by inhibiting neuronal function through the formation of glial scarring, which creates a physical barrier to the regrowth/function of axons.

Astrocytes as Immunocompetent Cells in the CNS. Recent studies have demonstrated that astrocytes are involved in immunological and inflammatory events occurring within the CNS [48]. Astrocytes have the capacity to respond to or secrete many immunoregulatory cytokines including interleukin (IL)-1,

Table 1. Astrocytes and cytokines

Cytokines produced	Response to cytokines						
	TNF-α	IL-1	IL-6	IFN-γ	TGF-β	IL-4	IL-10
IL-1	Proliferation	Proliferation	Proliferation	Proliferation	Inhibits proliferation	Inhibits proliferation	Inhibits proliferation
IL-6	Enhances ICAM-1,	Enhances ICAM-1	Inhibits ICAM-1	Enhances ICAM-1	Inhibits ICAM-1	Inhibits class II MHC	Inhibits ICAM-1
IL-8	VCAM-1, E-selectin	Inhibits class II MHC	Enhances	Induces class II	Inhibits class II MHC		Inhibits TNF-α
IL-10	Enhances class II	Enhances	complement	MHC	Inhibits complement		production
IL-12	MHC	complement	Inhibits TNF-α	Induces B7-1?	Induces cytokine		
TNF-α	Enhances	Induces cytokine	production	Enhances	production		
GM-CSF	complement	production	Enhances NGF	complement	IL-6		
M-CSF	Induces cytokine	TNF-α	production	Primes for	MCP-1		
G-CSF	production	IL-6		cytokine	Inhibits cytokine		
TGF-β	IL-6	TGF-β		production	production		
RANTES	GM-CSF	GM-CSF		TNF-α	TNF-α		
MCP-1	M-CSF	M-CSF		IL-6	GM-CSF		
CNTF	G-CSF	G-CSF					
NGF	IL-6	MCP-1					
	MCP-1	RANTES					
	RANTES						
	TNF-α						

IL-6, IL-8, IL-12, and IL-10; colony stimulating factors (CSFs) GM-CSF, M-CSF, and G-CSF; interferon (IFN)-γ; transforming growth factor-β (TGF-β); tumor necrosis factor-α (TNF-α), and chemokines (RANTES, MCP-1) (table 1). In addition, astrocytes are capable of expressing a variety of immunologically relevant proteins such as class I and II MHC antigens, complement components, costimulatory molecules (B7-1, B7-2), and adhesion molecules (ICAM-1, VCAM-1, E-selectin) upon cytokine stimulation [3]. The ability of astrocytes to both produce and respond to the above mentioned cytokines and chemokines contributes to the development of an inflamed state in the CNS and progression to disease.

Oligodendrocytes

Oligodendrocyte-Specific Antigens

Oligodendrocytes, the myelin-forming cells of the CNS, are identified for the most part by antisera directed against myelin-specific components [49]. Myelin is composed of 70–85% lipid and 15–30% protein [50, 51]. The most commonly used marker for oligodendrocyte identification is galactocerebroside (GalC), the major glycolipid of myelin. This antigen is unique to oligodendrocytes, and localized on the cell surface [52].

The major proteins of myelin include myelin basic protein (MBP), which makes up 30–35% of total myelin protein, and proteolipid protein (PLP), which accounts for 50% of total myelin protein [51]. MBP is associated with the cytoplasmic face of the myelin membrane, and is thought to mediate compaction between adjacent cytoplasmic membrane surfaces. PLP is an integral membrane protein thought to mediate interactions between opposing extracellular membrane surfaces. Myelin-associated glycoprotein (MAG) is closely associated with myelin, and makes up only 1% of total myelin proteins [51]. There is data to suggest that MAG may act as a cell-adhesion molecule [53]. The expression of all three myelin proteins, MBP, PLP and MAG, in tissue culture is indicative of oligodendrocyte maturation [54].

Oligodendrocyte Function

The function of the oligodendrocyte is myelin formation in the CNS [55]. Myelin is wrapped around axons, acts as insulation for nerve fibers, and allows for efficient nerve impulse conduction [56]. Cytoplasmic projections extend from the oligodendrocyte cell body to wrap around nerve fibers in a spiral fashion. Individual oligodendrocytes in white matter tracts provide myelin sheaths to numerous adjacent axons; in rat optic nerve, a single oligodendrocyte can myelinate up to 50 separate axons [57]. In disorders such as MS, damage to even a small number of oligodendrocytes can result in a dramatic functional change as action potential conduction in many axons can be slowed or totally blocked.

Microglia

Microglia, the resident macrophage of the brain, comprise 10–20% of all glial cells. Microglia were originally described by del Rio-Hortega [58]; he hypothesized that microglia were of mesodermal origin, had phagocytic functions, and exhibited changes in morphology following insult to the CNS. Most of the current evidence strongly suggests that microglia are derived from a bone marrow precursor of monocytic lineage [59, 60], and populate the CNS early in fetal development.

Microglial Subtypes

Parenchymal microglia represent a stable pool of cells with little to no turnover with bone marrow-derived cells [61]. At least three clearly identifiable states of parenchymal microglia have been defined based on developmental and pathophysiological studies. They are (1) the ramified, resting microglia present in the normal, nonpathologic adult CNS; (2) the activated, nonphagocytic microglia that is found in areas of secondary reaction due to nerve transection and CNS inflammation; and (3) the reactive, phagocytic microglia, found in areas of trauma, infection or neuronal degeneration. These different forms of parenchymal microglia are not independent from each other, but likely represent transformation of one cell type. Microglia exhibit plasticity in their morphology and appearance, particularly during injury or disease. Resting microglia are highly branched (ramified) cells with a small amount of perinuclear cytoplasm; however, upon pathologic insult, these cells become hypertrophied with short processes, and exhibit a 'bushy' appearance [62]. The term 'perivascular microglia' has been used to describe parenchymal microglia cells that are located in the vicinity of blood vessels. These perivascular microglia are found within the CNS parenchyma proper, and form part of the perivascular glia limitans [61]. These cells are often confused with 'perivascular cells' which are not part of the CNS parenchyma since they are separated from the brain tissue proper by a basal lamina. Perivascular cells have been shown to possess antigen presenting and phagocytic functions, and are thought to predominantly exist in an activated state [63].

Microglia Functions

Microglia are a class of brain mononuclear phagocytes, and are thought to be the principal immune cell resident to the CNS. Microglia have similar functions as other tissue macrophages including phagocytosis, antigen presentation, and production of cytokines, eicosanoids, complement components, excitatory amino acids (glutamate), proteinases, oxidative radicals and nitric oxide [61, 64, 65] (table 2). Production of these mediators is thought to contribute to CNS damage through a variety of mechanisms, some of which will be discussed in detail later. Microglia processes are incorporated in the layer of astrocytic foot processes of the perivascular glia limitans, and thus contribute to the structural integrity of the BBB [66].

Microglial Markers
There is a large amount of literature on the antigenic markers that microglia can express. These include class I and II MHC antigens, Fc receptors (FcRI-III), complement receptors (CR1, CR3, CR4), β2 integrins (LFA-1, LFA-3), ICAM-1, and the costimulatory molecules B7-1 and B7-2 [67–76]. Some of these markers are constitutively expressed by microglia, while others are inducible following injury, infection or inflammation of the nervous system. Currently, there are no unique histochemical markers that distinguish resting or activated microglia from monocytes/macrophages in the circulation, peripheral tissues or from macrophages which invade the brain [74].

Abnormal Glial Cell Function in Neurological Diseases

Although glial cell proliferation is critical in the development of the nervous system, these cells do not normally proliferate in the adult nervous system other than in response to injury, infection or trauma [77, 78]. An early response of the CNS to inflammation is the astrocytic reaction, astrogliosis, which is characterized by proliferation, hypertrophy and the increased synthesis of GFAP. This reaction is thought to contribute to the formation of dense glial scars in the CNS, leading to motor and sensory impairment. The mechanism(s) by which astrogliosis is induced is poorly understood at this time. Astrogliosis is associated with a number of neurologic disorders including MS, ADC, and EAE. A number of cytokines, including IL-1 [79, 80], TNF-α [81], and IL-6 [81], have been implicated in stimulating astrocyte proliferation.

Astrocyte function is also compromised in the disease of ADC, either by a nonproductive infection of astrocytes by HIV-1 [82–84]; modulation of astrocyte function by HIV-1 gene products; or by cell-cell interaction with HIV-1-infected macrophage/microglia [85–88]. Since disruption of astrocyte function can have serious consequences for ultimate neuronal functioning, the astrocyte is thought to act as an 'amplifier' in the disease of ADC.

Table 2. Microglia and cytokines

Cytokines produced	Response to cytokines								
	TNF-α	IL-1	IFN-γ	GM-CSF	M-CSF	IL-3	TGF-β	IL-4	IL-10
IL-1 IL-3 IL-6 IL-8 IL-10 IL-12 TNF-α MCP-1 MIP-1α RANTES TGF-β	Inhibits class II MHC Induces MCP-1 production MCP-1	Induces cytokine production TGF-β MCP-1	Enhances ICAM-1 Induces class II MHC Induces B7-1 Induces cytokine production TNF-α IL-6 IL-10 IL-15 MCP-1	Proliferation Enhances phagocytosis Inhibits class II MHC Induces IL-6 production	Proliferation Alters morphology Inhibits class II MHC Induces cytokine production MCP-1 IL-6	Proliferation Enhances phagocytosis	Inhibits class II MHC Chemotactic Inhibits cytokine production TNF-α IL-12	Inhibits class II MHC Induces cytokine production IL-1 IL-6	Inhibits ICAM-1 Inhibits class II MHC Inhibits cytokine production TNF-α IL-12

Table 3. Oligodendrocytes and cytokines

Cytokines produced	Response to cytokines					
	TNF-α	IL-1	IFN-γ	IL-2	NGF	CNTF
IL-1 TGF-β	Cell death Myelin damage	Induces TGF-β production	Inhibits proliferation Inhibits MBP expression Induces class I MHC	Induces proliferation Induces MBP expression Inhibits proliferation Cell death	Cell death	Prevents cell death

The fate of the myelin-producing cell, the oligodendrocyte, is much less well-defined in diseases such as MS and ADC. The oligodendrocyte has a critical role in the disease process of MS, as these cells and their membrane product (myelin) are destroyed, resulting in demyelination. In MS, there initially appears to be a burst of metabolic activity as evidenced by hyperplasia in the margin of active plaques, which is followed by an apparent loss of cells from the center of chronic lesions [77, 78]. There is evidence, however, that oligodendrocytes can survive active lesion formation, and can proliferate under these circumstances [89]. Additionally, it has been documented that remaining oligodendrocytes located at the margins of plaques are able to remyelinate to an extent denuded axons. These 'shadow plaques' are found primarily at the edge of MS lesions, and are composed of thinly remyelinated axons, with the myelin exhibiting aberrant layering [90, 91]. A correlation between oligodendrocyte proliferation and the extent of remyelination has been documented in the animal model of EAE [92], although this proliferative process may be abortive, incomplete, or transient. Oligodendrocytes do not appear to actively participate in immunological events during lesion formation in MS; however, they may be a target cell for a number of cytokines including IFN-γ [93], IL-2 [94, 95], and TNF-α [96, 97] (table 3).

Inappropriate activation of microglia in MS, EAE and ADC is thought to contribute directly to CNS damage through several mechanisms, including production of proinflammatory cytokines, matrix metalloproteinases and free radicals. Furthermore, activated microglia serve as the major APC in the CNS, likely contributing to aberrant immune reactivity within this site.

ADC occurs in the absence of recognized opportunistic pathogens, and is caused by direct infection of the CNS by HIV-1. Productive HIV-1 infection in the CNS is restricted to cells derived from the hematopoietic lineage, including infiltrating monocytes/macrophages and resident microglia [98, 99]. In vitro, HIV-1 is strongly tropic for microglial cells [100–104]. HIV-1 infection of microglia leads to the production of a number of neurotoxic substances, including nitric oxide and proinflammatory cytokines, which initiates the immunopathological events that eventually lead to neurotoxicity. As mentioned previously, infected microglia and astrocytes likely work together to cause neural damage.

The major pathological hallmark of MS is the presence of sclerotic plaques in the CNS that are characterized by demyelination, while axonal processes are generally unaffected. During active disease, demyelination is associated with an inflammatory reaction that is orchestrated by activated lymphocytes, macrophages and endogenous glial cells (astrocytes and microglia). Early MS lesions are characterized by the local accumulation of activated CD4+ and CD8+ T cells around small venules, with CD4+ cells predominating [8].

Later, there is myelin degeneration associated with perivascular inflammation consisting of T cells, B cells, plasma cells and activated macrophages [9, 78]. The primary demyelination observed in MS results from damage to the myelin sheath and/or oligodendrocytes. Macrophage/microglia are active participants in myelin breakdown; phagocytosis of myelin proteins in the lesions by these cells is a reliable indicator of ongoing demyelinating activity [105]. In addition, microglia become activated during MS to express molecules critical for antigen presentation, including class II MHC and B7-1 [106, 107]. Another immunologically relevant antigen expressed by macrophages/microglia in MS brain is CD40, a member of the TNF receptor family of cell surface proteins [108]. These CD40 positive macrophages/microglia colocalize with CD40 ligand (CD40L)-positive T-helper cells. CD40-CD40L interactions are thought to play a role in activation of cells of the monocytic lineage [109].

In vivo Expression of Cytokines in the CNS

A wide range of cytokines have been detected in the CNS of patients/ animals with neurological diseases such as MS, ADC, EAE and Alzheimer's disease. These include IL-1, -2, -3, -4, -6, -10 and -12, TNF-α, lymphotoxin (LT), IFN-α, -β and -γ, TGF-β, M-CSF, and chemokines [110–115] (table 4). IFN-γ is secreted by infiltrating activated T cells, while all the other cytokines/ chemokines can be produced by infiltrating leukocytes as well as activated endogenous astrocytes and microglia. TNF-α and LT have been implicated in the disease process of MS due to their ability to mediate myelin and oligodendrocyte damage, leading to the demyelination process observed in MS [96, 97, 116]. TNF-α and IL-1β induce astrocyte proliferation [79, 81], which could elicit the astrogliosis associated with MS and ADC and contribute to impairment of the BBB. In addition, some of these cytokines are thought to be involved in disease remission; these include IL-4, IL-10, IFN-β and TGF-β [110].

Cytokines

Cytokines play a major role in the initiation, propagation and regulation of immune and inflammatory responses. Cytokines are a diverse group of proteins, with a wide range of functions and target cells. The cytokines most relevant to inflammatory and immune responses will be briefly reviewed in this section, especially those involved with these events within the CNS. Numerous excellent review articles on cytokine function will be referenced for more detailed information.

Table 4. Cytokines present in CNS during disease states

Cytokine	Disease
Interleukin-1	MS, EAE, ADC, Alzheimer's
Interleukin-2	MS, EAE
Interleukin-3	EAE
Interleukin-4	MS, EAE
Interleukin-6	MS, EAE, ADC, Alzheimer's
Interleukin-10	MS, EAE
Interleukin-12	MS, EAE
Interferon-α/β	MS
Interferon-γ	MS, EAE, ADC
Tumor necrosis factor-α	MS, EAE, ADC, Alzheimer's
Lymphotoxin	MS, EAE
Chemokines (RANTES, MIP-1α, MIP-1β, IP-10, MCP-1)	EAE, ADC
Macrophage colony-stimulating factor	EAE
Transforming growth factor-β	MS, EAE, ADC

Although cytokines comprise a diverse group of proteins, they share a number of general properties. Cytokines are produced during the effector phases of immunity, and serve to mediate and regulate immune and inflammatory responses. Cytokine production is usually transient. Their expression is initiated by activation of gene transcription, the subsequent cytokine mRNA transcripts are unstable, and cytokines are rapidly secreted, resulting in a 'burst' of cytokine release. An individual cytokine can be produced by many different cell types, and have multiple effects on different cell types. Cytokines have also been shown to have redundant functions, i.e. several cytokines can mediate a common event due to the use of receptors with common signal transduction subunits. Thus, the cytokine system displays pleiotropism and redundancy. Cytokines often influence both the synthesis and function of other cytokines, resulting in complex regulatory pathways for immune and inflammatory responses. Cytokines initiate their action by binding to specific cell surface receptors on target cells. These receptors show high affinities for their ligands, with dissociation constants in the range of 10^{-10} to 10^{-12} M. This suggests that very small amounts of a cytokine need to be produced to elicit a biological response. The ultimate response of target cells to a particular cytokine is determined by the expression of the cytokine receptor, and the nature of the coupling between the receptor and the signal transduction pathways of the target cells.

Tumor Necrosis Factor-α

TNF-α is a cytokine synthesized by a wide variety of cells during host responses to microbial infection and neoplastic disease [117–119]. Within the CNS, astrocytes, microglia and neurons can be activated to secrete TNF-α [120–125]. TNF-α is the principal mediator of the host response to gram-negative bacteria, and also participates in inflammatory responses. TNF-α modulates immune reactivity by affecting the expression of class I and class II MHC molecules, adhesion molecules and costimulatory molecules on a variety of cell types, including astrocytes and microglia. In addition, TNF-α stimulates many cell types to produce cytokines, including IL-1, IL-6, IFN-β, CSFs, and TNF-α itself. In general, there is considerable evidence that overproduction of TNF-α contributes to various chronic inflammatory diseases. TNF-α is also an endogenous pyrogen that acts on cells in the hypothalamic regions of the brain to induce fever. Long-term systemic administration of TNF-α to animals causes cachexia, a state characterized by wasting of muscle and fat cells. TNF-α exists in both a transmembrane and secreted form. The transmembrane form is biologically active, and is thought to mediate its activity through the TNFR2 form of the TNF receptor (see below) [126].

There are two TNF receptors: TNFR1 (or TNFR55) and TNFR2 (or TNFR75) which exhibit specific and high-affinity binding to TNF-α. Both TNFR belong to the nerve growth factor (NGF)/TNF receptor superfamily, which also includes the low-affinity NGF receptor, *fas* antigen (or APO-1), CD40, CD30, CD27, and the TNF receptor-related protein (TNFRrp) [118, 119]. In addition to cell-membrane bound receptors, soluble forms have been described for most of the receptors. The TNFR2 is expressed primarily by endothelial cells and cells of the immune system, while TNFR1 is expressed by almost all cell types. TNFR1 is responsible for mediating most of the actions of TNF, including apoptosis, cytokine production, MHC expression, and antiviral activity, while TNFR2 transduces signals involved in proliferation of thymocytes, cytotoxicity, apoptosis and induction of NF-κB [117].

Interleukin-1

IL-1 is a cytokine produced by many cell types including activated macrophages, endothelial cells, B cells, epithelial cells, keratinocytes, microglia, astrocytes, and neurons [127–129]. IL-1 is produced in response to various inflammatory and infectious stimuli, and contributes to the development of the acute-phase response typical of inflammatory diseases. There are two forms of IL-1, IL-1α and IL-1β, which are the products of two different genes. Although these two forms of IL-1 have less than 30% structural homology to one another, they both bind to the same surface receptor, and have similar, although not completely overlapping biologic activities. Both IL-1α and IL-

1β are synthesized as precursor molecules. Pro-IL-1α is processed to the mature form by calpains, and, for the most part, remains intracellular or membrane-associated. Pro IL-1β can be processed by a variety of enzymes to the mature form, which is usually secreted and biologically active [129]. The IL-1 receptor antagonist (IL-1Ra) is a third member of the IL-1 family, and is a pure receptor antagonist [130]. The inhibitory action of the IL-1Ra results from binding to the IL-1R type I (see below), thus competing with IL-1α or IL-1β for binding to this receptor.

IL-1 is the major costimulator for T-cell activation via the augmentation of both IL-2 and IL-2 receptor expression. These effects allow antigen-stimulated T cells to rapidly proliferate and expand in number. IL-1, in cooperation with other cytokines, can enhance the growth and differentiation of B cells. IL-1 is a principal participant in inflammatory reactions through its induction of other inflammatory metabolites such as prostaglandins, collagenases, and phospholipase A_2. IL-1 stimulates numerous cell types to produce various cytokines, such as IL-6, TNF-α, CSFs and IL-1 itself. In the CNS, the effects of IL-1 include induction of fever and slow wave sleep.

IL-1α and IL-1β exert their effects by binding to specific receptors. There are two distinct receptors that bind both forms of IL-1. The IL-1R type I (80 kD) is expressed by a wide variety of cell types, and the IL-1R type II (68 kD) is found on B cells, neutrophils, and bone marrow cells. Both receptors belong to the Ig superfamily, and show approximately 28% homology in their extracellular domains. A major difference between the type I and II receptors is in the cytoplasmic domain; the type IIR has a cytoplasmic domain of only 29 amino acids whereas the type IR cytoplasmic domain consists of 213 amino acids [131]. Only the type IR is capable of transducing a biological signal following ligand binding, while the type IIR acts as a decoy target for IL-1, thus antagonizing the activity of IL-1 under appropriate conditions [132].

Interleukin-6

IL-6, along with IL-1 and TNF-α, is a pleiotropic cytokine involved in the regulation of inflammatory and immunologic responses [133]. IL-6 is secreted by a wide range of cells including fibroblasts, monocytes, B cells, endothelial cells, T cells, microglia, and astrocytes. Depending upon the cell type, synthesis of IL-6 is induced by a variety of agents including the cytokines IL-1, TNF-α and IFN-γ. IL-6 can stimulate hepatocytes to produce several plasma proteins such as fibrinogin and C-reactive protein, which contribute to the acute phase response. IL-6 has an important role in immune functions due to its effects on B-cell differentiation and antibody production, T-cell differentiation, and cytokine production.

IL-6 exerts its activity through binding to a receptor complex consisting of two membrane glycoproteins: an 80-kD IL-6 binding receptor protein (IL-6R) and a 130-kD signal-transducing protein (gp130) [133, 134]. IL-6 binds to IL-6R with low affinity, and in the absence of IL-6R, IL-6 does not bind to gp130. However, the presence of both IL-6R and gp130 will result in the formation of high-affinity IL-6 binding and subsequent signal transduction. IL-6 signaling involves the activation of three nonreceptor tyrosine kinases, JAK1, JAK2, and TYK2, and the transcription factors Signal Transducers and Activators of Transcription (STAT)-1 and STAT-3 [135–137].

Interferon-γ

IFN-γ is a 17-kD protein produced by a limited number of cell types that include T cells (both CD4+ and CD8+) and NK cells. Within the CD4+ T-cell population, IFN-γ is produced by the TH1 subset. IFN-γ is a pleiotropic cytokine that has physiological importance in regulating immune and inflammatory events. Some of the immune effects of IFN-γ include the ability to enhance the functional activity of macrophages, promotion of T and B-cell differentiation, and modulation of both class I and II MHC antigen expression on a variety of cells [138]. In this regard, IFN-γ is considered the most potent inducer of class II MHC expression on most cell types, except B cells [139]. IFN-γ also promotes inflammatory responses, largely through its ability to enhance TNF-α production. Two IFN-γ proteins self-associate to form a homodimer, and only the dimer displays biological activity due to its ability to mediate IFN-γ receptor dimerization [140].

The IFN-γ receptor bears little identity to any other known proteins, and structural analysis of the IFN-γ receptor's extracellular domain indicate that both the human and murine IFN-γ receptors belong to a family of cytokine receptors called the type II cytokine receptor family [140]. Functionally active IFN-γ receptors are composed of two distinct, species-specific polypeptides. A 90-kD α-chain is necessary and sufficient for ligand binding, but is not sufficient for induction of the biological response. The recently cloned IFN-γ receptor β-chain is essential for transmission of functional responses [141]. For a detailed description of the structural biology of IFN-γ and its receptor you may refer to the chapter by Walter [this vol.].

Binding of IFN-γ to its receptor results in the rapid induction of tyrosine phosphorylation of the transcription factor STAT-1α. Phosphorylated STAT-1α binds directly to the γ-activation sequence of a number of IFN-γ primary response genes, including guanylate-binding protein and the Fc receptor for IgG. The IFN-γ receptor does not contain intrinsic tyrosine kinase activity; rather, two nonreceptor tyrosine kinases, JAK1 and JAK2, become phosphorylated upon IFN-γ binding and then mediate the tyrosine phosphorylation of STAT-1α, resulting in the activation of primary response genes [142].

Chemokines

The chemokines are small molecular-weight (7–10 kD) secreted proteins that are expressed locally in response to inflammatory stimuli, and act to recruit inflammatory cells via their chemoattractant properties. Chemokines are the products of three related gene families, members of which exhibit sequence homology and structural similarities [143]. The CXC chemokines (α-chemokines) are chemotactic for neutrophils and T cells, while CC chemokines (β-chemokines) are chemotactic for monocyte/macrophage lineage cells. Members of the CXC family include IL-8, γIP-10, and GRO-α, β, γ; members of the CC family include macrophage inflammatory protein (MIP)-1α, MIP-1β, monocyte chemoattractant peptide-1 (MCP-1), and RANTES. A third chemokine subfamily (designated C) with a single cysteine near the N-terminus has been described on the basis of one member, lymphotactin [144].

Thus far, all functional chemokine receptors belong to the family of G protein-coupled, seven transmembrane receptors [145]. Multiple chemokine receptors with considerable overlapping ligand specificities have been identified, and in general, leukocytes express several different receptor types. This receptor 'promiscuity' may not be physiologically relevant in vivo, where expression may be highly restricted. There is currently a tremendous level of interest in the identification and characterization of chemokine receptors because of the recent studies identifying certain chemokine receptors as coreceptors for HIV-1 [146–148].

Interleukin-10

IL-10, a Th2-cytokine, is produced by numerous cell types including activated CD4+ Th2 cells, B cells, monocytes, astrocytes, and microglia. IL-10 generally exerts anti-inflammatory effects such as inhibition of proinflammatory cytokine production (IFN-γ, TNF-α, IL-1, IL-8), inhibition of class II MHC expression and antigen presentation ability, inhibition of macrophage activation, and inhibition of adhesion molecule expression [149].

The receptor for IL-10 is considered a member of the type II cytokine receptor family, and shares some similarity with the receptors for IFNα/β and IFN-γ. The signal transduction cascade initiated by IL-10 has not been well defined, but utilizes the tyrosine kinases TYK2 and JAK1, and the transcription factors STAT-1 and STAT-3.

Transforming Growth Factor-β

The TGF-β superfamily is a large group of cytokines that have diverse biological effects on cells derived from multiple cell lineages [150]. TGF-β is generally inhibitory for cells of the immune system, suppressing proliferation of B and T cells, preventing induction of IL-1 and IL-2 receptors, inhibiting production of proinflammatory cytokines such as TNF-α and IL-1, and inhibiting expression of class II MHC antigens [151]. Additionally, TGF-β promotes growth of new blood vessels, and serves as a chemotactic factor for macrophages.

TGF-β signaling involves both the type I (TβR-I) and type II (TβR-II) receptors. Wrana et al. [152] recently demonstrated that TGF-β binds directly to TβR-II, which is a constitutively active serine/threonine kinase. The bound TGF-β is then recognized by TβR-I, which is recruited into the complex, and becomes phosphorylated by TβR-II. This phosphorylation event of TβR-I is required for subsequent propagation of signals to substrates downstream of the TGF-β receptor complex. Although most cells express type I and II receptors for TGF-β, the specificity of the biological response to TGF-β in a given cell type depends on the state of differentiation of the cell, as well as the concentration of TGF-β to which cells are exposed.

Immune Cell-Derived Cytokines and Their Effect on Glial Cells

Studies in this field were initially directed towards investigating whether factors from immune cells may be contributing to astrocytic activation seen in the region of inflammatory infiltrates in diseases such as MS. Fontana et al. [153] tested this hypothesis by examining the ability of lymphocytes to produce glial-stimulating factors in vitro. Supernatants from activated rat lymphocytes were collected and tested for glial stimulating activity. Indeed, they found that these supernatants enhanced both RNA synthesis and DNA synthesis in rat astrocyte cultures [153]. This factor, named glial-stimulating factor, was produced by both activated T and B lymphocytes. A factor with similar activity was also derived from mitogen activated human T lymphocytes [154]. Merrill et al. [155] demonstrated that both rat astrocytes and oligodendrocytes could respond by increased proliferation to supernatants from activated human T cells. The supernatants tested were derived from a T-lymphoblast line (MO) which was infected with HTLV-II, human T lymphocytes transformed by HTLV-II, and human T lymphocytes activated by the mitogen phytohemagglutinin. A growth factor specific for oligodendrocytes was purified from the MO T-cell line [156]. This factor, termed glial growth-promoting factor, was constitutively produced by the MO T-cell line, and stimulated the proliferation of oligodendrocytes, with no apparent stimulatory activity on rat astrocytes.

The above-described studies indicated that soluble products from activated lymphoid cells could stimulate the growth of glial cells. An additional question to be addressed was whether glial cells could secrete soluble factors that would affect lymphocytes and/or monocytes. Fontana et al. [157] demonstrated that murine astrocytes, upon stimulation with LPS, secreted an IL-1-like factor, and that human astroglioma cell lines constitutively secreted an IL-1-like molecule. These early studies established that glial cells and lymphocytes could communicate through soluble mediators.

Cytokine Effects on Astrocytes

Proliferation

As mentioned previously, astrocyte proliferation (astrogliosis) is a hallmark of various neurological disease states. A number of cytokines have been identified that induce astrocyte proliferation both in vitro and in vivo; these include IL-1, TNF-α and IL-6. IL-1 was shown to have a stimulatory activity for astrocyte growth in vitro [79], while IL-1 injected into brain can stimulate astrogliosis [80, 158]. These results suggest that IL-1 may contribute to astroglial scarring in damaged mammalian brain. Recombinant IL-1 has also been shown to stimulate the proliferation of a human astrocytoma cell line, U373 [159]. This indicates that not only do cultures of rat astrocytes proliferate in response to IL-1, but a human GFAP+ astrocytoma cell line does as well. TNF-α has been shown to have a mitogenic effect on primary astrocytes [81] and human astroglioma cell lines [159, 160] in vitro, and induces astrogliosis when injected in vivo [158], again contributing to the astrogliosis associated with neurological diseases. Another cytokine with proinflammatory properties, IL-6, is mitogenic for astrocytes both in vitro and in vivo [81, 158]. Furthermore, transgenic expression of IL-6 in the CNS by using the rat neuron-specific enolase promoter (neurons) or murine GFAP promoter (astrocytes) induces astrogliosis [161, 162]. IFN-γ is also capable of promoting proliferation of fetal and adult human astrocytes in vitro, while having no effect on astrocytes derived from neonatal mouse brain [163, 164], suggesting a species-specific differential effect of IFN-γ on astrocyte proliferation. In addition, in vivo administration of IFN-γ into adult rat brain significantly enhanced the extent of reactive gliosis at the lesion site compared to saline controls [158, 163].

While TNF-α, IL-1β, IL-6 and IFN-γ are capable of promoting astrocyte proliferation, the cytokines TGF-β, IL-4, and IL-10 have been shown to inhibit proliferation of astrocytes in vitro and in vivo [165–171]. Thus, cytokines with proinflammatory properties can activate astrocytes in a manner leading to enhanced proliferation, while cytokines with immunosuppressive actions (TGF-β, IL-4, IL-10) can suppress this biological response (table 1).

Expression of Adhesion Molecules

Astrocyte expression of adhesion molecules can be influenced by various cytokines. Astrocytes can be induced by TNF-α, IL-1, and IFN-γ to express ICAM-1 [68, 172–174], and activated lymphocytes and monocytes bind to astrocytes in an ICAM-1-dependent manner [175]. Other adhesion molecules induced by TNF-α in astrocytes include VCAM-1 and E-selectin [172, 176]. The presence of ICAM-1, VCAM-1, E-selectin and other adhesion molecules in the vessel walls, as well as on astrocytes, may guide inflammatory leukocytes into and through the brain, thereby contributing to the neuropathology of disease states such as MS and ADC.

Cytokines with immunosuppressive properties, IL-10 and TGF-β, can inhibit expression of ICAM-1 on astrocytes, although they do so by different mechanisms. IL-10 inhibits TNF-α, IL-1β and IFN-γ induced ICAM-1 by blocking translation of ICAM-1 mRNA [68], while TGF-β inhibits ICAM-1 transcription induced by TNF-α and IL-1β [177]. In addition, TGF-β has a stimulus-specific inhibitory effect on ICAM-1 expression in astrocytes; TGF-β inhibits TNF-α and IL-1β induced ICAM-1 expression, but has no effect on IFN-γ-induced ICAM-1 expression in these cells [177]. Interestingly, astrocyte ICAM-1 transcription is also inhibited by IL-6 [68], while in other cell types (U937 cells, HepG2 cells, human breast cancer lines), IL-6 is a potent inducer of ICAM-1 expression [178–180]. These results suggest that IL-6 inhibition of ICAM-1 expression may be cell-type specific (table 1).

Class II MHC Expression

Class II MHC antigens have a critical role in regulating the immune response by presenting antigen to CD4+ T cells, leading to their activation and differentiation. The regulation of class II MHC genes occurs primarily at the transcriptional level, and recently, a non DNA-binding protein, class II transactivator (CIITA), has been shown to be *the* 'master control factor' for class II MHC transcription [139]. The appropriate constitutive and inducible expression of class II MHC antigens is essential for normal immune function, while aberrant expression has been correlated with various autoimmune diseases, including MS. In the inflamed CNS, class II MHC antigens are expressed by glial cells (both astrocytes and microglia), allowing them to function as APCs. This leads to activation of autoreactive CD4+ T cells, and subsequent inflammation and demyelination.

The local regulatory mechanisms that define how the pathogenic potential of autoreactive T cells is achieved as well as terminated has been an area of great interest over the past decade, and an area of controversy. At least two distinct signals are provided by APCs which leads to the generation of activated CD4+ T cells; an antigen-specific signal mediated through T-cell receptor ligation by antigen/class II MHC, and a second non-antigen-specific costimulatory signal [181]. Interactions between CD28 on T cells and its counterreceptors B7-1 (CD80) and B7-2 (CD86) on APCs are the most important for providing the costimulatory signals.

Astrocytes were the first CNS cell type shown to be inducible for class II MHC expression. In vitro, astrocytes can be induced to express class II upon exposure to IFN-γ or a combination of IFN-γ plus TNF-α [182–185]. As mentioned previously, astrocytes can respond to stimuli such as TNF-α, IL-1β, and IFN-γ with enhanced expression of adhesion molecules involved in antigen presentation such as ICAM-1 and VCAM-1 [68, 172, 173, 176, 186, 187]. Intrathecal injection of IFN-γ leads to class II MHC expression on astrocytes, although this expression occurs later and with less intensity than microglial expression of class II [188]. The documentation of class II MHC-positive astrocytes in disease states such as MS and EAE has been controversial, with some investigators finding such cells and others unable to detect them [106, 189–191]. Similarly, there is controversy as to whether astrocytes express the B7 costimulatory molecules; human astrocytes do not constitutively express either B7-1 or B7-2, nor are they inducible for expression of these molecules by IFN-γ [72, 192], while there is one report of constitutive B7-2 expression and IFN-γ inducible B7-1 expression by murine astrocytes [193]. There are conflicting reports on the ability of astrocytes to function as APCs. Class II MHC posistive astrocytes have been shown by some to function as APCs in vitro [183, 193–195], although other groups have reported that class II MHC positive astrocytes are unable to induce proliferation of T cells [196–199]. A recent study has demonstrated that IFN-γ-treated astrocytes which are induced to express B7-1 are in fact capable of activating *naive* T cells [193]. Other studies have shown that astrocytes can only activate T cells following priming by microglia [200], or upon coculture with microglia or the cytokine IL-1 [201]. There are also reports that class II MHC-positive astrocytes transmit a suppressive signal to CD4+ cells [196, 202–204], possibly due to the lack of B7 expression. Thus, the precise role of astrocytes as APCs is still unclear, i.e. whether they activate or inhibit T-cell function.

Many studies have focused on the regulation of class II MHC expression in astrocytes. As mentioned previously, IFN-γ is the strongest inducer for astrocytes, and TNF-α synergizes with IFN-γ for enhanced expression [185, 205, 206]. IFN-γ induction of class II MHC expression on astrocytes can be inhibited by a number of different factors including IL-1, TGF-β, IFN-β, IL-4, glutamate, cAMP agonists, norepinephrine, and nitric oxide, as well as direct contact with neurons [207–217]. We have been interested in the mechanism whereby TGF-β inhibits class II MHC expression in astrocytes, and have recently demonstrated that TGF-β suppresses IFN-γ-induced class II MHC expresssion by inhibiting the expression of CIITA [217]. Interestingly, IFN-β also inhibits class II MHC expression, but does not block CIITA expression, suggesting a possible inhibitory effect on CIITA protein function [218]. It will be important to understand the molecular mechanisms whereby the above mentioned factors inhibit class II MHC expression (table 1).

Production of Complement Components

The complement system is one of the main mediators of inflammation. It can be activated by immune complexes (classical pathway) or directly by microorganism surfaces (alternative pathway). Components of the complement cascade have been implicated in contributing to the pathology of several neurological autoimmune diseases such as MS, EAE and Guillain-Barré syndrome [219]. Recent studies have indicated that astrocytes can serve as a local endogenous source of many of the complement components, notably C3, the central component of the classical complement cascade [220]. Expression of C3 in astroglioma cells and astrocytes is enhanced by cytokines such as TNF-α, IL-1β, IFN-γ, IL-8 and IL-6 [221–225]. The observation that IFN-γ enhances C3 expression in astrocytes is of interest as IFN-γ has no effect on C3 expression in other cell types such as hepatocytes, monocytes and endothelial cells. Thus, the IFN-γ-mediated increase in C3 gene expression may be unique to astrocytes. Barnum and Jones [226] recently demonstrated that TGF-β could inhibit C3 production by astrocytes, indicating that cytokines can both stimulate and repress C3 expression in astrocytes.

Other components of the classical complement pathway, namely C1q, C1r, C1s, C2, C4 and C5, can also be produced by astrocytes, and expression is upregulated by IFN-γ and TNF-α [227, 228]. Astrocytes are also capable of synthesizing all of the components of the alternative activation pathway [225], as well as the components of the lytic terminal complement pathway [227]. These results indicate that astrocytes in the inflamed CNS can produce all the complement components necessary for the generation of a complete, lytic, complement system. This is relevant since both oligodendrocytes and neurons are susceptible to killing by the complement membrane attack complex [219, 229–231].

Complement fragments, in particular C5a, can function as powerful chemoattractants. Astrocytes express a functional C5a receptor, which enables C5a to cause activation of these cells [232, 233]. Thus, astrocytes are capable of both producing and responding to C5.

Cytokine/Chemokine Production

Astrocytes are capable of producing a wide array of cytokines/chemokines in response to cytokine stimulation and exposure to virus [48, 110, 234]. These cytokines/chemokines include IL-1, TNF-α, IL-6, IL-8, IL-12, IL-10, CSFs, MCP-1, and RANTES (table 1).

TNF-α is a potent inducer of the production of cytokines by astrocytes. Astrocytes produce three CSFs upon stimulation with TNF-α; GM-CSF, G-CSF, and M-CSF [235–236]. These CSFs can augment inflammatory responses due to their leukocyte chemotactic properties, which would promote migration of granulocytes and macrophages to inflammatory sites within the CNS. TNF-α also induces expression of IL-6 by astrocytes [237–239]. As discussed, IL-6 has both inflammatory and anti-inflammatory effects within the CNS. Expression of selected chemokines, MCP-1 and RANTES, is also induced by TNF-α in astrocytes [240–242]. MCP-1 expression within the CNS is likely to recruit monocytes to the site of inflammation, as well as activate those monocytes/microglia already present in an inflammatory lesion. In this regard, Fuentes et al. [243] generated transgenic mice overexpressing MCP-1 in the brain. There was a pronounced mononuclear cell infiltrate in the CNS of these animals, with the majority of cells identified as monocytes and macrophages. These cells were localized in a perivascular orientation with little infiltration into the parenchyma, which may reflect the accumulation of MCP-1 protein around blood vessels. These MCP-1 transgenic mice did not display any significant neurologic symptoms despite high transgene expression and the mononuclear cell infiltrate, indicating that the presence of monocytes/macrophages per se in the CNS is not sufficient to induce disease. RANTES expression by astrocytes can contribute to recruitment of monocytes as well as T lymphocytes to the CNS.

In addition to responding to TNF-α by the expression of cytokine/chemokines, TNF-α induces expression of its own gene in astrocytes, suggesting a positive feedback loop for TNF-α expression [244, 245]. We have recently described the molecular regulation of TNF-α-induced TNF-α gene expression in astrocytes, and our findings indicate that regulation of TNF-α expression in astrocytes differs from that previously described for monocytes, T cells and B cells, suggesting cell-type-specific mechanisms for control of this cytokine [245]. Specifically, our data demonstrated an involvement of 3′ NF-κB sites and modulation of the chromatin structure in TNF-α gene expression in astrocytes [245].

TNF-α gene expression is also susceptible to downregulation by cytokines such as TGF-β, IL-6 and IL-10 [171, 244, 246]. Of interest, these immunosuppressive cytokines act at different levels of TNF-α gene expression, i.e. TGF-β at the transcriptional level and IL-10/IL-6 at the translational level

[244, 246]. These results indicate a complex circuitry for the regulation of TNF-α expression in astrocytes; TNF-α induces expression of its own gene and can then go on to induce IL-6 and IL-10 [237], which ultimately act as negative regulators of TNF-α expression.

IL-1 also stimulates astrocytes to express cytokines/chemokines such as TNF-α [123], IL-6 [237–239], TGF-β [247], CSFs [248–250], MCP-1 [240], and RANTES [242]. Thus, IL-1 and TNF-α have the capacity to stimulate expression of similar cytokines/chemokines by astrocytes.

TGF-β stimulates astrocyte expression of IL–6, and synergizes with IL-1β and TNF-α for enhanced IL-6 production [244]. TGF-β also induces MCP-1 expression by astrocytes, and acts in an additive fashion with TNF-α for enhanced MCP–1 expression [241]. TGF-β induction of MCP–1 expression by astrocytes may be cell-type specific since endothelial cell expression of MCP-1 is inhibited by TGF-β [241].

These results collectively indicate that astrocytes have the capacity to produce both proinflammatory cytokines (TNF-α, IL-1, IL-6, MCP-1, RANTES, CSFs) as well as anti-inflammatory cytokines (TGF-β, IL-10, IL-6) upon activation. These cytokines/chemokines are involved in the activation as well as repression of immune reactivity and inflammatory responses within the CNS, thus their production by resident glial cells can contribute to these events in the inflamed CNS.

Microglia

Within the context of immune-mediated brain injury, microglia are considered as the main intrinsic immune effector cell of the CNS. In this section, some of the effector functions ascribed to microglia as determined by in vitro and in vivo studies will be described.

Activation
As activation of microglia, the macrophage of the brain, is an important early response to brain trauma, there has been interest in how the activation and differentiation of microglia is induced. In this regard, studies have focused on the effect of CSFs on microglia. CSFs have potent stimulatory effects on the growth and differentiation of bone marrow progenitor cells, and act to provide inflammatory leukocytes [251]. IL-3, also known as multi-CSF, acts on the most immature bone marrow progenitors to induce the expansion of cells that differentiate into all known mature cell types. GM-CSF is produced by a number of activated cells, including T cells, macrophages, endothelial cells, fibroblasts, and astrocytes. GM-CSF acts on bone marrow progenitor

cells already committed to differentiate into granulocytes and monocytes. GM-CSF can also interact with various mononuclear phagocytes, including microglia, to induce their activation. M-CSF, also called CSF-1, is made by macrophages, endothelial cells, and fibroblasts. M-CSF acts primarily on progenitor cells already committed to develop into monocytes; these progenitor cells are more mature than the targets for GM-CSF. G-CSF is made by the same cells that produce GM-CSF, and acts primarily on bone marrow progenitors already committed to develop into granulocytes.

Frei et al. [70] demonstrated that both IL-3 and GM-CSF induced murine microglia to proliferate. Further in vitro studies by Giulian et al. [252] also showed that rat microglia could proliferate in response to IL-3, GM-CSF, and M-CSF, and that both IL-3 and GM-CSF induced more rapid phagocytosis by microglia. They also performed in vivo experiments in which recombinant GM-CSF, IL-3, M-CSF, or G-CSF was infused into the cerebral cortex of rats. Both GM-CSF and IL-3 stimulated the appearance of microglia at the site of injection, and the phagocytic capability of these cells. Maysinger et al. [253] have utilized several strategies for the administration of M-CSF in vivo, including M-CSF in biodegradable spheres and microencapsulated fibroblasts producing M-CSF. The results from these studies demonstrated that in vivo administration of M-CSF altered the morphological appearance of microglia. Microglia have been shown to both produce and respond to the cytokine IL-3 [254, 255]. Within the brain, expression of the signal-transducing subunit of the IL-3 receptor shows restricted distribution, being expressed only by macrophages and/or microglia [256]. Chiang et al. [257] developed transgenic mice in which the expression of IL-3 was targeted to astrocytes using a GFAP fusion gene. In symptomatic transgenic mice, multifocal plaque-like lesions were detected in the cerebellum and brainstem. These lesions showed extensive primary demyelination and remyelination in association with the accumulation of large numbers of proliferating and activated macrophages/microglia. Lymphocytes were rarely present. This transgenic model exhibits many of the pathologic features of MS, and demonstrates that activation of macrophages/ microglia in a T-cell-independent manner is sufficient to induce demyelinating disease (table 2).

The major in vivo source of CSFs are astrocytes. Unstimulated astrocytes do not constitutively express GM-CSF and G-CSF, but are induced to by both TNF-α and LPS [235, 258]. Primary human astrocytes were recently shown to produce GM-CSF, M-CSF, and G-CSF in response to both IL-1 and TNF-α [248–250]. Unstimulated human astrocytes constitutively expressed mRNA for M-CSF, but had to be induced by IL-1 or TNF-α to express transcripts for GM-CSF or G-CSF. Similar observations have been made for murine astrocytes [259, 260] (table 1).

Adhesion Molecules

As mentioned previously, astrocytic end-feet on CNS capillaries contribute a major structural component of the BBB. There is also evidence that microglial processes also contribute to the structural integrity of the BBB [66]. Expression of ICAM-1 is enhanced in inflammatory diseases of the CNS such as MS and EAE [261–264], and expression has been localized to endothelial cells, astrocytes and microglia in these in vivo studies. ICAM-1 is a ligand for the β2 integrins LFA-1 (CD11a/CD18) and Mac-1 (CD11b/CD18), both of which are expressed by microglia [264, 265]. These results indicate the potential for homotypic interaction between microglia, which may be relevant in diseases such as ADC due to the formation of multinucleated giant cells (clusters of macrophages/microglia).

In vitro, microglia constitutively express low levels of ICAM-1, and only IFN-γ can enhance ICAM-1 gene expression [68]. This is in contrast to astrocytes, which express ICAM-1 in response to IFN-γ, TNF-α and IL-1β [68, 174]. Other cell types such as hepatocytes, epithelial cells, monocytes and keratinocytes also show a selective response to IFN-γ for ICAM-1 expression [266–268], as do microglia, demonstrating that there are cell-specific differences in how the ICAM-1 gene is regulated. ICAM-1 expression in microglia is inhibited by IL-10 and IL-6, but not TGF-β, again demonstrating differences in how ICAM-1 gene expression is regulated in astrocytes and microglia [68, 177] (table 2).

Class II MHC Expression

Much of the literature suggests that microglia are the most efficient APCs within the brain parenchyma. In vitro, microglia can be induced to express class II MHC antigens upon exposure to IFN-γ [69–71]. In vivo infusion or intrathecal injection of IFN-γ leads to rapid, robust expression of class II antigens on microglia [184, 188, 269]. In numerous CNS diseases such as EAE, MS, ADC, Alzheimer's disease, and Parkinson's disease, prominent expression of class II molecules has been detected on microglia [106, 270, 271]. Microglia can be activated to express other molecules critical for effective antigen presentation, including LFA-3, ICAM-1 and B7-1 [68, 72, 73]. Microglia expression of B7-1 is detected in vivo in the disease state of MS, particularly in acute plaques [72, 73, 107]. Since B7 expression is critical for delivery of the costimulatory signal required for complete activation of T cells [181, 272], this suggests that microglia are fully equipped to function as APCs for both naive and memory T cells. This has been borne out by in vitro experiments documenting that activated microglia are able to initiate and perpetuate CD4+ T-cell activation [70, 72, 195, 199, 273–277]. Many of these studies demonstrated the ability of activated microglia to both prime naive CD4+ T cells, as well as activate memory CD4+ T cells in an antigen-specific, class II MHC-restricted manner. Recent studies have also suggested that the B7-1 isoform induces naive T cells to undergo differentiation into a Th1 effector phenotype in vivo, contributing to disease progression of EAE [278]. Thus, expression of B7-1 by microglia may be a critical event in disease initiation by providing the costimulatory signal for generation of an autoreactive TH1 type T-cell response. In addition to activating an autoreactive T-cell response, microglia also have the ability to eliminate effector T cells. Ford et al. [279] recently demonstrated that class II MHC positive microglia support only an incomplete form of autoreactive CD4+ T-cell activation by inducing expression of IFN-γ and TNF-α, but not IL-2. After this interaction, apoptosis was detected in ~20% of the T cells. Thus, microglia can potentially control and/or eliminate T-cell responses in the CNS through apoptotic death.

IFN-γ-induced class II MHC expression in microglia is subject to inhibition by a number of mediators including GM-CSF, M-CSF, IL-4, TGF-β, TNF-α, and IL-10 [195, 249, 280–283], but is insensitive to many of the factors that inhibit class II MHC expression in astrocytes, such as IL-1, glutamate, cAMP agonists and neuronal contact [208–211]. The molecular mechanism(s) by which microglial class II MHC expression is inhibited is currently unknown (table 2).

Cytokine Production

Microglia can be activated to express a broad array of cytokines, including IL-1, IL-3, IL-6, IL-8, IL-10, IL-12, TNF-α, MCP-1, MIP-1α, RANTES, and TGF-β [67, 70, 235, 239, 240, 250, 254, 280, 284–302] (table 2). For production of many of these cytokines/chemokines, LPS is the most potent inducer. However, other cytokines such as IL-1, IL-6, TNF-α, M-CSF, GM-CSF, IL-4, and IL-13 can activate expression of cytokine genes in microglia, as can viruses and fragments of amyloid β-protein (Aβ(25–35)).

Many of these cytokines (IL-1, IL-6, IL-8, IL-12, TNF-α, MIP-1α, MCP-1, RANTES) have proinflammatory properties that can mediate inflammation and demyelination within the CNS. TNF-α has been documented to contribute to the demyelination process in the CNS by damaging oligodendrocytes, and activated microglia are involved in this event by production of both secreted and membrane-bound TNF-α [303]. Interestingly, secreted TNF-α produced by microglia was capable of killing oligodendrocytes, but the membrane bound form of TNF-α was more effective in this process [303], indicating a requirement for cell-cell contact between microglia and oligodendrocytes.

The cytokine IL-12 is recognized as being the key cytokine in determining the T-helper phenotype; IL-12 increases IFN-γ production by T cells, driving the immune response toward the TH1 profile [304]. Production of IL-12 by microglia represents another mechanism whereby these cells can function as regulators of immune activity within the CNS [292, 293].

Microglia also have the capacity to produce cytokines with immuno-suppressive actions such as IL-10 and TGF-β [280, 290, 300]. Lodge and Sriram [293] recently demonstrated that IL-10 and TGF-β inhibit TNF-α and IL-12 production by microglia, suggesting that microglia have intrinsic control mechanisms for regulating cytokine production.

Oligodendrocytes

Proliferation
IL-2 is the product of activated T cells and, thus, would only be present in the CNS during pathological disease states associated with lymphoid infiltration. IL-2 has been shown to influence the proliferation and differentiation of oligodendrocytes [305]. GalC+ oligodendrocytes are increased approximately 3-fold in cultures containing IL-2. Additionally, IL-2 appears to stimulate the maturation of oligodendrocytes, assessed as the enhanced expression of MBP in IL-2-treated oligodendrocytes. Both MBP mRNA and protein levels are increased in IL-2 stimulated oligodendrocytes [306]. MBP mRNA levels increase within 8 h after IL-2 stimulation, while MBP protein levels increase 24 h after stimulation. These findings provide evidence that an important step in oligodendrocyte differentiation – MBP mRNA and protein expression – can be amplified in part by IL-2. Human glioblastoma cell lines with an oligodendroglial phenotype (GalC+, GFAP–) proliferate in the presence of IL-2 [307, 308]. These findings indicate that both GalC+ primary oligodendrocytes and GalC+ glioblastoma cell lines can respond in a mitogenic fashion to IL-2. Interestingly, IL-2 appears to have an opposite effect on oligodendrocyte progenitor cells [95]. Purified IL-2 inhibited the proliferation of rat oligodendrocyte progenitor cells. These results suggest that IL-2 can have varying biological effects on oligodendrocytes depending on the maturational stage of these cells. Several recent studies have identified a substance produced by regenerating optic nerves from fish which is cytotoxic to oligodendrocytes [309]. The cytotoxic factor was identified as IL-2, and had the molecular weight of an IL-2 dimer. Apparently, only dimerized IL-2, but not monomeric IL-2, is cytotoxic to oligodendrocytes [310].

IFN-γ has a direct inhibitory effect on both the proliferation and differentiation of oligodendrocyte precursors [93]. IFN-γ treatment caused a change in cell morphology, a 50% reduction in GalC+ cells, and a decrease in MBP and MAG mRNA expression. TNF-α alone had no effect on any of the above parameters, but synergized with IFN-γ for a more pronounced effect (table 3). The authors propose that IFN-γ may have an important role in preventing remyelination in diseases such as MS.

Cell Death

Most relevant to CNS disease is the ability of TNF-α to mediate myelin and oligodendrocyte damage in vitro [96, 97, 311]. Lymphotoxin (LT), the cytokine which is genetically and functionally related to TNF-α [312], exerts a more potent cytotoxic effect toward oligodendrocytes than does TNF-α, and mediates its effect via apoptosis [313]. These aspects of TNF-α/LT activity may contribute directly to myelin damage and/or the demyelination process observed in MS. Human oligodendrocytes express both types of TNF receptors (TNFR1 and TNFR2) [314, 315]. The cytotoxicity mediated by TNF-α may occur through activation of either receptor since both soluble and membrane-bound TNF-α can kill oligodendrocytes.

The importance of TNF-α in demyelinating diseases was recently highlighted by the generation of transgenic mice constitutively expressing TNF-α in the CNS. These animals spontaneously developed a chronic inflammatory demyelinating disease with 100% penetrance from ~3 to 8 weeks of age [316]. Histopathological analysis revealed infiltration of the meninges and CNS parenchyma by CD4+ and CD8+ T cells, widespread astrogliosis and microgliosis, and focal demyelination. The direct effect of TNF-α in this disease was documented by administration of a neutralizing antibody against TNF-α, which prevented the development of neurological symptoms, T-cell infiltration, astrogliosis, microgliosis and demyelination. These results strongly support the hypothesis that within the CNS, TNF-α functions as a potent proinflammatory cytokine and a major effector of immune-mediated demyelination. In addition, transgenic mice expressing bioactive transmembrane TNF-α protein on astrocytes develop a similar neurologic disorder as described above [317]. Interestingly, transgenic mice producing a high level of transmembrane TNF-α in their neurons did not develop any phenotypic abnormalities [317]. The authors suggest that only astrocytes can form the intercellular contacts that are necessary for TNF-α to trigger CNS inflammation.

The cytokine ciliary neurotropic factor (CNTF) is produced by astrocytes, and promotes the generation, maturation and survival of oligodendrocytes [318]. CNTF has been shown to rescue oligodendrocytes from TNF-α-mediated and serum-deprivation-induced death [319, 320]. Interestingly, CNTF does not protect oligodendrocytes from injury induced by activated CD4+ T cells, which occurs by a TNF-α-independent effector mechanism [320, 321].

The neurotrophic factor nerve growth factor (NGF) is essential for the survival and differentiation of neurons, and astrocytes serve as one source of

NGF in the CNS [322, 323]. Recently, NGF was shown to induce the death of mature oligodendrocytes by interaction with the p75 neurotrophin receptor [324]. The p75 receptor belongs to the NGF/TNF receptor superfamily, and has similarity to the TNFR1, which mediates apoptosis of a variety of cell types [119]. Thus, two cytokines with death-inducing properties for oligodendrocytes (TNF-α, NGF), utilize receptors that can generate a cell-death signal (table 3).

Class I MHC Expression

Oligodendrocytes do not constitutively express class I MHC antigens; however, IFN-γ induces expression of class I MHC on oligodendrocytes in vivo and in vitro [184, 325, 326]. Increased expression of class I MHC is detected in the CNS in association with diseases such as MS and EAE. Transgenic mice expressing the class I MHC gene under control of the MBP promoter display dysmyelination without immune involvement, and develop a severe neurological disorder [327]. In addition, the CNS of such transgenic mice contain hypertrophic microglia and astrocytes [328]. The clinical and pathological features of the transgenic mice are likely due to class I MHC-induced alterations in oligodendrocyte function (table 3).

Cytokine Production

Oligodendrocyte function is modulated by numerous cytokines; however, oligodendrocytes themselves have a limited capacity to produce cytokines (table 3). Human oligodendroglioma cell lines are capable of producing IL-1 [329], and primary rat oligodendrocytes can secrete TGF-β upon stimulation with IL-1 [330].

Conclusion

This article highlights the fact that cells of the immune system and CNS can share similar functions: (1) secretion of immunoregulatory cytokines; (2) response to cytokines; and (3) antigen presentation. These properties allow for both physical contact between the two systems, i.e. microglia and/or astrocytes presenting antigen to T cells, as well as communication by soluble factors such as cytokines. There is a complex circuitry of interactions mediated by cytokines, especially in the event of lymphoid/mononuclear cell infiltration into the CNS. The secretion of IFN-γ by infiltrating activated T cells could initially induce astrocytes and microglia to express class I and class II MHC antigens, as well as prime these cells for subsequent cytokine production. The activation of astrocytes and microglia may contribute to either the initiation and/or propagation of intracerebral immune responses. A number of inflammatory mediators such as PGE_2, cytokines such as IFN-α/β, TGF-β, IL-10, and IL-4, and endogenous molecules like norepinephrine and glutamate, can act to ultimately suppress an immune response by inhibiting class II MHC expression, adhesion molecule expression, and cytokine production by glial cells.

The induction and ultimate repression of immune responses and cytokine production within the CNS is dependent upon: (1) the activational status of immune and glial cells; (2) the extent of cytokine receptor expression on these cells; (3) the concentration and location of these cytokines in the CNS; and (4) the temporal sequence in which a particular cell responds to the cytokines. The ultimate outcome of immunological and inflammatory events in the CNS will be determined, in part, by an interplay of the above parameters.

Future studies on the cellular and molecular mechanisms involved with cytokine expression by glial cells, specifically: (1) the nature of the signal transduction pathways utilized by astrocytes, microglia, and oligodendrocytes; (2) characterizing cytokine receptor expression on glial cells and modulation during disease states; and (3) transgenic expression or deletion of cytokines/chemokines in the CNS, will aid us in better understanding bidirectional communication between the immune system and nervous system.

Acknowledgements

I thank Sue B. Wade for her expert secretarial assistance in preparing this manuscript. Studies cited in this manuscript were supported by grants 2269-B-5 and 2205-B-5 from the National Multiple Sclerosis Society (NMSS), and by NIH Grants NS-29719, NS-31096, MH 50421, and MH-55795.

References

1   Baker CF, Billingham RF: Immunologically privileged sites. Adv Immunol 1977;25:1–49.
2   Nathanson JA, Chun LLY: Immunological function of the blood-cerebrospinal fluid barrier. Proc Natl Acad Sci USA 1989;86:1684–1688.
3   Shrikant P, Benveniste EN: The central nervous system as an immunocompetent organ: Role of glial cells in antigen presentation. J Immunol 1996;157:1819–1822.
4   Hickey WF, Hsu BL, Kimura H: T-lymphocyte entry into the central nervous system. J Neurosci Res 1991;28:254–260.
5   Prineas JW: Multiple sclerosis: Presence of lymphatic capillaries and lymphoid tissue in the brain and spinal cord. Science 1979;203:1123–1125.
6   Moench TR, Griffin DE: Immunocytochemical identification and quantitation of the mononuclear cells in the cerebrospinal fluid, meninges, and brain during acute viral meningoencephalitis. J Exp Med 1984;159:77–88.

7   Traugott U, Reinherz EL, Raine CS: Multiple sclerosis: Distribution of T-cells, T-cell subsets and Ia-positive macrophages in lesions of different ages. J Neuroimmunol 1983;4:201–221.
8   Hauser SL, Bhan AK, Gilles FH, et al: Immunohistochemical staining of human brain with monoclonal antibodies that identify lymphocytes, monocytes and the Ia antigen. J Neuroimmunol 1983;5:197–205.
9   Prineas JW, Wright RG: Macrophages, lymphocytes and plasma cells in the perivascular compartment in chronic multiple sclerosis. Lab Invest 1978;38:409–421.
10   Navia BA, Jordan BD, Price RW: The AIDS dementia complex. Ann Neurol 1986;19:517–524.
11   Raine CS: Biology of disease: Analysis of autoimmune demyelination: Its impact upon multiple sclerosis. Lab Invest 1984;50:608–635.
12   Virchow R: Cellular Pathology as Based upon Physiological and Pathological Histology (edited and translated by F Chance). London, Churchill, 1860.
13   Eddleston M, Mucke L: Molecular profile of reactive astrocytes: Implications for their role in neurologic disease. Neuroscience 1993;54:15–36.
14   Bignami A, Eng LF, Dahl D, Uyeda CT: Localization of the glial fibrillary acidic protein in astrocytes by immunofluorescence. Brain Res 1972;43:429–435.
15   McCall MA, Gregg RG, Behringer RR, et al: Targeted deletion in astrocyte intermediate filament (*Gfap*) alters neuronal physiology. Proc Natl Acad Sci USA 1996;93:6361–6366.
16   Pekny M, Levéen P, Pekna M, et al: Mice lacking glial fibrillary acidic protein display astrocytes devoid of intermediate filaments but develop and reproduce normally. EMBO J 1995;14:1590–1598.
17   Norenberg MD: The distribution of glutamine synthetase in the rat central nervous system. J Histochem Cytochem 1979;27:756–762.
18   Norenberg MD, Martinez-Hernandez A: Fine structural localization of glutamine synthetase in astrocytes in rat brain. Brain Res 1979;161:303–310.
19   Sadasivudu B, Rao TL, Murthy CR: Acute metabolic effects of ammonia in mouse brain. Neurochem Res 1977;2:639–645.
20   Ghandour MS, Langley OK, Labourdette G, Vencendon G, Gombos G: Specific and artifactual cellular localization of S-100 protein: An astrocyte marker in rat cerebellum. Dev Neurosci 1981; 4:66–78.
21   Herschman HR, Levine L, de Vellis J: Appearance of a brain-specific antigen (S–100 protein) in the developing rat brain. J Neurochem 1971;18:629–633.
22   Selinfreund RH, Barger SW, Welsh MJ, Van Eldik LJ: Antisense inhibition of glial S100β production results in alterations in cell morphology, cytoskeletal organization, and cell proliferation. J Cell Biol 1990;111:2021–2028.
23   Selinfreund RH, Bager SW, Pledger WJ, Van Eldik LJ: Neurotrophic protein S100β stimulates glial cell proliferation. Proc Natl Acad Sci USA 1991;88:3554–3558.
24   Kojima K, Berger T, Lassmann H, et al: Experimental autoimmune panencephalitis and uveoretinitis transferred to the Lewis rat by T lymphocytes specific for the S100β molecule, a calcium binding protein of astroglia. J Exp Med 1994;180:817–829.
25   Selmaj K: Pathophysiology of the blood-brain barrier. Springer Semin Immunopathol 1996;18: 57–73.
26   Abbott NJ, Revest PA, Romero IA: Astrocyte-endothelial interaction: Physiology and pathology. Neuropathol Appl Neurobiol 1992;18:424–433.
27   Wolburg H, Risau W: Formation of the blood-brain barrier; in Ransom BR, Kettenmann H (eds): Neuroglia. London, Oxford University Press, 1995, pp 763–776.
28   Rubin LL, Hall DE, Porter S, et al: A cell culture model of the blood-brain barrier. J Cell Biol 1991;115:1725–1735.
29   Janzer RC, Raff MC: Astrocytes induce blood-brain barrier properties in endothelial cells. Nature 1987;325:253–257.
30   Hurwitz AA, Berman JW, Rashbaum WK, Lyman WD: Human fetal astrocytes induce the expression of blood-brain barrier specific proteins by autologous endothelial cells. Brain Res 1993;625: 238–243.
31   Isobe I, Watanabe T, Yotsuyanagi T, et al: Astrocytic contributions to blood-brain barrier (BBB) formation by endothelial cells: A possible use of aortic endothelial cell for in vitro BBB model. Neurochem Int 1996;28:523–533.

32 Rakic P: Guidance of neurons migrating to the fetal monkey neocortex. Brain Res 1971;33:471–476.

33 Rakic P: Neuron-glial relationship during granule cell migration in developing cerebellar cortex: A Golgi and electronmicroscopic study in *Maccacus rhesus*. J Comp Neurol 1971;141:238–312.

34 Schmechel DE, Rakic P: A Golgi study of radial glial cells in developing monkey telencephalon: Morphologenesis and transformation into astrocytes. Anat Embryol 1979;156:115–152.

35 Rakic P: Radial glial cells: Scaffolding for brain construction; in Ransom BR, Kettenmann H (eds): Neuroglia. London, Oxford University Press, 1995, pp 746–762.

36 Hatten ME: Riding the glial monorail: A common mechanism for glial guided neuronal migration in different regions of the developing mammalian brain. Trends Neurosci 1990;13:179–184.

37 Choi BH, Lapham LW: Interactions of neurons and astrocytes during growth and development of human fetal brain in vitro. Exp Molec Pathol 1976;24:110–125.

38 Zheng C, Heintz N, Hatten ME: CNS gene encoding astrotactin, which supports neuronal migration along glial fibers. Science 1996;272:417–419.

39 Newman EA: Glial cell regulation of extracellular potassium; in Ransom BR, Kettenmann H (eds): Neuroglia. London, Oxford University Press, 1995, pp 717–731.

40 Erecinska M, Silver IA: Metabolism and role of glutamate in mammalian brain. Prog Neurobiol 1990;35:245–296.

41 Lipton SA, Rosenberg PA: Excitatory amino acids as a final common pathway for neurologic disorders. N Engl J Med 1994;330:613–622.

42 Martin DL: The role of glia in the activation of neurotransmitters, in Ransom BR, Kettenmann H (eds): Neuroglia. London, Oxford University Press, 1995, pp 732–745.

43 Nicholls D, Attwell D: The release and uptake of excitatory amino acids. Trends Pharmacol Sci 1990;11:462–468.

44 Rothstein JD, Dykes-Hoberg M, Pardo CA, et al: Knockout of glutamate transporters reveals a major role for astroglial transport in excitotoxicity and clearance of glutamate. Neuron 1996;16:675–686.

45 Mennerick S, Zorumski CF: Glial contributions to excitatory neurotransmission in cultured hippocampal cells. Nature 1994;368:59–62.

46 Balazs R, Machiyama Y, Hammond BJ, Julian T, Richter D: The operation of the γ-aminobutyrate bypath of the tricarboxylic acid cycle in brain tissue in vitro. Biochem J 1970;116:445–467.

47 Hatten ME, Liem RKH, Shelanski ML, Mason CA: Astroglia in CNS injury. Glia 1991;4:233–243.

48 Benveniste EN: Cytokine production; in Ransom BR, Kettenmann H (eds): Neuroglia. London, Oxford University Press, 1995, pp 700–716.

49 Miller R: Oligodendrocyte origins. Trends Neurosci 1996;19:92–96.

50 Norton WT, Cammer W: Isolation and characterization of myelin; in Morrel P (ed): Myelin. New York, Plenum Press, 1984, pp 147–180.

51 Lees MB, Brostoff SW: Proteins of myelin; in Morrel P (ed): Myelin. New York, Plenum Press, 1984, pp 197–217.

52 Raff MC, Mirsky R, Fields KL, et al: Galactocerebroside is a specific cell-surface antigenic marker for oligodendrocytes in culture. Nature 1978;274:813–815.

53 Bloom FE, Battenberg EL, Milner RJ, Sutcliffe JG: Immunocytochemical mapping of 1B236. A brain-specific neuronal polypeptide deduced from the sequence of a cloned mRNA. J Neurosci 1985;5:1781–1802.

54 Ranscht B, Clapshaw PA, Pride J, Noble M, Seifert W: Development of oligodendrocytes and Schwann cells studied with a monoclonal antibody against galactocerebroside. Proc Natl Acad Sci USA 1982;79:2709–2713.

55 Pfeiffer SE, Warrington AE, Bansal R: The oligodendrocyte and its many cellular processes. Trends Cell Biol 1993;3:191–197.

56 Morell P, Norton WT: Myelin. Scient Am 1980;242:88–118.

57 Bunge RP: Glial cells and the central myelin sheath. Physiol Rev 1968;48:197–251.

58 del Rio-Hortega P: Microglia; in Penfield W (ed): Cytology and Cellular Pathology of the Nervous System. New York, Hoeber, 1932, pp 481–584.

59 Hickey WF, Kimura H: Perivascular microglial cells of the CNS are bone marrow-derived and present antigen in vivo. Science 1988;239:290–292.

60 Perry VH, Gordon S: Macrophages and microglia in the nervous system. Trends Neurosci 1988; 11:273–277.

61 Gehrmann J, Matsumoto Y, Kreutzberg GW: Microglia: Intrinsic immuneffector cell of the brain. Brain Res Rev 1995;20:269–287.

62 Kreutzberg GW: Microglia: A sensor for pathological events in the CNS. Trends Neurosci 1996; 19:312–318.

63 Graeber MB, Streit WJ, Kreutzberg GW: Identity of ED2-positive perivascular cells in rat brain. J Neurosci Res 1989;22:103–106.

64 Banati RB, Gehrmann J, Schubert P, Kreutzberg GW: Cytotoxicity of microglia. Glia 1993;7:111–118.

65 Gordon S: The macrophage. BioEssays 1995;17:977–986.

66 Lassmann H, Vass FZK, Hickey WF: Microglial cells are a component of the perivascular glia limitans. J Neurosci Res 1991;28:236–243.

67 Walker DG, Kim SU, McGeer PL: Complement and cytokine gene expression in cultured microglia derived from postmortem human brains. J Neurosci Res 1995;40:478–493.

68 Shrikant P, Weber E, Jilling T, Benveniste EN: ICAM-1 gene expression by glial cells: Differential mechanisms of inhibition by interleukin-10 and interleukin-6. J Immunol 1995;155:1489–1501.

69 Panek RB, Benveniste EN: Class II MHC gene expression in microglia: Regulation by the cytokines IFN-γ, TNF-α and TGF-β. J Immunol 1995;154:2846–2854.

70 Frei K, Siepl C, Groscurth P, Bodmer S, Schwerdel C, Fontana A: Antigen presentation and tumor cytotoxicity by interferon-γ-treated microglial cells. Eur J Immunol 1987;17:1271–1278.

71 Suzumura A, Mezitis SGE, Gonatas NK, Silberberg DH: MHC antigen expression on bulk isolated macrophage-microglia from newborn mouse brain: Induction of Ia antigen expression by γ-interferon. J Neuroimmunol 1987;15:263–278.

72 Williams K, Ulvestad E, Antel JP: B7/BB-1 antigen expression on adult human microglia studied in vitro and in situ. Eur J Immunol 1994;24:3031–3037.

73 De Simone R, Giampaolo A, Giometto B, et al: The costimulatory molecule B7 is expressed on human microglia in culture and in multiple sclerosis acute lesions. J Neuropathol Exp Neurol 1995;54:175–187.

74 Ulvestad E, Williams K, Bjerkvig R, Tiekotter K, Antel J, Matre R: Human microglial cells have phenotypic and functional characteristics in common with both macrophages and dendritic antigen-presenting cells. J Leukoc Biol 1994;56:732–740.

75 Korotzer AR, Watt J, Cribbs D, et al: Cultured rat microglia express C1q and receptor for C1q: Implications for amyloid effects on microglia. Exp Neurol 1995;134:214–221.

76 Williams K, Bar-Or A, Ulvestad E, Olivier A, Antel JP, Yong VW: Biology of adult human microglia in culture: Comparisons with peripheral blood monocytes and astrocytes. J Neuropathol Exp Neurol 1992;51:538–549.

77 Adams CWM: Pathology of multiple sclerosis: Progression of the lesion. Br Med J 1977;33:15–20.

78 Prineas JW: Pathology of the early lesion in multiple sclerosis. Hum Pathol 1975;6:531–554.

79 Giulian D, Lachman LB: Interleukin 1 stimulation of astroglial proliferation after brain injury. Science 1985;228:497–499.

80 Giulian D, Woodward J, Young DG, Krebs JF, Lachman LB: Interleukin-1 injected into mammalian brain stimulates astrogliosis and neovascularization. J Neurosci 1988;8:2485–2490.

81 Selmaj KW, Farooq M, Norton WT, Raine CS, Brosnan CF: Proliferation of astrocytes in vitro in response to cytokines. A primary role for tumor necrosis factor. J Immunol 1990;144:129–135.

82 Ranki A, Nyberg M, Ovod V, et al: Abundant expression of HIV Nef and Rev proteins in brain astrocytes in vivo is associated with dementia. AIDS 1995;9:1001–1008.

83 Tornatore C, Chandra R, Berger JR, Major EO: HIV-1 infection of subcortical astrocytes in the pediatric central nervous system. Neurology 1994;44:481–487.

84 Saito Y, Sharer LR, Epstein LG, et al: Overexpression of *nef* as a marker for restricted HIV-1 infection of astrocytes in postmortem pediatric central nervous tissues. Neurology 1994;44:474–481.

85 Nottet HSLM, Jett M, Flanagan CR, et al: A regulatory role for astrocytes in HIV-1 encephalitis: An overexpression of eicosanoids, platelet-activating factor, and tumor necrosis factor-α by activated HIV-1-infected monocytes is attenuated by primary human astrocytes. J Immunol 1995;154:3567–3581.

86 Nottet HSLM, Gendelman HE: Unraveling the neuroimmune mechanisms for the HIV-1 associated cognitive/motor complex. Immunol Today 1995;16:441–448.

87 Nath A, Power C, Geiger JD: Interactions of the human immunodeficiency virus with astrocytes. Persp Drug Disc Design 1996;5:30–42.

88 Patton HK, Benveniste EN, Benos DJ: Astrocytes and the AIDS dementia complex. J Neuro-AIDS 1996;1:111–131.

89 Raine CS, Scheinberg CC, Waltz JM: Multiple sclerosis: Oligodendrocyte survival and proliferation in an active, established lesion. Lab Invest 1981;45:534–546.

90 Raine CS: Neurons, astrocytes and ependyma; in Davis RL, Robertson DM (eds): Textbook of Neuropathology. Baltimore, Williams & Wilkins, 1985, pp 468–547.

91 Prineas JW, Connell F: Remyelination in multiple sclerosis. Ann Neurol 1979;5:22–31.

92 Raine CS, Moore GRW, Hintzen R, Traugott U: Induction of oligodendrocyte proliferation and remyelination after chronic demyelination: Relevance to multiple sclerosis. Lab Invest 1988;59: 467–476.

93 Agresti C, D'Urso D, Levi G: Reversible inhibitory effects of interferon-γ and tumour necrosis factor-α on oligodendroglial lineage cell proliferation and differentiation in vitro. Eur J Neurosci 1996;8:1106–1116.

94 Benveniste EN, Kutsunai S, Merrill JE: Immunoregulatory molecules modulate glial cell growth; in Oppenhem JJ (ed): Leukocytes and Host Defense. New York, Liss, 1986, pp 221–226.

95 Saneto RP, Altman A, Knobler R, Johnson HM, de Vellis J: Interleukin 2 mediates the inhibition of oligodendrocyte progenitor cell proliferation in vitro. Proc Natl Acad Sci USA 1986;83:9221–9225.

96 Robbins DS, Shirazi Y, Drysdale BE, Lieberman A, Shin HS, Shin ML: Production of cytotoxic factor for oligodendrocytes by stimulated astrocytes. J Immunol 1987;139:2593–2597.

97 Selmaj KW, Raine CS: Tumor necrosis factor mediates myelin and oligodendrocyte damage in vitro. Ann Neurol 1988;23:339–346.

98 Eilbott DJ, Peress N, Burger H, et al: Human immunodeficiency virus type 1 in spinal cords of acquired immunodeficiency syndrome patients with myelopathy: Expression and replication in macrophages. Proc Natl Acad Sci USA 1989;86:3337–3341.

99 Koenig S, Gendelman HE, Orenstein TM, et al: Detection of AIDS virus in macrophages in brain tissue from AIDS patients with encephalopathy. Science 1986;233:1089–1093.

100 Sharpless NE, O'Brien WA, Verdin E, Kufta CV, Chen ISY, Dubois-Dalcq M: Human immuno-deficiency virus type 1 tropism for brain microglial cells is determined by a region of the env glycoprotein that also controls macrophage tropism. J Virol 1992;66:2588–2593.

101 Watkins BA, Dorn HH, Kelly WB, et al: Specific tropism of HIV-1 for microglial cells in primary human brain cultures. Science 1990;249:549–553.

102 Peudenier S, Hery C, Montagnier L, Tardieu M: Human microglial cells: Characterization in cerebral tissue and in primary culture, and study of their susceptibility to HIV-1. Ann Neurol 1991;29: 152–161.

103 Ioannidis JPA, Reichlin S, Skolnik PR: Long-term productive human immunodeficiency virus-1 infection in human infant microglia. Am J Pathol 1995;147:1200–1206.

104 Lee SC, Hatch WC, Liu W, Brosnan CF, Dickson DW: Productive infection of human fetal microglia in vitro by HIV-1. Ann NY Acad Sci 1993;693:314–316.

105 Bauer J, Sminia T, Wouterlood FG, Dijkstra CD: Phagocytic activity of macrophages and microglial cells during the course of acute and chronic relapsing experimental autoimmune encephalomyelitis. J Neurosci Res 1994;38:365–375.

106 Hofman FM, VonHanwher R, Dinarello C, Mizel S, Hinton D, Merrill JE: Immunoregulatory molecules and IL-2 receptors identified in multiple sclerosis brain. J Immunol 1986;136:3239–3245.

107 Winghagen A, Newcombe J, Dangond F, et al: Expression of costimulatory moleculels B7-1 (CD80), B7-2 (CD86), and interleukin 12 cytokine in multiple sclerosis lesions. J Exp Med 1995;182:1985–1996.

108 Gerritse K, Laman JD, Noelle RJ, et al: CD40-CD40 ligand interactions in experimental allergic encephalomyelitis and multiple sclerosis. Proc Natl Acad Sci USA 1996;93:2499–2504.

109 Alderson MR, Armitage RJ, Tough TW, Strockbine L, Fanslow WC, Spriggs MK: CD40 expression by human monocytes: Regulation by cytokines and activation of monocytes by the ligand for CD40. J Exp Med 1993;178:669–674.

110   Benveniste EN: Role of cytokines in multiple sclerosis, autoimmune encephalitis, and other neurolo-
       gical disorders; in Aggarawal B, Puri R (eds): Human Cytokines: Their Role in Research and
       Therapy. Boston, Blackwell, 1995, pp 195–216.

111   Merrill JE, Benveniste EN: Cytokines in inflammatory brain lesions: Helpful and harmful. Trends
       Neurosci 1996;19:331–338.

112   McArthur JC, Hoover DR, Bacellar H, et al: Dementia in AIDS patients: Incidence and risk factors.
       Neurology 1993;43:2245–2252.

113   Glass JD, Johnson RT: Human immunodeficiency virus and the brain. Ann Rev Neurosci 1996;
       19:1–26.

114   Stanley LC, Mrak RE, Woody RC, et al: Glial cytokines as neuropathogenic factors in HIV infection:
       Pathogenic similarities to Alzheimer's disease. J Neuropathol Exp Neurol 1994;53:231–238.

115   Sheng JG, Mrak RE, Griffin WST: Microglial interleukin-1α expression in brain regions in Alzheimer's
       disease: Correlation with neuritic plaque distribution. Neuropathol Appl Neurobiol 1995;21:290–301.

116   Selmaj K, Raine CS, Cross AH: Anti-tumor necrosis factor therapy abrogates autoimmune demy-
       elination. Ann Neurol 1991;30:694–700.

117   Aggarwal BB, Natarajan K: Tumor necrosis factors: Development during the last decade. Eur
       Cytokine Net 1996;7:93–124.

118   Bazzoni F, Beutler B: The tumor necrosis factor ligand and receptor families. N Engl J Med 1996;
       334:1717–1725.

119   Lotz M, Setareh M, von Kempis J, Schwarz H: The nerve growth factor/tumor necrosis factor
       receptor family. J Leukoc Biol 1996;60:1–7.

120   Hetier E, Ayala J, Bousseau A, Denefle P, Prochiantz A: Amoeboid microglial cells and not astrocytes
       synthesize TNF-α in swiss mouse brain cell cultures. Eur J Neurosci 1990;2:762–768.

121   Sawada M, Kondo N, Suzumura A, Marunouchi T: Production of tumor necrosis factor-alpha by
       microglia and astrocytes in culture. Brain Res 1989;491:394–397.

122   Lieberman AP, Pitha PM, Shin HS, Shin ML: Production of tumor necrosis factor and other
       cytokines by astrocytes stimulated with lipopolysaccharide or a neurotropic virus. Proc Natl Acad
       Sci USA 1989;86:6348–6352.

123   Chung IY, Benveniste EN: Tumor necrosis factor-α production by astrocytes: Induction by lipopoly-
       saccharide, IFN-γ and IL-1β. J Immunol 1990;144:2999–3007.

124   Breder CD, Dinarello CA, Saper CB: Interleukin-1 immunoreactive innervation of human hypothal-
       amus. Science 1988;240:321–324.

125   Tchélingérian J-L, Quinonero J, Booss J, Jacque C: Localization of TNFα and IL-1α immunoreactivi-
       ties in striatal neurons after surgical injury to the hippocampus. Neuron 1993;10:213–224.

126   Grell M, Douni E, Wajant H, et al: The transmembrane form of tumor necrosis factor is the prime
       activating ligand of the 80 kDa tumor necrosis factor receptor. Cell 1995;83:793–802.

127   de Giovine FS, Duff GW: Interleukin 1: The first interleukin. Immunol Today 1990;11:13–14.

128   Arai K, Lee F, Miyajima A, Miyatake S, Arai N, Yokota T: Cytokines: Coordinators of immune
       and inflammatory responses. Annu Rev Biochem 1990;59:783–836.

129   Dinarello CA: The interleukin-1 family: 10 years of discovery. FASEB J 1994;8:1314–1325.

130   Dripps DJ: Interleukin-1 (IL-1) receptor antagonist binds to the 80-kDa IL-1 receptor but does
       not initiate IL-1 signal transduction. J Biol Chem 1991;266:10331–10336.

131   Kuno K, Matsushima K: The IL-1 receptor signaling pathway. J Leukoc Biol 1994;56:542–547.

132   Colotta F, Re F, Muzio M, et al: Interleukin-1 type II receptor: A decoy target for IL-1 that is
       regulated by IL-4. Science 1993;261:472–475.

133   Kishimoto T, Akira S, Narazaki M, Taga T: Interleukin-6 family of cytokines and gp130. Blood
       1995;86:1243–1254.

134   Kishimoto T, Taga T, Akira S: Cytokine signal transduction. Cell 1994;76:253–262.

135   Stahl N, Boulton TG, Farruggella T, et al: Association and activation of Jak-Tyk kinases by CNTF-
       LIF-OSM-IL-6 β receptor components. Science 1994;263:92–95.

136   Zhong Z, Wen Z, Darnell JE Jr: Stat3: A STAT family member activated by tyrosine phosphorylation
       in response to epidermal growth factor and interleukin-6. Science 1994;264:95–98.

137   Akira S, Nishio Y, Inoue M, et al: Molecular cloning of APRF, a novel IFN-stimulated gene factor 3
       p91-related transcription factor involved in the gp130-mediated signaling pathway. Cell 1994;77:63–71.

138 Billiau A: Interferon-γ: Biology and role in pathogenesis. Adv Immunol 1996;61–130.

139 Rohn WM, Lee Y-J, Benveniste EN: Regulation of class II MHC expression. Crit Rev Immunol 1996;16:311–330.

140 Farrar MA, Schreiber RD: The molecular cell biology of interferon-γ and its receptor. Annu Rev Immunol 1993;11:571–611.

141 Greenlund AC, Farrar MA, Viviano BL, Schreiber RD: Ligand-induced IFNγ receptor tyrosine phosphorylation couples the receptor to its signal transduction system (p91). EMBO J 1994;13: 1591–1600.

142 Darnell JE Jr, Kerr IM, Stark GR: Jak-STAT pathways and transcriptional activation in response to IFNs and other extracellular signaling proteins. Science 1994;264:1415–1421.

143 Baggiolini M, Dahinden CA: CC chemokines in allergic inflammation. Immunol Today 1994;15: 127–133.

144 Kelner GS, Kennedy J, Bacon KB, et al: Lymphotactin: A cytokine that represents a new class of chemokine. Science 1994;266:1395–1399.

145 Power CA, Wells TNC: Cloning and characterization of human chemokine receptors. Trends Pharmacol Sci 1996;17:209–213.

146 Doranz BJ, Rucker J, Yi Y, et al: A dual-tropic primary HIV-1 isolate that uses fusin and the β-chemokine receptors CKR-5, CKR-3, and CKR-2b as fusion cofactors. Cell 1996;85:1149–1158.

147 Alkhatib G, Combadiere C, Broder CC, et al: CC CKR5: A RANTES, MIP-1α, MIP-1β receptor as a fusion cofactor for macrophage-tropic HIV-1. Science 1996;272:1955–1958.

148 Deng H, Liu R, Ellmeier W, et al: Identification of a major co-receptor for primary isolates of HIV-1. Nature 1996;381:661–666.

149 Moore KW, O'Garra A, de Waal Malefyt M, Vieira P, Mosmann TR: Interleukin-10. Annu Rev Immunol 1993;11:165–190.

150 Miyazono K, Hidenori I, Heldin CH: Transforming growth factor-β: Latent forms, binding proteins and receptors. Growth Factors 1993;8:11–22.

151 Wahl SM: Transforming growth factor-β: The good, the bad, the ugly. J Exp Med 1994;180: 1587–1590.

152 Wrana JL, Attisano L, Wieser R, Ventura F, Massagué J: Mechanism of activation of the TGF-β receptor. Nature 1994;370:341–347.

153 Fontana A, Dubs R, Merchant R, Balsiger S, Grob PJ: Glia cell stimulating factor (GSF): A new lymphokine. I. Cellular sources and partial purification of murine GSF, role of cytoskeleton and protein synthesis in its production. J Neuroimmunol 1982;2:55–71.

154 Fontana A, Otz U, DeWeck AL, Grob PJ: Glia cell stimulating factor (GSF): A new lymphokine. 2. Cellular sources and partial purification of human GSF. J Neuroimmunol 1982;2:73–81.

155 Merrill JE, Kutsunai S, Mohlstrom C, Hofman F, Groopman J, Golde DW: Proliferation of astroglia and oligodendroglia in response to human T-cell derived factors. Science 1984;224:1428–1431.

156 Benveniste EN, Merrill JE, Kaufman SE, Golde DW, Gasson JC: Purification and characterization of human T-lymphocyte derived glial growth promoting factor. Proc Natl Acad Sci USA 1985;82: 3930–3934.

157 Fontana A, Kristensen F, Dubs R, Gemsa D, Weber E: Production of prostaglandin E and an interleukin-1-like factor by cultured astrocytes and C6 glioma cells. J Immunol 1982;129:2413–2419.

158 Balasingam V, Tejada-Berges T, Wright E, Bouckova R, Yong VW: Reactive astrogliosis in the neonatal mouse brain and its modulation by cytokines. J Neurosci 1994;14:846–856.

159 Lachman LB, Brown DC, Dinarello CA: Growth promoting effect of recombinant interleukin-1 and tumor necrosis factor for a human astrocytoma cell line. J Immunol 1987;138:2913–2916.

160 Bethea JR, Gillespie GY, Chung IY, Benveniste EN: Tumor necrosis factor production and receptor expression by a human astroglioma cell line. J Neuroimmunol 1990;30:1–13.

161 Campbell IL, Abraham CR, Masliah E, et al: Neurologic disease induced in transgenic mice by cerebral overexpression of interleukin 6. Proc Natl Acad Sci USA 1993;90:10061–10065.

162 Fattori E, Lazzaro D, Musiani P, Modesti A, Alonzi T, Ciliberto G: IL-6 expression in neurons of transgenic mice causes reactive astrocytosis and increase in ramified microglial cells but no neuronal damage. Eur J Neurosci 1995;7:2441–2449.

163 Yong VW, Moumdjian R, Yong FP, et al: γ-Interferon promotes proliferation of adult human astrocytes in vitro and reactive gliosis in the adult mouse brain in vivo. Proc Natl Acad Sci USA 1991;88:7016–7020.

164 Yong VW, Tejada-Berges T, Goodyer CG, Antel JP, Yong FP: Differential proliferative response of human and mouse astrocytes to gamma-interferon. Glia 1992;6:269–280.

165 Lindholm D, Castren E, Kiefer R, Zafra F, Thoenen H: Transforming growth factor-β1 in the rat brain: Increase after injury and inhibition of astrocyte proliferation. J Cell Biol 1992;117:395–400.

166 Morganti-Kossmann MC, Kossmann T, Brandes ME, Mergenhagen SE, Wahl SM: Autocrine and paracrine regulation of astrocyte function by transforming growth factor-β. J Neuroimmunol 1992; 39:163–174.

167 Hunter KE, Sporn MB, Davies AM: Transforming growth factor-βs inhibit mitogen-stimulated proliferation of astrocytes. Glia 1993;7:203–211.

168 Iwasaki K, Rogers LR, Estes ML, Barna BP: Modulation of proliferation and antigen expression of a cloned human glioblastoma by interleukin-4 alone and in combination with tumor necrosis factor-α and/or interferon γ. Neurosurgery 1993;33:489–494.

169 Xiao B-G, Zhang G-X, Ma C-G, Link H: Transforming growth factor-beta1 (TGF β1)-mediated inhibition of glial cell proliferation and down-regulation of intercellular adhesion molecule-1 (ICAM-1) are interrupted by interferon-gamma (IFN-γ). Clin Exp Immunol 1996;103:475–481.

170 Estes ML, Iwasaki K, Jacobs BS, Barna BP: Interleukin-4 down-regulates adult human astrocyte DNA synthesis and proliferation. Am J Pathol 1993;143:337–341.

171 Balasingam V, Yong VW: Attenuation of astroglial reactivity by interleukin-10. J Neurosci 1996; 16:2945–2955.

172 Hurwitz AA, Lyman WD, Guida MP, Calderon TM, Berman JW: Tumor necrosis factor α induces adhesion molecule expression on human fetal astrocytes. J Exp Med 1992;176:1631–1636.

173 Frohman EM, Frohman TC, Dustin ML, et al: The induction of intercellular adhesion molecule 1 (ICAM-1) expression on human fetal astrocytes by interferon-γ, tumor necrosis factor-α, lymphotoxin, and interleukin-1: Relevance to intracerebral antigen presentation. J Neuroimmunol 1989;23:117–124.

174 Shrikant P, Chung IY, Ballestas M, Benveniste EN: Regulation of intercellular adhesion molecule-1 gene expression by tumor necrosis factor-α, interleukin–1β, and interferon-γ in astrocytes. J Neuroimmunol 1994;51:209–220.

175 Héry C, Sebire G, Peudenier S, Tardieu M: Adhesion to human neurons and astrocytes of monocytes: The role of interaction of CR3 and ICAM-1 and modulation by cytokines. J Neuroimmunol 1995; 57:101–109.

176 Rosenman SJ, Shrikant P, Dubb L, Benveniste EN, Ransohoff RM: Cytokine-induced expression of vascular cell adhesion molecule-1 (VCAM-1) by astrocytes and astrocytoma cell lines. J Immunol 1995;154:1888–1899.

177 Shrikant P, Lee SJ, Kalvakalanu I, Ransohoff RM, Benveniste EN: Stimulus-specific inhibition of ICAM-1 gene expression by TGF-β. J Immunol 1996;157:892–900.

178 Caldenhoven E, Coffer P, Yuan J, et al: Stimulation of the human intercellular adhesion molecule-1 promoter by interleukin-6 and interferon-γ involves binding of distinct factors to a palindromic response element. J Biol Chem 1994;269:21146–21154.

179 Duits A, Dimjati W, Van de Winkel JGJ, Capel PJA: Synergism of interleukin 6 and 1α,25-dihydroxyvitamin D₃ in induction of myeloid differentiation of human leukemic cell. J Leukoc Biol 1992;51:237–243.

180 Hutchins D, Steel CM: Regulation of ICAM-1 (CD54) expression in human breast cancer cell lines by interleukin 6 and fibroblast-derived factors. Int J Cancer 1994;58:80–84.

181 June CH, Bluestone JA, Nadler LM, Thompson CB: The B7 and CD28 receptor families. Immunol Today 1994;15:321–331.

182 Hirsch MR, Wietzerbin J, Pierres M, Goridis C: Expression of Ia antigens by cultured astrocytes treated with interferon-γ. Neurosci Lett 1983;41:199–204.

183 Fontana A, Fierz W, Wekerle H: Astrocytes present myelin basic protein to encephalitogenic T-cell lines. Nature 1984;307:273–276.

184 Wong GHW, Bartlett PF, Clark-Lewis I, Battye F, Schrader JW: Inducible expression of H-2 and Ia antigens on brain cells. Nature 1984;310:688–691.

185 Vidovic M, Sparacio SM, Elovitz M, Benveniste EN: Induction and regulation of class II MHC mRNA expression in astrocytes by IFN-γ and TNF-α. J Neuroimmunol 1990;30:189–200.

186 Aloisi F, Borsellino G, Samoggia P, et al: Astrocyte cultures from human embryonic brain: Characterization and modulation of surface molecules by inflammatory cytokines. J Neurosci Res 1992;32: 494–506.

187 Shrikant P, Benos DJ, Tang L-P, Benveniste EN: HIV gp120 enhances ICAM-1 gene expression in glial cells: Involvement of JAK/STAT and protein kinase C signaling pathways. J Immunol 1996; 156:1307–1314.

188 Vass K, Lassmann H: Intrathecal application of interferon gamma. Am J Pathol 1990;137:789–800.

189 Lee SC, Moore GRW, Golenwsky G, Raine CS: Multiple sclerosis: A role for astroglia in active demyelination suggested by class II MHC expression and ultrastructural study. J Neuropathol Exp Neurol 1990;49:122–136.

190 Hickey WF, Osborn JP, Kirby WM: Expression of Ia molecules by astrocytes during acute experimental allergic encephalmyelitis in the Lewis rat. Cell Immunol 1985;91:528–535.

191 Matsumoto Y, Kawai K, Fujiwara M: In situ Ia expression on brain cells in the rat: Autoimmune encephalomyelitis-resistant strain (BN) and susceptible strain (Lewis) compared. Immunology 1989; 66:621–627.

192 Satoh J-I, Lee YB, Kim SU: T-cell costimulatory molecules B7-1 (CD80) and B7-2 (CD86) are expressed in human microglia but not in astrocytes in culture. Brain Res 1995;704:92–96.

193 Nikcevich KM, Gordon KB, Tan L, Hurst SD, Kroepfl JF, Gardinier M, Barrett TA, Miller SM: IFN-γ-activated primary murine astrocytes express B7 costimulatory molecules and prime naive antigen-specific T cells. J Immunol 1997;158:614–621.

194 Fierz W, Endler B, Reske K, Wekerle H, Fontana A: Astrocytes as antigen presenting cells. I. Induction of Ia antigen expression on astrocytes by T cells via immune interferon and its effect on antigen presentation. J Immunol 1985;134:3785–3793.

195 Frei K, Lins H, Schwerdel C, Fontana A: Antigen presentation in the central nervous system: The inhibitory effect of IL-10 on MHC class II expression and production of cytokines depends on the inducing signals and the type of cell analyzed. J Immunol 1994;152:2720–2728.

196 Matsumoto Y, Ohmori K, Fujiwara M: Immune regulation by brain cells in the central nervous system: Microglia but not astrocytes present myelin basic protein to encephalitogenic T cells under in vivo mimicking conditions. Immunology 1992;76:209–216.

197 Weber F, Meinl E, Aloisi F, et al: Human astrocytes are only partially competent antigen presenting cells. Brain 1994;117:59–69.

198 Williams K Jr, Ulvestad E, Cragg L, Blain M, Antel JP: Induction of primary T cell responses by human glial cells. J Neurosci Res 1993;36:382–390.

199 Cash E, Rott O: Microglial cells qualify as the stimulators of unprimed CD4+ and CD8+ T lymphocytes in the central nervous system. Clin Exp Immunol 1994;98:313–318.

200 Sedgwick JD, Möbner R, Schwender S, ter Meulen V: Major histocompatibility complex-expressing nonhematopoietic astroglial cells prime only CD8+ T lymphocytes: Astroglial cells as perpetuators but not initiators of CD4+ T cell responses in the central nervous system. J Exp Med 1991;173:1235–1246.

201 Williams KC, Dooley NP, Ulvestad E, et al: Antigen presentation by human fetal astrocytes with the cooperative effect of microglia or the microglial-derived cytokine IL-1. J Neurosci 1995;15: 1869–1878.

202 Takiguchi M, Frelinger JA: Induction of antigen presentation ability in purified cultures of astroglia by interferon-γ. J Mol Cell Immunol 1986;2:269–280.

203 Wekerle H: Antigen presentation by central nervous system glia; in Ransom BR, Kettenmann H (eds): Neuroglia. London, Oxford University Press, 1995, pp 685–699.

204 Meinl E, Aloisi K, Ertl B, et al: Multiple sclerosis: Immunomodulatory effects of human astrocytes on T cells. Brain 1994;117:1323–1332.

205 Panek RB, Moses H, Ting JP-Y, Benveniste EN: Tumor necrosis factor α response elements in the HLA-DRA promoter: Identification of a tumor necrosis factor α-induced DNA-protein complex in astrocytes. Proc Natl Acad Sci USA 1992;89:11518–11522.

206 Panek RB, Lee Y-J, Lindstrom-Itoh Y, Ting JP-Y, Benveniste EN: Characterization of astrocyte nuclear proteins involved in IFN-γ and TNF-α mediated class II MHC gene expression. J Immunol 1994;153:4555–4564.

207 Panek RB, Lee Y-J, Benveniste EN: TGF-β suppression of IFN-γ induced class II MHC gene expression does not involve inhibition of phosphorylation of JAK1, JAK2 or STAT1α or modification of IFNEX expression. J Immunol 1995;154:610–619.

208 Lee SC, Collins M, Vanguri P, Shin ML: Glutamate differentially inhibits the expression of class II MHC antigens on astrocytes and microglia. J Immunol 1992;148:3391–3397.

209 Sasaki A, Levison SW, Ting JPY: Differential suppression of interferon γ-induced Ia antigen expression on cultured rat astroglia and microglia by second messengers. J Neuroimmunol 1990;29: 213–222.

210 Smith ME, McFarlin DE, Dhib Jalbut S: Differential effect of interleukin-1β on Ia expression in astrocytes and microglia. J Neuroimmunol 1993;46:97–104.

211 Tontsch U, Rott O: Cortical neurons selectively inhibit MHC class II induction in astrocytes but not in microglial cells. Inter Immunol 1993;5:249–254.

212 Heuschling P: Nitric oxide modulates γ-interferon-induced MHC class II antigen expression on rat astrocytes. J Neuroimmunol 1995;57:63–69.

213 Devajyothi C, Kalvakolanu I, Babcock GT, Vasavada HA, Howe PH, Ransohoff RM: Inhibition of interferon-γ-induced major histocompatibility complex class II gene transcription by interferon-β and type β1 transforming growth factor in human astrocytoma cells: Definition of cis-element. J Biol Chem 1993;268:18794–18800.

214 Schluesener HJ: Transforming growth factors type β1 and β2 suppress rat astrocyte autoantigen presentation and antagonize hyperinduction of class II major histocompatibility complex antigen expression by interferon-γ and tumor necrosis factor-α. J Neuroimmunol 1990;27:41–47.

215 Jiang H, Milo R, Swoveland P, Johnson KP, Panitch H, Dhib-Jalbut S: Interferon β-1b reduces interferon γ-induced antigen-presenting capacity of human glial and B cells. J Neuroimmunol 1995; 61:17–25.

216 Morga E, Heuschling P: Interleukin 4 down-regulates MHC class II antigens on cultured rat astrocytes. Glia 1996;17:175–179.

217 Lee Y-J, Han Y, Lu H-T, et al: Transforming growth factor-β suppresses induction of class II MHC gene expression by inhibiting class II transactivator mRNA expression. J Immunol 1997; 158:2065–2075.

218 Lu H-T, Riley JL, Babcock GT, et al: Interferon (IFN) β acts downstream of IFN-γ-induced class II transactivator messenger RNA accumulation to block major histocompatibility complex class II gene expression and requires the 48-kD DNA-binding protein, ISGF3-γ. J Exp Med 1995;182: 1517–1525.

219 Shin ML, Koski CL: The complement system in demyelination; in Martenson R (ed): Myelin: Biology and Chemistry. Boca Raton, CRC Press, 1992, pp 801–831.

220 Levi-Strauss M, Mallat M: Primary cultures of murine astrocytes produce C3 and factor B, two components of the alternative pathway of complement activation. J Immunol 1987;139:2361–2366.

221 Rus HG, Kim LM, Niculescu FI, Shin ML: Induction of C3 expression in astrocytes is regulated by cytokines and Newcastle disease virus. J Immunol 1992;148:928–933.

222 Barnum SR, Jones JL, Benveniste EN: Interferon-gamma regulation of C3 gene expression in human astroglioma cells. J Neuroimmunol 1992;38:275–282.

223 Barnum SR, Jones JL: Differential regulation of C3 gene expression in human astroglioma cells by interferon-γ and interleukin-1β. Neurosci Lett 1995;197:121–124.

224 Barnum SR, Jones JL, Müller Ladner U, Samimi A, Campbell IL: Chronic complement C3 gene expression in the CNS of transgenic mice with astrocyte targeted interleukin-6 expression. Glia 1996;18:107–117.

225 Gasque P, Julen N, Ischenko AM, et al: Expression of complement components of the alternative pathway by glioma cell lines. J Immunol 1992;149:1381–1387.

226 Barnum SR, Jones JL: Transforming growth factor-β1 inhibits inflammatory cytokine-induced C3 gene expression in astrocytes. J Immunol 1994;152:765–773.

227 Gasque P, Fontaine M, Morgan BP: Complement expression in human brain. J Immunol 1995; 154:4726–4733.

228 Barnum SR, Ishii Y, Agrawal A, Volanakis JE: Production and interferon-γ-mediated regulation of complement C2 and factors B and D by the astroglioma cell line U105-MG. Biochem J 1992; 287:595–601.

229 Rus HG, Niculescu F, Shin ML: Sublytic complement attack induces cell cycle in oligodendrocytes. J Immunol 1996;156:4892–4900.

230 Koski CL, Estep AE, Sawant Mane S, Shin ML, Highbarger L, Hansch GM: Complement regulatory molecules on human myelin and glial cells: Differential expression affects the deposition of activated complement proteins. J Neurochem 1996;66:303–312.

231 Shirazi Y, McMorris FA, Shin ML: Arachidonic acid mobilization and phosphoinositide turnover by the terminal complement complex, C5b–9, in rat oligodendrocyte X C6 glioma cell hybrids. J Immunol 1989;142:4385–4391.

232 Gasque P, Chan P, Fontaine M, et al: Identification and characterization of the complement C5a anaphylatoxin receptor on human astrocytes. J Immunol 1995;155:4882–4889.

233 Lacy M, Jones J, Whittemore SR, Haviland DL, Wetsel RA, Barnum SR: Expression of the receptors for the C5a anaphylatoxin, interleukin-8 and FMLP by human astrocytes and microglia. J Neuroimmunol 1995;61:71–78.

234 Benveniste EN: Cytokine expression in the nervous system; in Keane RW, Hickey WF (eds): Immunology of the Nervous System. London, Oxford University Press, 1997, pp 419–459.

235 Malipiero UV, Frei K, Fontana A: Production of hemopoietic colony-stimulating factors by astrocytes. J Immunol 1990;144:3816–3821.

236 Tweardy DJ, Glazer EW, Mott PL, Anderson K: Modulation by tumor necrosis factor-α of human astroglial cell production of granulocyte-macrophage colony-stimulating factor (GM-CSF) and granulocyte colony stimulating factor (G-CSF). J Neuroimmunol 1991;32:269–278.

237 Norris JG, Tang L-P, Sparacio SM, Benveniste EN: Signal transduction pathways mediating astrocyte IL–6 induction by IL-1β and tumor necrosis factor-α. J Immunol 1994;152:841–850.

238 Benveniste EN, Sparacio SM, Norris JG, Grenett HE, Fuller GM: Induction and regulation of interleukin-6 gene expression in rat astrocytes. J Neuroimmunol 1990;30:201–212.

239 Frei K, Malipiero UV, Leist TP, Zinkernagel RM, Schwab ME, Fontana A: On the cellular source and function of interleukin-6 produced in the central nervous system in viral diseases. Eur J Immunol 1989;19:689–694.

240 Hayashi M, Luo Y, Laning J, Strieter RM, Dorf ME: Production and function of monocyte chemoattractant protein-1 and other β-chemokines in murine glial cells. J Neuroimmunol 1995;60: 143–150.

241 Hurwitz AA, Lyman WD, Berman JW: Tumor necrosis factor α and transforming growth factor β upregulate astrocyte expression of monocyte chemoattactant protein-1. J Neuroimmunol 1995; 57:193–198.

242 Barnes DA, Huston M, Holmes R, et al: Induction of RANTES expression by astrocytes and astrocytoma cell lines. J Neuroimmunol 1996;71:207–214.

243 Fuentes ME, Durham SK, Swerdel MR, et al: Controlled recruitment of monocytes and macrophages to specific organs through transgenic expression of monocyte chemoattractant protein-1. J Immunol 1995;155:5769–5776.

244 Benveniste EN, Kwon JB, Chung WJ, Sampson J, Pandya K, Tang L-P: Differential modulation of astrocyte cytokine gene expression by TGF-β. J Immunol 1994;153:5210–5221.

245 Kwon J, Lee SJ, Benveniste EN: A 3′ cis-acting element is involved in tumor necrosis factor-α gene expression in astrocytes. J Biol Chem 1996;271:22383–22390.

246 Benveniste EN, Tang LP, Law RM: Differential regulation of astrocyte TNF-α expression by the cytokines TGF-β, IL-6 and IL-10. Int J Dev Neurosci 1995;13:341–349.

247 da Cunha A, Vitkovic L: Transforming growth factor-beta (TGF-β1) expression and regulation in rat cortical astrocytes. J Neuroimmunol 1992;36:157–169.

248 Aloisi F, Care A, Borsellino G, et al: Production of hemolymphopoietic cytokines (IL-6, IL-8, colony-stimulating factors) by normal human astrocytes in response to IL-1β and tumor necrosis factor-α. J Immunol 1992;149:2358–2366.

249 Lee SC, Liu W, Roth P, Dickson DW, Berman JW, Brosnan CF: Macrophage colony-stimulating factor in human fetal astrocytes and microglia: Differential regulation by cytokines and lipopolysaccharide, and modulation of class II MHC on microglia. J Immunol 1993;150:594–604.

250 Lee SC, Liu W, Dickson DW, Brosnan CF, Berman JW: Cytokine production by human fetal microglia and astrocytes: Differential induction by lipopolysaccharide and IL-1β. J Immunol 1993; 150:2659–2667.

251 Golde DW, Gasson JC: Hormones that stimulate the growth of blood cells. Scient Am 1988;July:62–70.

252 Giulian D, Ingeman JE: Colony stimulating factors as promoters of ameboid microglia. J Neurosci 1988;8:4707–4717.

253 Maysinger D, Berezovskaya O, Fedoroff S: The hematopoietic cytokine colony stimulating factor 1 is also a growth factor in the CNS. II. Microencapsulated CSF-1 and LM-10 cells as delivery systems. Exp Neurol 1996;141:47–56.

254 Appel K, Honegger P, Gebicke-Haerter PJ: Expression of interleukin-3 and tumor necrosis factor-β mRNAs in cultured microglia. J Neuroimmunol 1995;60:83–91.

255 Gebicke-Haerter PJ, Appel K, Taylor GD, et al: Rat microglial interleukin–3. J Neuroimmunol 1994;50:203–214.

256 Appel K, Buttini M, Sauter A, Gebicke-Haerter PJ: Cloning of rat interleukin-3 receptor β-subunit from cultured microglia and its mRNA expression in vivo. J Neurosci 1995;15:5800–5809.

257 Chiang C-S, Powell HC, Gold LH, Samimi A, Campbell IL: Macrophage/microglial-mediated primary demyelination and motor disease induced by the central nervous system production of interleukin-3 in transgenic mice. J Clin Invest 1996;97:1512–1524.

258 Ohno K, Suzumura A, Sawada M, Marunouchi T: Production of granulocyte/macrophage colony-stimulating factor by cultured astrocytes. Biochem Biophys Res Commun 1990;169:719–724.

259 Hao C, Guilbert LJ, Fedoroff S: Production of colony-stimulating factor-1 (CSF-1) by mouse astroglia in vitro. J Neurosci Res 1990;27:314–323.

260 Thery C, Hetier E, Evrard C, Mallat M: Expression of macrophage colony-stimulating factor gene in the mouse brain during development. J Neurosci Res 1990;26:129–133.

261 Sobel RA, Mitchell ME, Fondren G: Intercellular adhesion molecule-1 (ICAM-1) in cellular immune reactions in the human central nervous system. Am J Pathol 1990;136:1309–1316.

262 Cannella B, Cross AH, Raine CS: Adhesion-related molecules in the central nervous system: Upregulation correlates with inflammatory cell influx during relapsing experimental autoimmune encephalomyelitis. Lab Invest 1991;65:23–31.

263 O'Neill JK, Butter C, Baker D, et al: Expression of vascular addressins and ICAM-1 by endothelial cells in the spinal cord during chronic relapsing experimental allergic encephalomyelitis in the Biozzi AB/H mouse. Immunology 1991;72:520–525.

264 Bö L, Peterson JW, Mork S, et al: Distribution of immunoglobulin superfamily members ICAM-1, -2, -3, and the β2 integrin LFA-1 in multiple sclerosis lesions. J Neuropathol Exp Neurol 1996;55: 1060–1072.

265 Lee TT, Martin FC, Merrill JE: Lymphokine induction of rat microglia multinucleated giant cell formation. Glia 1993;8:51–61.

266 Satoh S, Nüssler AK, Liu Z-Z, Thomson AW: Proinflammatory cytokines and endotoxin stimulate ICAM-1 gene expression and secretion by normal human hepatocytes. Immunology 1994;82:571–576.

267 Look DC, Rapp SR, Keller BT, Holtzman MJ: Selective induction of intercellular adhesion molecule-1 by interferon-γ in human airway epithelial cells. Am J Physiol 1992;L79–L87.

268 Möst J, Schwaeble W, Drach J, Sommerauer A, Dierich MP: Regulation of the expression of ICAM-1 on human monocytes and monocytic tumor cell lines. J Immunol 1992;148:1635–1642.

269 Steiniger B, Falk P, Van der Meide PH: Interferon-γ in vivo. Induction and loss of class II MHC antigens and immature myelomonocytic cells in rat organs. Eur J Immunol 1988;18:661–669.

270 McGeer PL, Kawamata T, Walker DG, Akiyama H, Tooyama I, McGeer E: Microglia in degenerative neurological disease. Glia 1993;7:84–92.

271 Dickson DW, Lee SC, Mattiace LA, Yen S-HC, Brosnan C: Microglia and cytokines in neurological disease, with special reference to AIDS and Alzheimer's disease. Glia 1993;7:75–83.

272 Wingren AG, Parra E, Varga M, et al: T cell activation pathways: B7, LFA-3, and ICAM-1 shape unique T cell profiles. Crit Rev Immunol 1995;15:235–253.

273   Woodroofe MN, Hayes GM, Cuzner ML: Fc receptor density, MHC antigen expression and superoxide production are increased in interferon-gamma treated microglia isolated from adult rat brain. Immunology 1989;68:421–426.

274   Cash E, Zhang Y, Rott O: Microglia present myelin antigens to T cells after phagocytosis of oligodendrocytes. Cell Immunol 1993;147:129–138.

275   Walker WS, Gatewood J, Olivas E, Askew D, Havenith CEG: Mouse microglial cell lines differing in constitutive and interferon-γ-inducible antigen presenting activities for naive and memory CD4+ and CD8+ T cells. J Neuroimmunol 1995;63:163–174.

276   Dhib-Jalbut S, Gogate N, Jiang H, Eisenberg H, Bergey G: Human microglia activate lymphoproliferative responses to recall viral antigens. J Neuroimmunol 1996;65:67–73.

277   Ford AL, Goodsall AL, Hickey WF, Sedgwick JD: Normal adult ramified microglia separated from other cental nervous system macrophages by flow cytometric sorting. J Immunol 1995;154:4309–4321.

278   Kuchroo VK, Das MP, Brown JA, et al: B7-1 and B7-2 costimulatory molecules activate differentially the Th1/Th2 developmental pathways: application to autoimmune disease therapy. Cell 1995;80:707–718.

279   Ford AL, Foulcher E, Lemckert FA, Sedgwick JD: Microglia induce CD4 T lymphocyte final effector function and death. J Exp Med 1996;184:1737–1745.

280   Mizuno T, Sawada M, Marunouchi T, Suzumura A: Production of interleukin-10 by mouse glial cells in culture. Biochem Biophys Res Commun 1994;205:1907–1915.

281   Hayashi M, Dorf ME, Abromson Leeman S: Granulocyte-macrophage colony stimulating factor inhibits class II major histocompatibility complex expression and antigen presentation by microglia. J Neuroimmunol 1993;48:23–32.

282   Loughlin AJ, Woodroofe MN, Cuzner ML: Modulation of interferon-γ-induced major histocompatibility complex class II and Fc receptor expression on isolated microglia by transforming growth factor-β1, interleukin-4, noradrenaline and glucocorticoids. Immunology 1993;79:125–130.

283   Suzumura A, Sawada M, Itoh Y, Marunouchi T: Interleukin-4 induces proliferation and activation of microglia but suppresses their induction of class II major histocompatibility complex antigen expression. J Neuroimmunol 1994;53:209–218.

284   Briers TW, Desmaretz C, Vanmechelen E: Generation and characterization of mouse microglial cell lines. J Neuroimmunol 1994;52:153–164.

285   Murphy GM, Jr., Jia X-C, Song Y, et al: Macrophage inflammatory protein 1-α mRNA expression in an immortalized microglial cell line and cortical astrocyte cultures. J Neurosci Res 1995;40:755–763.

286   Giulian D, Baker TJ, Shih LC, Lachman LB: Interleukin-1 of the central nervous system is produced by ameboid microglia. J Exp Med 1986;164:594–604.

287   Righi M, Mori L, De Libero G, et al: Monokine production by microglial cell clones. Eur J Immunol 1989;19:1443–1448.

288   Gottschall PE, Yu X, Bing B: Increased production of gelatinase B (matrix metalloproteinase-9) and interleukin-6 by activated rat microglia in culture. J Neurosci Res 1995;42:335–342.

289   Chao CC, Hu S, Sheng WS, Peterson PK: Tumor necrosis factor-alpha production by human fetal microglial cells: Regulation by other cytokines. Dev Neurosci 1995;17:97–105.

290   Chao CC, Hu S, Sheng WS, Tsang M, Peterson PK: Tumor necrosis factor-α mediates the release of bioactive transforming growth factor-β in murine microglial cell cultures. Clin Immunol Immunopathol 1995;77:358–365.

291   Norris JG, Benveniste EN: Interleukin-6 production by astrocytes: Induction by the neurotransmitter norepinephrine. J Neuroimmunol 1993;45:137–146.

292   Becher B, Dodelet V, Fedorowicz V, Antel JP: Soluble tumor necrosis factor receptor inhibits interleukin 12 production by stimulated human adult microglial cells in vitro. J Clin Invest 1996;98:1539–1543.

293   Lodge PA, Sriram S: Regulation of microglial activation by TGF-β, IL-10, and CSF-1. J Leukoc Biol 1996;60:502–508.

294   Clavo CF, Yoshimura T, Gelman M, Mallat M: Production of monocyte chemotactic protein-1 by rat brain macrophages. Eur J Neurosci 1996;8:1725–1734.

295 Lafortune L, Nalbantoglu J, Antel JP: Expression of tumor necrosis factor α (TNFα) and interleukin 6 (IL-6) mRNA in adult human astrocytes: Comparison with adult microglia and fetal astrocytes. J Neuropathol Exp Neurol 1996;55:515–521.

296 Meda L, Bernasconi S, Bonaiuto C, et al: β-amyloid (25–35) peptide and IFN-γ synergistically induce the production of the chemotactic cytokine MCP-1/JE in monocytes and microglial cells. J Immunol 1996;157:1213–1218.

297 Meda L, Bonaiuto C, Szendrei GI, Ceska M, Rossi F, Cassatella MA: β-Amyloid (25–35) induces the production of interleukin-8 from human monocytes. J Neuroimmunol 1995;59:29–33.

298 Meda L, Cassatella MA, Szendrel GI, et al: Activation of microglial cells by β-amyloid protein and interferon-γ. Nature 1995;374:647–650.

299 Fisher SN, Vanguri P, Shin HS, Shin ML: Regulatory mechanisms of murantes and CRG–2 chemokine gene induction in central nervous system glial cells by virus. Brain Behavior Immun 1995;9:331–344.

300 Williams K, Dooley N, Ulvestad E, Becher B, Antel JP: IL-10 production by adult human derived microglial cells. Neurochem Int 1996;29:55–64.

301 Suzumura A, Sawada M, Marunouchi T: Selective induction of interleukin-6 in mouse microglia by granulocyte-macrophage colony-stimulating factor. Brain Res 1996;713:192–198.

302 Sebire G, Delfraissy J, Demotes-Mainard J, Oteifeh A, Emilie D, Tardieu M: Interleukin-13 and interleukin-4 act as interleukin-6 inducers in human microglial cells. Cytokine 1996;8:636–641.

303 Zajicek JP, Wing M, Scolding NJ, Compston DAS: Interactions between oligodendrocytes and microglia. Brain 1992;115:1611–1631.

304 Trinchieri G: Interleukin-12: A proinflammatory cytokine with immunoregulatory functions that bridge innate resistance and antigen-specific adaptive immunity. Ann Rev Immunol 1995;13:251–276.

305 Benveniste EN, Merrill JE: Stimulation of oligodendroglial proliferation and maturation by interleukin-2. Nature 1986;321:610–613.

306 Benveniste EN, Herman PK, Whitaker JN: Myelin basic protein-specific RNA levels in interleukin-2-stimulated oligodendrocytes. J Neurochem 1987;49:1274–1279.

307 Benveniste EN, Tozawa H, Gasson JC, Quan S, Golde DW, Merrill JE: Response of human glioblastoma cells to recombinant interleukin-2. J Neuroimmunol 1988;17:301–314.

308 Okamoto Y, Minamoto S, Shimizu K, Mogami H, Taniguchi T: Interleukin 2 receptor β chain expressed in an oligodendroglioma line binds interleukin 2 and delivers growth signal. Proc Natl Acad Sci USA 1990;87:6584–6588.

309 Eitan S, Zisling R, Cohen A, et al: Identification of an interleukin 2-like substance as a factor cytotoxic to oligodendrocytes and associated with central nervous system regeneration. Proc Natl Acad Sci USA 1992;89:5442–5446.

310 Eitan S, Schwartz M: A transglutaminase that converts interleukin-2 into a factor cytotoxic to oligodendrocytes. Science 1993;261:106–108.

311 Merrill JE, Ignarro LJ, Sherman MP, Melinek J, Lane TE: Microglial cell cytotoxicity of oligodendrocytes is mediated through nitric oxide. J Immunol 1993;151:2132–2141.

312 Paul NL, Ruddle NH: Lymphotoxin. Annu Rev Immunol 1988;6:407–438.

313 Selmaj K, Raine CS, Farooq M, Norton WT, Brosnan CF: Cytokine cytotoxicity against oligodendrocytes: Apoptosis induced by lymphotoxin. J Immunol 1991;147:1522–1529.

314 Wilt SG, Milward E, Zhou JM, et al: In vitro evidence for a dual role of tumor necrosis factor-α in human immunodeficiency virus type 1 encephalopathy. Ann Neurol 1995;37:381–394.

315 Tchélingérian J-L, Monge M, Le Saux F, Zalc B, Jacque C: Differential oligodendroglial expression of the tumor necrosis factor receptors in vivo and in vitro. J Neurochem 1995;65:2377–2380.

316 Probert L, Akassoglou K, Pasparakis M, Kontogeorgos G, Kollias G: Spontaneous inflammatory demyelinating disease in transgenic mice showing central nervous system-specific expression of tumor necrosis factor α. Proc Natl Acad Sci USA 1995;92:11294–11298.

317 Akassoglou K, Probert L, Kontogeorgos G, Kollias G: Astrocyte-specific but not neuron specific transmembrane TNF triggers inflammation and degeneration in the central nervous system of transgenic mice. J Immunol 1997;158:438–445.

318 Mayer M, Bhakoo K, Noble M: Ciliary neurotrophic factor and leukemia inhibitory factor promote the generation, maturation and survival of oligodendrocytes in vitro. Development 1994;120:143–153.

319 Louis J-C, Magal E, Takayama S, Varon S: CNTF protection of oligodendrocytes against natural and tumor necrosis factor-induced death. Science 1993;259:689–692.
320 D'Souza SD, Alinauskas KA, Antel JP: Ciliary neurotrophic factor selectively protects human oligodendrocytes from tumor necrosis factor-mediated injury. J Neurosci Res 1996;43:289–298.
321 D'Souza S, Alinauskas K, McCrea E, Goodyer C, Antel JP: Differential susceptibility of human CNS-derived cell populations to TNF dependent and independent immune-mediated injury. J Neurosci 1995;15:7293–7300.
322 Saad B, Constam DB, Ortmann R, Moos M, Fontana A, Schachner M: Astrocyte-derived TGF-β2 and NGF differentially regulate neural recognition molecule expression by cultured astrocytes. J Cell Biol 1991;115:473–484.
323 Awatsuji H, Furukawa Y, Hirota M, et al: Interleukin-4 and -5 as modulators of nerve growth factor synthesis/secretion in astrocytes. J Neurosci Res 1993;34:539–545.
324 Casaccia-Bonnefil P, Carter BD, Dobrowsky RT, Chao MV: Death of oligodendrocytes mediated by the interaction of nerve growth factor with its receptor p75. Nature 1996;383:716–719.
325 Turnley AM, Miller JFAP, Bartlett PF: Regulation of MHC molecules on MBP positive oligodendrocytes in mice by IFN-γ and TNF-α. Neurosci Lett 1991;123:45–48.
326 Suzumura A, Silberberg DH, Lisak RP: The expression of MHC antigens on oligodendrocytes: Induction of polymorphic H-2 expression by lymphokines. J Neuroimmunol 1986;11:179–190.
327 Turnley AM, Morahan G, Okano H, et al: Dysmyelination in transgenic mice resulting from expression of class I histocompatibility molecules in oligodendrocytes. Nature 1991;353:566–569.
328 Power C, Kong P-A, Trapp BD: Major histocompatibility complex class I expression in oligodendrocytes induces hypomyelination in transgenic mice. J Neurosci Res 1996;44:165–173.
329 Merrill JE, Matsushima K: Production of and response to interleukin-1 by cloned human oligodendroglioma cell lines. J Biol Regul Homeost Agents 1988;2:77–86.
330 de Cunha A, Jefferson JA, Jackson RW, Vitkovic L: Glial cell-specific mechanisms of TGF-β1 induction by IL-1 in cerebral cortex. J Neuroimmunol 1993;42:71–86.

Etty N. Benveniste, PhD, University of Alabama at Birmingham, Department of Cell Biology, 350 Basic Health Sciences Bldg., Birmingham, AL 35294-0005 (USA)
Tel. (205) 934 7667, Fax (205) 975 6748

Blalock JE (ed): Neuroimmunoendocrinology, 3rd rev ed.
Chem Immunol. Basel, Karger, 1997, vol 69, pp 76–98

....

Structural Biology of Cytokines, Their Receptors, and Signaling Complexes: Implications for the Immune and Neuroendocrine Circuit

Mark R. Walter

Department of Microbiology and Center for Macromolecular Crystallography,
University of Alabama at Birmingham, Ala., USA

Introduction

The complex biological processes of cellular defense, metabolism, and growth require an efficient commmunication network to coordinate and control the responses of huge numbers of different cells. Many of the signals which regulate the growth and metabolism of muscle, bone and cartilage, hematopoiesis, and neuropoiesis are delivered by a family of small α-helical extracellular signaling proteins. The diverse functions of these proteins, now collectively called cytokines, are reflected in their many names which include colony stimulating factors, hormones, growth factors, interferons, interleukins, lymphokines, and neurotrophic factors. This general nomenclature may be more descriptive since, as discussed in earlier chapters, many of these molecules and their receptors are shared among the endocrine, immune, and nervous systems. Cellular communication occurs when a cytokine produced by one cell is subsequently recognized by specific receptors on another cell. The cell surface receptors transduce the binding of the extracellular proteins into cytoplasmic signals which trigger the appropriate cellular responses. This chapter will compare and contrast the structural features of cytokines and cytokine receptor complexes that are more classically associated with the immune system with those more classically associated with the neuroendocrine system.

The goal of cytokine structural biology is to determine how the receptors specifically recognize and respond to their ligands. While structures of the cytokines have progressed remarkably well, data on the receptors and the cytokine receptor complexes have been hard to obtain. Despite over twenty different signaling proteins in the cytokine receptor family, detailed three-dimensional structure data is only available for three cytokine-receptor complexes: growth hormone (GH):growth hormone receptor (GHR) [1], growth hormone:prolactin receptor (PRLR) [2], and interferon-γ (IFN-γ):interferon-γ receptor-α (IFN–γRα) [3]. Recently, a fourth complex structure has been elucidated of the erythropoietin receptor (EPOR) in complex with a 20-residue cyclic peptide [4]. This chapter will attempt to show the importance of three-dimensional structure for promoting high-affinity binding in the cytokine receptor family. This will be accomplished by a review of cytokine and receptor folds followed by an analysis of the crystal structures of the GH and IFN-γ receptor complexes.

The Cytokine Receptor Family

The cytokine receptor superfamily is comprised of two distinct subclasses: class 1 and class 2 (fig. 1). The class 1 family members include the receptors for growth hormone (GH), prolactin (PL), erythropoietin (EPO), granulocyte-, macrophage-, and granulocyte macrophage-colony-stimulating factors (G-CSF, M-CSF, and GM-CSF, respectively), interleukins (IL) -2, -3, -4, -5, -6, -7, leukemia inhibitory factor (LIF), and cilliary neutrophic factor (CNTF). The class 2 cytokine family is currently limited to the interferons (IFN) -α, -β, -γ, IL-10, and the functionally unrelated membrane-bound receptor for coagulation factor protease VII, tissue factor (TF). Most of the transmembrane cytokine receptors are composed of an extracellular domain (ECD) involved in cytokine binding (~220 residues), a single membrane spanning peptide, and a cytoplasmic domain. The class 1 and class 2 receptors are distinguished by limited primary sequence homology among the extracellular domains including distinct cysteine sequence patterns. An additional feature of the class 1 receptors is the presence of a Trp-Ser-X-Trp-Ser (WSXWS, where X is any amino acid) homology box. Despite these sequence differences, the extracellular portions of each receptor class shares a modular architecture consisting of a tandem set of fibronectin type III (FBN-III) domains [6]. In some cases, this architecture is repeated (e.g. IFN-αR) or additional non-FBN-III domains form part of the receptor sequence [7].

In contrast to the extracellular regions of the receptors, the cytoplasmic domains show almost no amino acid sequence similarity and exhibit large differences in their chain lengths, ranging from about 54 (huGM-CSFR) to 569 amino acids (huIL-4R) [8, 9]. Unlike the transmembrane receptor-tyrosine kinases (e.g. PDGF receptor), the cytoplasmic domains of the cytokine recep-

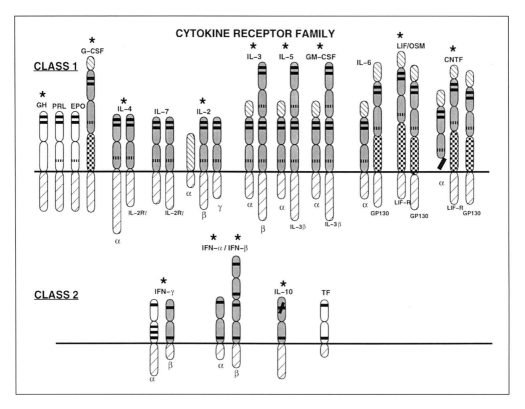

Fig. 1. Schematic diagram of the cytokine receptor family. The abbreviations of each family member is found in the text. The cell membrane is shown as a horizontal bar. Each extracellular domain is shown as a distinct unit. FBN-III domains are gray, immunoglobulin domains are represented by slashes, FBN-III spacer modules are checked. Crystal structures have been completed for the receptors colored white. Disulfide bonds are shown as black lines on the domains. The WSXWS motif is denoted by a dashed horizontal line on the receptors. A star denotes that the crystal structure of the ligand has been determined. Figure adapted from Kossiakoff et al. [47].

tors lack intrinsic kinase domains or any other sequences with catalytic activity. However, cytokine stimulation leads to rapid tyrosine phosphorylation which has now been attributed to several nonreceptor-tyrosine kinases, including Tyk2 and the JAK kinases, which associate with the cytoplasmic domains of the receptors [10]. Thus, the intracellular domains appear to act as tethers for various inactive kinases. Activation of the kinases requires cytokine binding induced oligomerization of the receptors which leads to the interaction and activation of the cytoplasmic domain associated kinases.

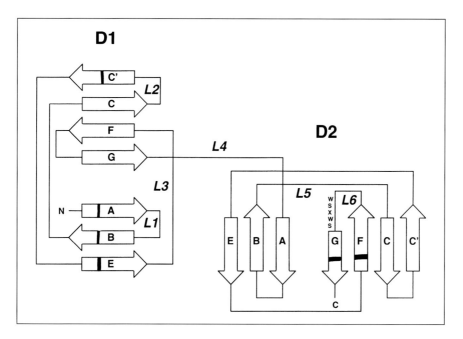

Fig. 2. Schematic diagram of the extracellular portion of the cytokine receptor. The FBN-III domains are labeled D1 and D2. β-Strands are shown by arrows (arrowhead denotes the C-terminal end of the β-strand) and labeled as discussed in the text. Cysteine residues are represented as black lines in the arrows. The cytokine binding loops are labeled. Figure adapted from Livnah et al. [4].

Structural Characterization of the Cytokine Receptors

Due to the difficulty of crystallizing transmembrane proteins, all crystallographic studies on the cytokine receptors have analyzed the extracellular domains of the receptors rather than the intact molecules. Since soluble truncated forms of many of the cytokine receptors (such as GH) have been isolated from cells and maintained their high binding affinity, it is unlikely that these analyses alter their three-dimensional structures [11].

To date, the crystal structures of the cytokine receptors (GHR, PLR, IFN-γRα, EPOR) have been determined as part of cytokine or peptide receptor complexes. The extracellular receptors are comprised of two domains which most closely resemble fibronectin type-III (FBN-III) domains (fig. 2). The N-terminal domain is denoted D1 while the C-terminal domain, which is located near the cell membrane is labeled D2. The domains are connected by a short helical linker. Based on the last residue of D2 and the predicted start of the transmembrane helix, the extracellular portion of the receptors are thought to be attached to the membrane by a flexible stretch of amino acids ('the stalk').

The FBN-III domain is comprised of two antiparallel β-sheets formed from β-strands A, B, and E, and G, F, C and C'. The FBN-III fold differs from immunoglobulin constant domains due to the 'switch' of β-strand C' which is part of the G, F, C β-sheet rather than the A, B, E β-sheet. In addition to the domains of the cytokine receptors, equivalent folds have been observed for domain 2 of CD2 [12] and CD4 [13, 14], and the chaperone protein pap D [15]. Each cytokine receptor forms at least two disulfide bonds which differ between the class 1 and class 2 receptors. The class 1 disulfide bonds link β-strands A to B and C' to E in D1 while the conserved disulfides in the class 2 receptors are found between β-strands C' and E in D1 and F and G in D2. The WSXWS homology motif of the class 1 receptors is located just prior to β-strand G in D2. The tryptophans in the sequence form part of a ladder of alternating aromatic and charged amino acids. The serine residues maintain a common set of hydrogen bonds between their side chain hydroxyls and the main chain carbonyls of β-strand F. Mutagenesis studies suggest that the WSXWS sequences are important for proper folding and transport of receptors to the cell surface in the class 1 receptors [4]. It is interesting that a similar motif of alternating aromatic and charged residues is found in D1 of the class 2 receptors which participate in ligand binding [3].

Comparison of the Class 1 and Class 2 Cytokine Receptors

The largest differences in the structures of the class 1 and class 2 receptors are the unique interdomain angles of 90 and 120°, respectively (fig. 3). Changes in the interdomain angles are accompanied by significant translations (~5–8 Å) of the domains with respect to one another. Smaller changes are also observed between the structures of receptors within the same receptor class (class 1: GHR, PRLR, EPOR; class 2: IFN-γRα, TF) [16, 17]. These rigid body domain shifts provide a mechanism for altering the cytokine binding site which is located at the D1-D2 interface. In the GHR and PRLR, the binding site is formed from six exposed loops which connect the β-strands of the β-sandwich. Loops 1–3 (L1–L3) are formed from the AB, C'C, and EF β-strand connections in D1, Loop 4 (L4) from the helical domain linker, and loops 5 and 6 (L5,L6) from the segments linking β-strands B to C and F to G in D2. The 120° interdomain angle in IFN-γRα significantly changes the location of surface loops at the domain interface. As a result of the different domain orientations, the surface loop corresponding to L1 in the GHR is buried in the IFN-γRα

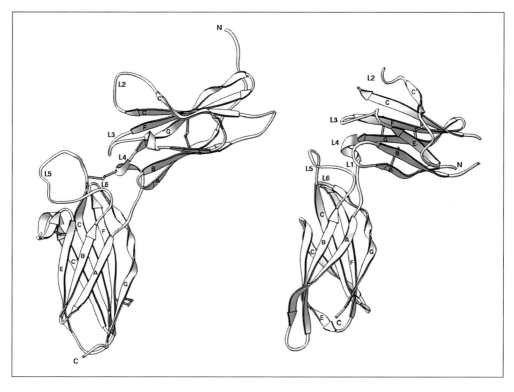

Fig. 3. Ribbon diagram of the IFN-γ (left) and GH (right) receptors. β-Strands are shown as arrows. Disulfide bonds are shown as balls and sticks. The cytokine-binding loops are labeled.

domain interface. The remaining five binding loops (L2–L6) are conserved between class 1 and class 2 receptors. The flexibility between the domains of the receptors is restricted by hydrogen bonding and hydrophobic interactions in the domain interface. The total buried surface area between the D1 and D2 domains is about 1,000 Å². Based on these observations it is thought that the domains are 'locked' into preformed orientations.

The Cytokine Four-Helix Bundle Motif

When the cytokines were first being identified, the tremendous amino acid sequence diversity observed among the different molecules suggested that each molecule might exhibit a unique three-dimensional structure. The theory also suggested that each distinct cytokine fold would be able to activate a

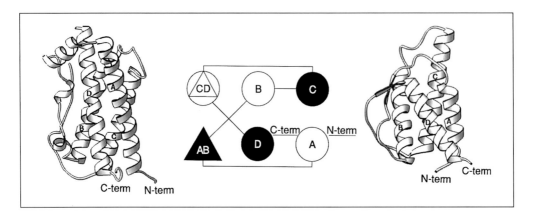

Fig. 4. Ribbon diagram of the long chain cytokine, GH (left) and the short chain cytokine, IL-4 (right). The figures are separated by a schematic diagram of the cytokine fold. In this diagram, α-helices are represented as circles, loops as lines, and extended or β-structure as triangles. Open circles or triangles denote that the N-terminus of the segment is below the plane of the figure. Dark circles or triangles denote that the N-terminus is above the plane of the figure.

different biological function. However, the crystal structures of 13 cytokines have revealed an amazing structural redundancy among the molecules. Each cytokine may be grouped into one of two closely related protein folds which each exhibit a four-helix bundle topology first observed in the structure of porcine growth hormone [18]. The four helices in the bundle are labeled consecutively (A–D) from the N-terminus (fig. 4). The unique feature of the fold is the presence of two long loops which pack against one edge of the bundle and link consecutive helices (A and B, C and D) such that they are parallel to one another. Despite the unique topology observed only among the cytokines, the helix bundle maintains an antiparallel left-handed topology observed in other four helix bundle proteins lacking the long connecting loops.

The structural characteristics of the four-helix bundle are best described by the packing angle (Ω) between the antiparallel helix pairs A-D and B-C [15]. The Ω angle, along with helix lengths, and the structure of the long crossover loops, provide a basis for dividing the cytokine structures into distinct subgroups: short-chain (SC) and long-chain (LC) cytokines [19] (fig. 4). The SC cytokines consist of 105–140 amino acid residues. Each α-helix in the four-helix bundle is comprised of about 15 amino acids in length and display large packing angles ($\Omega\sim35°$). The overhand loops of the SC cytokines contain two short antiparallel β-strands near the N-terminus of helix D. Furthermore, the AB-loop passes between the CD-loop and helix D. Crystal structures exhibiting these features include GM-CSF [20, 21], IL-2 [22], IL-3 [23], IL-4 [24, 25],

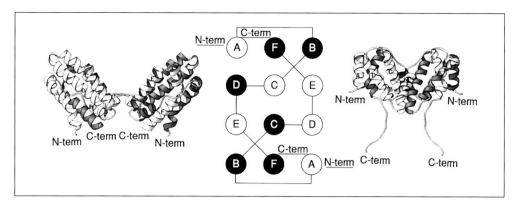

Fig. 5. The intercalated dimer cytokine fold. Ribbon diagram of IL-10 (left) and IFN-γ (right). IL-5 also displays an intercalated dimer structure but is not shown. The figures are separated by a schematic diagram of the intercalated dimer cytokine fold. In the schematic diagram, α-helices are represented as circles. Open circles denote that the N-terminus of the segment is below the plane of the figure. Dark circles denote that the N-terminus is above the plane of the figure.

IL-5 [26], and M-CSF [27]. Other molecules which are predicted to adopt the SC fold include IL-7, IL-9, IL-13, and stem cell factor. The helices of the LC cytokines are significantly longer than the SC cytokines (~25 amino acids) and pack at angles nearly parallel to one another (Ω~18°). The length of the peptide chain for the LC cytokines range from 160 to 200 amino acids. In contrast to the SC cytokines, the overhand loops of the LC cytokines are devoid of β-strands but contain various nonequivalent helical segments. A notable difference in this region is observed for IFN-α and IFN-β which replace the CD loop with a long α-helix that packs against the bundle. Also unique to the LC cytokines is location of the AB-loop which encircles the exterior face of helix D. The LC cytokine fold is exhibited by the structures of GH [18], IFN-α [28], IFN-β [29], G-CSF [30], LIF [31], IL-10 [32, 33], and CNTF [34]. Molecules predicted to adopt this fold include PRL, EPO, IL-6, IL-11, and OSM.

Although most of the cytokines exist as monomers, four of the molecules (IL-5, M-CSF, IL-10 and IFN-γ [35]) form unique dimers. The M-CSF dimer is formed from two of the SC monomers linked by a disulfide bond between Cys-31 from the twofold related monomer. Additional molecular interactions are formed between the AB-loop and CD-loop regions of the molecule. For IL-5, IFN-γ, and IL-10, each twofold related domain of the dimer is formed from the intercalation of two peptide chains (fig. 5). In IL-5, helix D from one peptide chain packs into a cleft formed from helices A, B, and C from the other chain. The same topology is observed for IFN-γ and IL-10 although each peptide chain contains two additional helices that are located in their overhand loop regions. It is interesting that the domain characteristics of IL-5 (SC topology), IL-10 (LC topology) and IFN-γ (SC/LC topology) are each distinct. Also unique to each molecule is the angle separating the twofold related domains of IL-5, IFN-γ, and IL-10 is approximately 180, 120 and 90°, respectively. The different domain orientations of the molecules likely play an important role in properly positioning the cytoplasmic domains of the receptors for subsequent signal transduction events.

Cytokine Receptor Complexes

Cytokine-induced receptor oligomerization is a sequential process where each step is dependent on a prior protein-protein interaction [36]. In most cases, the process begins with a specific high affinity interaction between a cytokine and a receptor. This initial complex provides a new modified protein surface (the receptor-cytokine complex) which will have affinity for additional receptors. Studies have shown that some cytokines oligomerize two copies of the same receptor (homodimerization), while others interact with two or three distinct receptor chains (hetero-oligomerization). Examples of receptor homo-dimerization are observed for GH, PL, EPO, and G-CSF where a single receptor binds two distinct surfaces on the cytokine ligand [37]. For each example above, a single cytokine specific receptor is able to play a role as the binding and/or the signal transducing receptor chain. In other cases, such as IL-3, IL-5, and GM-CSF, two distinct receptors are required for signal transduction [38]. The first α receptor confers specificity to the particular cytokine (IL-3, IL-5, or GM-CSF) while the second is required for high affinity ligand binding and signal transduction. For IL-3, IL-5, and GM-CSF, each specific α-receptor:cytokine complex interacts with the same signal transducing receptor. More complicated interactions are observed for CNTF where at least three unique receptors participate in the transmission of the signal across the cell membrane [39]. While many details of each interaction are still unknown, crystallographic studies on the GH-GHR, PRL-PRLR, and IFN-γRα/IFNγ complexes provide initial insights into the structural basis for molecular recognition.

The Growth Hormone and Prolactin Receptor System

Human GH and PRL share overlapping biological activities in the growth and differentiation of muscle, bone, and cartilage cells, as well as in lactation

[40]. As mentioned in the previous section, GH and PRL activate their receptors by dimerization of one specific receptor (homodimerization). A unique feature of this system is the ability of GH to bind and activate cellular responses through either the GH or PRL receptors. In contrast, PRL can only bind to the PRLR and not the GHR. Thus, the endocrine hormones have adopted a highly specific binding mechanism which allows the receptors to discriminate between the GH and PRL hormones. Furthermore, this fine specificity is maintained although the GHR and PRLR share only 28% amino acid sequence homology and interact with the same surfaces on GH [2]. The combination of X-ray structure data and detailed mutagenesis studies for this system provides a number of important insights into class 1 cytokine-receptor interactions.

The Structure of Growth Hormone

Growth hormone (GH) is a long-chain cytokine comprised of 191 amino acids. The four helices in the bundle range from 21 to 30 amino acids in length. As a result of the close packing of the helices as well as the long overhand connecting loops, the molecule resembles a cylinder with a diameter of 30 Å and a length of 50 Å. Many of the cytokines contain disulfide bonds which stabilize portions of their three-dimensional structures. Growth hormone contains two disulfide bonds which connect the AB loop to helix D (Cys-53:Cys-165) and the C-terminus to helix D (Cys182-Cys189). The AB crossover loop contains two short α-helices which are formed from residues 38–47 (minihelix 1) and 64–70 (minihelix 2) in the long AB-loop. While the connection between helices A and B adopts an ordered conformation, most of the CD loop is not visible in the X-ray crystal structure of the molecule and believed to be extremely flexible.

Additional structural information on GH has been obtained by the structure determination of affinity-matured (Amat) GH variant [41]. Especially important, the structure provides additional data about the conformational flexibility of the hormone. AmatGH contains 15 amino acid changes that were introduced by phage display mutagenesis techniques. These mutations improve the affinity of AmatGH for the GHR by about 400-fold. In spite of the 15 mutations, comparison of the AmatGH with the receptor bound wild type GH revealed a conserved structure with the exception of minihelix 1 which had undergone a rigid body shift consisting of a 2 Å translation and 23° rotation. In the AmatGH crystals, minihelix 1 is involved in numerous crystal contacts. This data suggests that minihelix 1 may alter its position in response to its environment. Thus, in solution it is likely minihelix 1 can assume multiple positions relative to the four-helix bundle core.

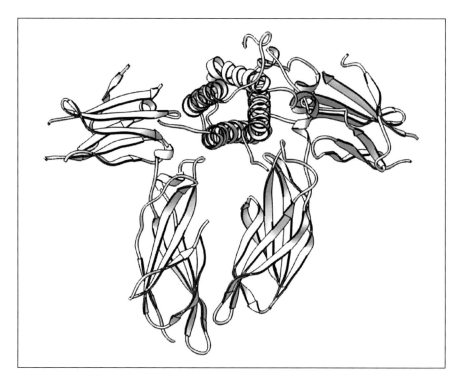

Fig. 6. Ribbon diagram of the GH receptor complex.

The GH Receptor Complex

The crystal structure of the growth hormone receptor complex revealed two GH receptors bound to one molecule of GH (fig. 6). The complex exhibits pseudo twofold symmetry (~159°) around an axis approximately parallel to the helical axes of the GH bundle. This is especially remarkable, since GH contains no internal amino acid sequence repeats nor does the molecule display any internal twofold symmetry. Thus, two identical receptor molecules using identical binding loops are interacting with two chemically and structurally distinct sites on the hormone. The first binding site (site 1) on GH is concave shaped and comprised of residues from helix D, and the AB-loop. Approximately 1,300 Å^2 of hormone molecular surface area is buried in this interaction site. The second receptor binding site (site 2) is relatively flat and formed from helices A and C. The total surface area buried in this interface is about 900 Å^2. In addition to site 2 on GH, the 1:1 GH:GHR complex provides another interaction site (site 3) for the second GHR. Site 3 is formed between the membrane proximal domains (AB-loop of D2) of the receptors and contributes

Table 1. Intermolecular hydrogen bonds observed in the crystal structures of the cytokine receptor complexes.

GH	PRLR	GH	GHR	IFN-γ	IFN-γRα
Ser-62 O	Met-103 N	Pro-61 O	Ile-103 N	Gln-1 Nε2	Trp-210 O
Lys-168 Nζ	Trp-104 O	Lys-168Nζ	Trp-104 O	Glu-9 Oε1	Arg-109 NH2
Ser-51 Oγ	Glu-75 Oε2	Lys-41 Nζ	Glu-127 Oε2	Gly-18 O	Trp-85 Nε1
Tyr-164 Oη	Glu-75 Oε1	Arg-167 Nη1	Glu-127 Oε1	Ala-23 O	Gly-53 N
Arg-167 Nη2	Asp-124 Oδ2	Arg-167 Nη2	Glu-127 Oε1	Ala-23 O	Val-54 N
Arg-178 Nη1	Thr-171 Oγ1	Arg-178 Nη2	Il3-165 O	Asp-24 Oδ1	Lys-50 Nζ
Arg-178 Nη1	Phe-170 O	Thr-175 Oγ1	Arg-43 Nη1	Asn-25 N	Val-54 O
Arg-178 Nη2	Gln-193 Oε2	Glu-46 Nε2	Gly-120 Oε2	Gly-26 N	Val-54 O
Asp-171 Oδ1	Tyr-127 Oη	Asp-171 Oδ2	Arg-43 Nη2	His-111 Nδ2	Glu-104 Oε1
				Glu-112 Oε1	Tyr-52 OH
				Gln-115 Nε	Asn-82 Oδ1

an additional 500 Å^2 to the surface area of the second receptor interaction. The structure of the complex is consistent with a sequential mechanism of receptor activation proposed from mutagenesis studies [36]. The larger interaction area of site 1 with the receptor (1,300 vs. 900 Å^2) likely promotes the high affinity interaction at site 1. The second receptor-binding site requires the formation of the 1:1 GH:GHR complex to create the second GHR binding epitope composed of sites 2 and 3.

Despite the fact that the two binding sites on the hormone are structurally and chemically distinct, the residues on the receptor which interact with GH are largely the same. The overall structures of the two GHRs are very similar as revealed by a root mean square (rms) deviation of 1 Å. Each GH-binding site is formed from the six receptor loops (L1-L6). Key residues which form hydrogen bonds or salt bridges in the interface are listed in table 1. Other residues which bury significant amounts of surface area in both hormone-binding interfaces are Arg-43, Trp-104, and Trp-169. In both interfaces, Trp-104 buries the most surface area with a decrease in solvent accessibility of 170 Å^2 in site 1 and 210 Å^2 in site 2. Comparison of the GHR binding loops reveals small local conformational changes that allow the receptor to adapt to the different hormone surfaces. The greatest structural changes occur in the orientationn of Trp-104 (~3 Å) on the L3 loop, and the mainchain residues 163–168 (~2–4 Å) on the L5 binding loop in D2.

Based on the crystal structure of the GHR complex, thirty two residues were found to contribute to the 1,300 Å^2 of buried surface area in GH:GHR site 1 interface. Prior to the structure determination of the GHR complex,

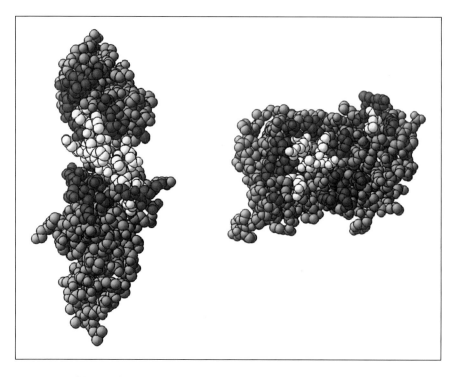

Fig. 7. GHR and GH structural and functional epitopes. Space filling models of the GH receptor (left) and GH (right) are shown. Residues which make up the cytokine-binding interface in the GHR complex crystal structure are shown in black and white (32 residues). The subset of contact residues which contribute ~85% of the binding energy is shown in white.

residues on GH which are important for receptor binding at site 1 were elucidated by alanine scanning mutagenesis [42, 43]. This technique replaces the amino acid residue to be studied with an alanine residue. The alanine substitution should identify the specific contribution of sidechain atoms after Cβ towards the binding energy of the interaction. Surprisingly, over half of the 32 GH contact residues identified in the GHR complex crystal structure had essentially no effect on receptor binding affinity. Further analysis revealed that only eight of the 32 sidechains accounted for almost 85% of the binding free energy. This subset of contact residues is referred to as the functional epitope of GH and forms a small patch on the GH surface of about 420 Å² (fig. 7). Similar experiments identified a small functional epitope consisting of eleven residues on the GHR while the remaining residues made no substantial contribution to the binding affinity [44]. For the GHR, Trp-104 and Trp-169 were shown to contribute more than three-quarters of the binding free energy.

Comparison of the GH and GHR functional epitopes reveals a striking complementarity where energetically important and unimportant residues on one molecule match those on the other. The overall picture of the binding interfce may be likened to a cross-section through the center of a folded protein with hydrophobic residues inside and hydrophilic residues outside. The site 1 interface consists of a tightly packed hydrophobic core, surrounded by five intermolecular salt bridges and hydrogen bonds. While this data provides tremendous insight into residues which are critical for the binding free energy, it explains the function of only a small number of residues in the entire binding interface. What is the function of the other 23 residues in the binding interface? These peripheral contact residues may play roles in solubilizing the receptor, as well as contributing to the specificity of the interaction by electrostatic and steric interactions. The binding free energy for site 1 from GH:GHR complex is regulated by a few strong interactions that are clustered together rather than many weaker contacts spread over the entire surface of the interface. This data suggests that designing small molecules which prevent or promote the interaction of these large protein surfaces may be possible. The possibility that this observation is general for all of the cytokines in the family is strengthened by the reent identification of a 20-residue agonist of the EPOR [45].

1:1 Prolactin Receptor Complex

Biochemical analysis of the PRL system has shown that it activates cells through a sequential receptor-binding mechanism similar to that described for the GH:GHR system. Unlike the GH:GHR complex, the 1:2 GH:PRLR complex is highly unstable in solution. As a result, only the 1:1 GH:PRLR complex has been isolated, crystallized, and its structure determined [2]. This result actually is quite fortuitous since it provides a view of an inactive intermediate of the endocrine hormone signaling process which is poised for interaction with the signal transducing second receptor.

As in the GH:GHR complex, GH interacts with the PRLR through site 1 comprised of helix-D and the AB loop. The PRLR binds GH through the equivalent receptor loops L1-L6. Comparison of the structures of GH from the two complexes (GH:GHR and GH:PRLR) reveals a conserved four-helix bundle core. The largest structural differences in GH occur in mini-helix 1 (residues 38–47) which is found in the AB loop. The position of this segment of the hormone differs by about 2.5 Å depending on the receptor (GHR or PRLR). This observation is consistent with the crystal structure of AmatGH described above.

Despite only 28% sequence identity, the overall structures of the GHR and PRLR are similar. The individual domains of the PRLR can be superimposed with an rms deviation of ~0.85 Å onto the domains of the GHR. This superposition reveals that the L1-L6 binding loops have similar conformations in the GHR and PRLR structures. Although the individual domains are structurally equivalent (including the binding loops), the relative orientation of the D1 and D2 domains has undergone a significant shift (~5 Å translation, 8° rotation) which is centered at the D1D2 linker. The result of this domain shift is to change the relative positions of the binding loops by about 3.5 Å. Despite the change in position of the receptor loops, many of the same residues used by the GHR are also used by the PRLR to bind GH. Thus, the GHR and PRLR make use of different structural rearrangement mechanisms to engage the hormone. The GHR adopts to the different surfaces of GH (sites 1 and 2) by local conformational changes of the binding loops while the PRLR makes use of a rigid body movement of its domains to reposition its binding loops for interaction with the GH.

As found for the GH receptor complex, the amount of buried surface area in the 1:1 PRL complex is about 1,300 Å². While structural information is extremely useful for identifying residues in the binding interface, it is difficult to distinguish between residues which are energetically important and those which are not. The GH:GHR and GH:PRLR structures combined with detailed mutagenesis studies provide several insights into the energetic importance of similar interactions in the two complexes [46, 47]. Based on these studies, the identified mechanisms which modulate the strength of side-chain interactions in the interface include local and domain structural changes as well as sequence variations between the receptors. A simple example of a conformational change effecting the ion pair strength is the interaction between Arg-64 of GH and Asp-164 of the GHR and PRLR. In the GH:GHR complex, Arg-64 forms a salt bridge with Asp-164 of the GHR. Replacement of Arg-64 with alanine results in a large decrease in affinity for the GHR but has no effect on the affinity of GH for the PRLR. Comparison of the receptor structures shows that the Cα atom of Asp-164 in the PRLR has moved about 3.5 Å which moves the carboxylate side chain away from Arg-64 of the hormone. Thus, the energetic importance of the salt-bridge interaction in the GH:PRLR complex has been greatly reduced due to the increased distance between the side-chain residues.

Sequence variation can also change the importance of residues in the receptor-ligand interaction. An example of this is found between Asp-171 of GH and Arg-43 of the GHR which contribute significantly to the complex binding energy. However, in the PRLR, Arg-43 is replaced by Lys-43 which is too short to form an interaction with Asp-171. Instead, Lys-43 interacts with the OH of Tyr-127. These hydrogen-bonding differences observed in the crystal structures are consistent with the mutagenesis data which shows that replacing Asp-171 in the PRLR with alanine has little effect on binding.

The different interactions in the GH:GHR and GH:PRLR involving Arg-167 provides striking evidence that a salt bridge does not necessarily contribute substantially to binding energy. In the GH: GHR complex, Arg-167 forms a salt bridge with Glu-127. Surprisingly, this interaction has little influence on binding. However, the interaction between Arg-167 and Asp-124 makes a significant contribution to binding energy of the GH:PRLR complex. Comparison of the structures of the complexes provides some insight into these energetic differences. In the GH:GHR complex, the side chains of the amino acids are not involved in any additional interactions. The situation is very different for the GH:PRLR complex, where Asp-124 forms a hydrogen bond with Thr-106 which restricts the position of the carboxylate oxygens. Furthermore, Arg-167 stacks between Tyr-28 from GH and Tyr-127 from the receptor. Based on the structures, the energetics of the system may be explained by entropic and desolvation factors. In the case of the GH:GHR Arg-167:Glu-127 interaction, the enthalpy gain for the salt bridge is likely offset by the loss in side-chain entropy for each residue. The hydrogen bond between Thr-106 and Asp-124 in the PRLR removes the entropic penalty by preordering the aspartate prior the GH binding. Furthermore, the close stacking of Tyr-127 with Arg-167 shields the residue from solvent further promoting the entropic benefits of the interaction. These examples of how structure influences the energetics of binding affinity are likely working in other cytokine-receptor interactions.

Interferon-γ Receptor System

IFN-γ is produced by T cells and natural killer cells [48, 49]. Although originally isolated based on its antiviral properties, IFN-γ also displays powerful antiproliferative and immunomodulatory activities. In contrast to the GH and PRL systems, IFN-γ interacts with class 2 cytokine receptors. IFN-γ signals by sequential interactions with the high affinity ligand binding chain (IFN-γRα) followed by the signal transducing IFN-γRβ receptor chain [50, 51]. Additional studies suggest that there may be several different IFN-γRβ chains which may confer different signals to cells [52]. Like the GH:PLR complex, the IFN-γ:IFN-γRα complex is an inactive intermediate complex consisting of one IFN-γ dimer and two IFN-γRαs.

The Structure of IFN-γ

The three-dimensional structure of IFN-γ is very distinct from GH. IFN-γ is a homodimer composed of two identical peptide chains of 143 amino acids. The amino acid sequence of the C-terminus is highly basic consisting of the sequence (KTGKRKR, 6 residues, RR). Each domain of the dimer is comprised of six helices which range from 9 to 21 amino acids in length. The helices are labeled consecutively A-F from the N- to C-terminus. The two carboxy-terminal helices (E and F) from one chain associate with helices A, B, C, and D from the twofold related chain. Unique to helix F is a pronounced bend of 129° centered on Glu-112. With the exception of the AB-loop, the helices are connected by short connections of 3–5 residues. The AB-loop consists of 13 residues which, like GH, encircles the C-terminal helix (helix F in IFN-γ, D in GH). Residues following Ala-120 (the C-terminal 23 residues) extend away from the core of the molecule. Based on the crystallographic and nuclear magnetic resonance (NMR) studies on IFN-γ, the AB loop and the highly basic C-terminus are flexible [53].

The IFN-γ Receptor Complex

The crystal structure of the IFN-γ receptor complex provided the first view of a class 2 cytokine-receptor complex (fig. 8). In the crystal, two IFN-γRα molecules bind the identical twofold related surfaces of the IFN-γ dimer. The orientation of IFN-γ and GH on their receptors differs by approximately 60° with IFN-γ assuming the more upright position. The twofold axis of IFN-γ is oriented approximately perpendicular to the putative position of the cell membrane. While the stalk regions of the receptors are thought to be flexible, binding of the two receptors to IFN-γ is expected to form a fairly rigid ternary complex. In contrast to the GH receptor complex, the two IFN-γRαs do not interact with one another and are separated by 27 Å. An analysis of the surface loops of D2 from the IFN-γR and GHR revealed that the IFN-γRα BC and C′E loops have been extended by 10 and 9 residues, respectively, compared to the GHR. The increased lengths of these segments results in a shorter AB and CC′ loops compared to the GHR. The result of the shorter AB loop in the IFN-γRα is to remove residues which could form a receptor-receptor interaction analogous to site 3 in the GHR complex.

The receptor binding surface on IFN-γ is comprised of helices A, the AB-loop, and helix F (equivalent to helix D in GH). As a result of the 120° domain orientation, only the receptor loops L2 through L6 are used by the receptor to bind IFN-γ. IFN-γ is oriented with its N- and C-termini near the D1D2 receptor interface with the AB-loop interacting with L2 from D1. A total of 25 residues participate in complex formation and bury a total of 960 Å². The aromatic receptor residues Tyr-52 (144 Å²), Trp-85 (95 Å²) and Trp-210 (75 Å²) contribute approximately one-third of the buried surface area.

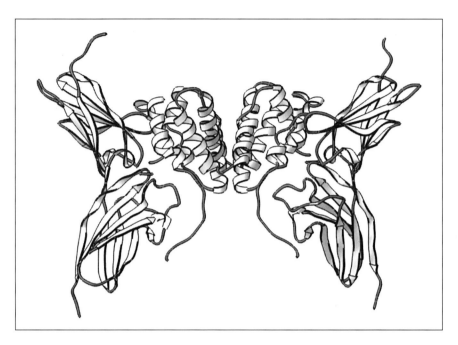

Fig. 8. Ribbon diagram of the IFN-γ receptor complex. The position of the C-terminus of IFN-γ is modeled into the acidic patch as discussed in the text.

Tyr-52 and Trp-85 form a protruding surface which makes extensive contacts with the AB loop, and His-111 and Glu-112 on helix F in IFN-γ. Of the 11 hydrogen bonds and salt bridges identified in the interface, 5 involve mainchain atoms of the AB loop. On the opposite side of the molecule, IFN-γ residues Val 5, Ile-114, and Ala-118 pack against Trp-210 and Val-209 of the receptor.

Although data on the importance of each residue in the IFN-γ complex interaction has not been completed, mutagenesis data from the GH system suggests that the tryptophan residues and Tyr-52 in the IFN-γRα are likely energetically important residues in the IFN-γ binding site. This is consistent with receptor binding assays using IFN-γ mutants and synthetic peptide studies identifying His-111, AB-loop residues, and the C-terminus of IFN-γ as critical for receptor binding [54–59]. Analysis of the crystallographically determined binding interface of the complex correlates well with biochemical studies, except in the C-terminus. It is especially interesting that two of these critical regions (AB loop and C-terminus) were found to be flexible in the NMR and X-ray structures of IFN-γ. However, due to extensive interactions with the receptor the AB loop becomes well ordered upon receptor binding. Residues in the center of the AB loop (residues 20–23) form a well-defined turn of 3_{10}

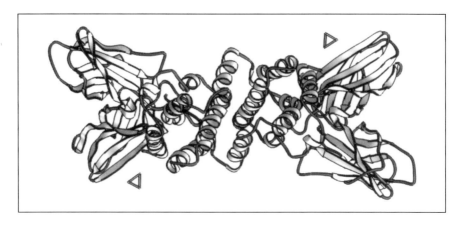

Fig. 9. Ribbon diagram of the IFN-γ receptor complex. The view is parallel to the twofold axis of IFN-γ. The likely interaction surface with the IFN-γRβ is denoted with arrows.

helix that is not observed in the structure of unbound IFN-γ. Based on this data, it is likely that receptor binding induces the formation of the 3_{10} helix and ordering of the loop. A rigid body conformational change was also observed for the AB loop of GH (minihelix 1) based on the structural comparison of GH in the GH and PRL receptor complexes. In contrast to the AB-loop, the C-terminal residues 122–138 extend into the solvent in the IFN-γ receptor complex structure. Analysis of the D2 of the IFN-γRα reveals an acidic patch which is a likely binding site for the basic C-terminus of IFN-γ. The patch is formed from residues 178–183 of β-strand D which display five solvent accessible glutamic and aspartic acid residues on the receptor surface. An additional five acidic residues are contributed from the BC loop of D2. In the crystal structure of the IFN-γ receptor complex, the interaction of the C-terminus with the acidic patch is prevented by a crystal contact.

Possible Places of Interaction of the IFN-γRβ Chain

Signaling by IFN-γ requires the interaction of at least one additional receptor molecule (IFN-γRβ) which binds to the inactive 1 (IFN-γ dimer):2 (IFN-γRα) complex. Receptor-binding studies have shown that the IFN-γRβ has no affinity for IFN-γ until it binds to the IFN-γRα. From this data, two models may be proposed for IFN-γRβ binding. IFN-γ might undergo a conformational change upon IFN-γRα binding that is recognized by the IFN-γRβ. This model is unlikely since comparison of the structures of bound and unbound IFN-γ does not show any significant conformational changes except in the AB loop which binds to the IFN-γRα. More likely, the high affinity IFN-γRβ binding site is formed from the surfaces of IFN-γ and the IFN-γRα. Based on IFN-γ mutant studies, the C-terminus of IFN-γ may be involved in the IFN-γRβ binding site. Without any concrete biochemical data, the best model of the IFN-γRβ binding site is found by placing D2 of the GHR 1 (site 1) from the GHR complex onto D2 of the IFN-γRα. The location of the second GHR in this superposition suggests the likely binding surface for the IFN-γRβ (fig. 9).

Acknowledgments

I would like to thank Maxine Rice for help in preparation of the manuscript and Leigh J. Walter for help with the figures. The figures were generated using the program RIBBONS [60]. This work was supported in part by grants AI36871-02 and PO1 NS29719-05 from NIH, as well as Grant-in-Aids from the American Heart Association and Schering Plough Research Institute.

References

1   de Vos AM, Ultsch M, Kossiakoff AA: Human growth hormone and extracellular domain of its receptor: Crystal structure of the complex. Science 1992;255:306.
2   Somers W, Ultsch M, de Vos AM, Kossiakoff AA: The x-ray structure of a growth hormone-prolactin receptor complex. Nature 1994;372:478.
3   Walter MR, Windsor WT, Nagabhushan TL, Lundell DJ, Lunn CA, Zauodny PJ, Narula SK: Crystal structure of a complex between interferon-γ and its soluble high-affinity receptor. Nature 1995;376:230.
4   Livnah O, Stura EA, Johnson DL, Middleton SA, Mulcahy LS, Wrighton NC, Dower WJ, Jolliffe LK, Wilson IA: Functional mimicry of a protein hormone by a peptide agonist: The EPO receptor complex at 2.8 Å. Science 1996;273:464.
5   Bazan JF, McKay DB: Structural design and molecular evolution of a cytokine receptor superfamily. Proc Natl Acad Sci USA 1990;87:6934.
6   Leahy DJ, Hendrickson WA, Aukhil I, Erickson HP: Structure of a fibronectin type III domain from tenascin phased by MAD analysis of the selenomethionyl protein. Science 1992;257:987.
7   Cosman D: The hematopoietin receptor superfamily. Cytokine 1993;5:95.
8   Gearing DP, King JA, Goough NM, Nicola NA: Expression cloning of a receptor for human granulocyte-macrophage colony-stimulating factor. EMBO J 1989;8:3667.
9   Galizzi JP, Zuber CE, Harada N, Gorman DM, Djossou O, Kastelein R, Banchereau J, Howard M, Miyajima A: Molecular cloning of a cDNA encoding the human interleukin 4 receptor. Int Immunol 1990;2:669.
10 Ihle JN, Witthuhn BA, Quelle FW, Yamamoto K, Thierfelder WE, Kreider B, Silvennoinen O: Signaling by the cytokine receptor superfamily: JAKs and STATs. Trends Biol Sci 1994;19:222.
11 Baumann G, Lowman HB, Mercado M, Wells JA: The stoichiometry of growth hormone-binding protein complexes in human plasma: Comparison with cell surface receptors. J Clin Endocrinol Metab 1994;78:1113.

12   Jones EY, Davis SJ, Williams AF, Harlos K, Stuart DI: Crystal structure at 2.8 Å resolution of a soluble form of the cell adhesion molecule CD2. Nature 1992;360:232.

13   Wang J, Yan Y, Garrett TPJ, Liu J, Rodgers DW, Garlick RL, Tarr GE, Husain Y, Reinherz EL, Harrison SC: Atomic structure of a fragment of human CD4 containing two immunoglobulin-like domains. Nature 1990;348:411.

14   Ryu S-E, Kwong PD, Truneh A, Porter TG, Arthos J, Rosenberg M, Dai X, Xuong N-H, Axel R, Sweet RW, Hendrickson WA: Crystal structure of an HIV-binding recombinant fragment of human CD4. Nature 1990;348:419.

15   Holmgren A, Branden CI: Crystal structure of chaperone protein PapD reveals an immunoglobulin fold. Nature 1989;342:248.

16   Harlos K, Martin DMA, O'Brien DP, Jones EY, Stuart DI, Polikarpov I, Miller A, Tuddenham EGD, Boys CWG: Crystal structure of the extracellular region of human tissue factor. Nature 1994; 370:662.

17   Muller YA, Ultsch MH, Kelley RF, de Vos AM: Structure of the extracellular domain of human tissue factor: Location of the factor VIIa binding site. Biochemistry 1994;33:10864.

18   Abdel-Meguid SS, Shieh H-S, Smith WW, Dayringer HE, Violand BN, Bentle LA: Three-dimensional structure of a genetically engineered variant of porcine growth hormone. Proc Natl Acad Sci USA 1987;84:6434.

19   Sprang SR, Bazan JF: Cytokine structural taxonomy and mechanisms of receptor engagement. Curr Opin Struct Biol 1993;3:815.

20   Diederichs K, Boone T, Karplus PA: Novel fold and putative receptor binding site of granulocyte-macrophage colony-stimulating factor. Science 1991;254:1779.

21   Walter MR, Cook WJ, Ealick SE, Nagabhushan TL, Trotta PP, Bugg CE: Three-dimensional structure of recombinant human granulocyte-macrophage colony–stimulating factor. J Mol Biol 1992;224:1075.

22   Bazan JF, McKay DB: Unraveling the structure of IL-2. Science 1992;257:410.

23   Feng Y, Klein BK, Vu L, Aykent S, McWherter CA: ^{1}H, ^{13}C, and ^{15}N NMR resonance assignments, secondard structure, and backbone topology of a variant of human interleukin-3. Biochemistry 1995;34:6540.

24   Walter MR, Cook WJ, Zhao BG, Cameron RP Jr, Ealick SE, Walter RL Jr, Reichert P, Nagabhushan TL, Trotta PP, Bugg CE: Crystal structure of recombinant human interleukin-4. J Biol Chem 1992; 267:20371.

25   Smith LJ, Redfield C, Smith RAG, Dobson CM, Clore GM, Groneborn AM, Walter MR, Naganbushan TL, Wlodawer A: Comparison of four independently determined structures of human recombinant interleukin-4. Struct Biol 1994;1:301.

26   Milburn MV, Hassell AM, Lamber MH, Jordan SR, Proudfoot AEI, Graber P, Wells TNC: A novel dimer configuration revealed by the crystal structure at 2.4 Å resolution of human interleukin-5. Nature 1993;363:172.

27   Pandit J, Bohm A, Jancarik J, Halenbeck R, Koths K, Kim S-H: Three-dimensional structure of dimeric human recombinant macrophage colony-stimulating factor. Science 1992;258:1358.

28   Radhakrishnan R, Walter LJ, Hruza A, Reichert P, Trotta PP, Nagabhushan TL, Walter MR: Zinc mediated dimer of human interferon-α_{2b} revealed by x-ray crystallography. Structure 1996;4:1.

29   Senda T, Saitoh S, Mitsui Y: Refined crystal structure of recombinant murine interferon-β at 2.15 Å resolution. J Mol Biol 1995;253:187.

30   Hill CP, Osslund TD, Eisenberg D: The structure of granulocyte-colony-stimulating factor and its relationship to other growth factors. Proc Natl Acad Sci USA 1993;90:5167.

31   Robinson RC, Grey LM, Staunton D, Vankelecom H, Vernallis AB, Moreau J-F, Stuart DI, Heath JK, Jones EY: The crystal structure and biological function of leukemia inhibitory factor: Implications for receptor binding. Cell 1994;77:1101.

32   Walter MR, Nagabhushan TL: Crystal structure of interleukin 10 reveals an interferon γ-like fold. Biochemistry 1995;34:12118.

33   Zdanov A, Schalk-Hihi C, Gustchina A, Tsang M, Weatherbee J, Wlodawer A: Crystal structure of interleukin-10 reveals the functional dimer with an unexpected topological similarity to interferon γ. Structure 1995;3:591.

34 McDonald NQ, Panayotatos N, Hendrickson WA: Crystal structure of dimeric human ciliary neurotrophic factor determined by MAD phasing. EMBO J 1995;14:2689.

35 Ealick SE, Cook WJ, Vijay-Kumar S, Carson M, Nagabhushan TL, Trotta PP, Bugg CE: Three-dimensional structure of recombinant human interferon-γ. Science 1991;252:698.

36 Cunningham BC, Wells JA: Rational design of receptor-specific variants of human growth hormone. Proc Natl Acad Sci USA 1991;88:3407.

37 Cunningham BC, Ultsch M, de Vos AM, Mulkerrin MG, Glauser KR, Wells JA: Dimerization of the extracellular domain of the human growth hormone receptor by a single hormone molecule. Science 1991;254:821.

38 Sato N, Miyajima A: Multimeric cytokine receptors: Common versus specific functions. Curr Opin Cell Biol 1994;6:174.

39 Davis S, Aldrich TH, Stahl N, Pan L, Taga T, Kishimoto T, Ip NY, Yancopoulos GD: LIFRβ and gp130 as heterodimerizing signal transducers of the tripartite CNTF receptor. Science 1993;260: 1805.

40 Nicoll CS, Mayer GL, Russell SM: Structural featuares of prolactins and growth hormones that can be related to the biological properties. Endocr Rev 1987;8:43.

41 Ultsch MH, Somer W, Kossiakoff AA, de Vos AM: The crystal structure of affinity-matured human growth hormone at 2 Å resolution. J Mol Biol 1994;236:286.

42 Cunningham BC, Wells JA: High-resolution epitope mapping of hGH-receptor interactions by alanine-scanning mutagenesis. Science 1989;244:1081.

43 Cunningham BC, Wells JA: Comparison of a structural and a functional epitope. J Mol Biol 1993; 234:554.

44 Clackson T, Wells JA: A hot spot of binding energy in a hormone-receptor interface. Science 1995; 267:383.

45 Wrighton NC, Farrell FX, Chang R, Kashyap AK, Barbone FP, Mulcahy LS, Johnson DL, Barrett RW, Jolliffe LK, Dower WJ: Small peptides as potent mimetics of the protein hormone erythropoietin. Science 1996;273:458.

46 Cunningham BC, Wells JA: Rational design of receptor-specific variants of human growth hormone. Proc Natl Acad Sci USA 1991;88:3407.

47 Kossiakoff AA, Somers W, Ultsch M, Andow K, Muller YA, de Vos AM: Comparison of the intermediate complexes of human growth hormone bound to the human growth hormone and prolactin receptors. Prot Sci 1994;3:1697.

48 Farrar MA, Schreiber RD: The molecular cell biology of interferon-gamma and its receptor. Annu Rev Immunol 1993;11:571.

49 Pestka S, Langer JA, Zoon KC, Samuel CE: Interferons and their actions. Annu Rev Biochem 1987;56:727.

50 Sohn J, Donnelly RJ, Kotenko S, Mariano TM, Cook JR, Wang N, Emanuel S, Schwartz B, Miki T, Pestka S: Identification and sequence of an accessory factor required for activation of the human interferon γ receptor. Cell 1994;78:793.

51 Marsters S, Pennica D, Back E, Schreiber R, Ashkenazi A: Interferon γ signals via a high-affinity multisubunit receptor complex that contains two types of polypeptide chain. Proc Natl Acad Sci USA 1995;92:5401.

52 Soh J, Donnelly RJ, Mariano TM, Cook JR, Schwartz B, Pestka S: Identification of a yeast artificial chromosome clone encoding an accessory factor for the human interferon γ receptor: Evidence for multiple accessory factors. Proc Natl Acad Sci USA 1993;90:8737.

53 Grzesiek S, Dobeli H, Gentz R, Garotta G, Labhardt AM, Bax A: 1H, 13C, and 15N NMR backbone assignments and secondary structure of human interferon-gamma. Biochemistry 1992; 31:8180.

54 Jarpe MA, Johnson HM: Stable conformation of an interferon-gamma receptor binding peptide in aqueous solution is required for interferon-gamma antagonist activity. J Interferon Res 1993;13: 99.

55 Lundell D, Lunn CA, Senior NM, Zavodny PJ, Narula SK: Importance of the loop connecting A and B helices of human interferon-gamma in recognition by interferon-gamma receptor. J Biol Chem 1994;269:16159.

56 Lunn CA, Fossetta J, Dalgarno D, Murgolo N, Windsor W, Zavodny PJ, Narula SK, Lundell D: A point mutation of human interferon gamma abolishes receptor recognition. Protein Eng 1992; 5:253.

57 Lundell D, Lunn C, Dalgarno D, Fossetta J, Greenberg R, Reim R, Grace M, Narula S: The carboxyl-terminal region of human interferon gamma is important for biological activity: Mutagenic and NMR analysis. Protein Eng 1991;4:335.

58 Wetzel R, Perry LJ, Veilleux C, Chang G: Mutational analysis of the C-terminus of human interferon-gamma. Protein Eng 1990;3:611.

59 Griggs ND, Jarpe MA, Pace JL, Russell SW, Johnson HM: The N-terminus and C-terminus of IFN-gamma are binding domains for cloned soluble IFN-gamma receptor. J Immunol 1992;149: 517.

60 Carson M: RIBBONS 2.0. J Appl Cryst 1991;24:958–961.

Mark R. Walter, Department of Microbiology and Center for Macromolecular Crystallography, University of Alabama at Birmingham, Birmingham, AL 35294 (USA)
Tel. (205) 934 9279, Fax (205) 934 0480, E-Mail: Walter@mimas.cmc.uab.edu

Blalock JE (ed): Neuroimmunoendocrinology, 3rd rev ed.
Chem Immunol. Basel, Karger, 1997, vol 69, pp 99–131

....
Noradrenergic and Peptidergic Innervation of Lymphoid Organs

Suzanne Y. Stevens-Felten, Denise L. Bellinger

Department of Neurobiology and Anatomy, Department of Psychiatry, and
Center for PsychoNeuroImmunology Research, University of Rochester School of
Medicine, Rochester, N.Y., USA

Introduction

Anatomical studies from our laboratories [4, 20, 23, 25, 63, 65, 66, 68, 74–79, 87, 121, 163, 200, 201] and other laboratories [41, 42, 90, 113, 157, 177, 194, 197, 205] have revealed the presence of autonomic nerve fibers, mainly noradrenergic (tyrosine hydroxylase-positive sympathetic fibers), in both primary and secondary lymphoid organs, as well as mucosal associated lymphoid tissue. These fibers distribute into specific compartments of these organs (fig. 1–4), and are associated with both smooth muscle and specific cellular elements of the immune system, including lymphocytes, macrophages, associated cells such as mast cells, and supporting cells such as reticular cells. Norepinephrine (NE), the postganglionic sympathetic neurotransmitter present in these fibers, appears to be available for release, both from sites immediately adjacent to lymphocytes, such as those in the periarteriolar lymphatic sheath (PALS) [77, 78, 80], and from more distant sites that provide a paracrine-like diffusion through widespread regions of the lymphoid organs. In view of past evidence for adrenergic receptors on lymphocytes and other lymphoid cells, and a functional role for NE in modulation of immune function, it is now clear that NE fulfills the criteria for neurotransmission with cells of the immune system as targets. Evidence for this hypothesis is extensively reviewed elsewhere [10, 62, 67, 68, 71, 135].

NE is not the only neurotransmitter that influences immune responses. Neuropeptides, including vasoactive intestinal polypeptide (VIP), somatostatin, substance P (SP), opioid peptides, and others can modulate some aspects of immune function through specific receptors on lymphocytes and other cells

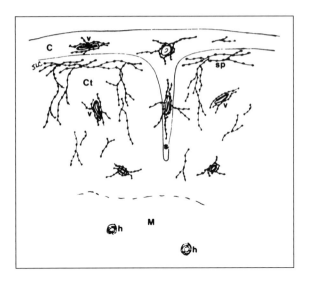

Fig. 1. Schematic drawing of noradrenergic innervation of the thymus. Varicose fibers with blood vessels and in the capsule (C) and associated septa (s) form a subcapsular plexus (sp) and give rise to scattered varicosities in the cortex (Ct), associated with blood vessels (v) and found as free profiles in the parenchyma. The medullary region (M) and Hassall's corpuscles (h) have only sparse innervation. [From 121, with permission.]

of the immune system [1, 44, 91, 140, 156, 158, 186]. Several neuropeptides, such as SP, somatostatin, VIP, calcitonin gene-related peptide (CGRP), neuro-peptide Y (NPY) and opioid peptides, have been identified in nerves in spleen, lymph nodes, thymus, and other lymphoid tissue [31, 32, 45, 50, 57, 66, 72, 79, 83, 113, 117, 124, 125, 148, 157, 159, 161, 171, 177, 187, 197, 198, 205]. These neuropeptide-containing nerve fibers have distinct patterns of distribution and termination, often in association with cells of the immune system. Some neuropeptides appear to be colocalized with each other (e.g. SP and CGRP) or with a classical amine (e.g. NPY and NE), but these relationships are not invariable, and may differ from species to species, organ to organ, and compartment to compartment. Since lymphocytes, macrophages, and other cells of the immune system also possess receptors for many of these neuropeptides, and respond functionally to the neuropeptides, it is likely that they also can be viewed as neurotransmitters with cells of the immune system as targets [62; for review see chap by Carr, this vol.].

Neuropeptide-containing fibers each possess their own distinct pattern of distribution in lymphoid organs. In general, NPY follows the pattern of

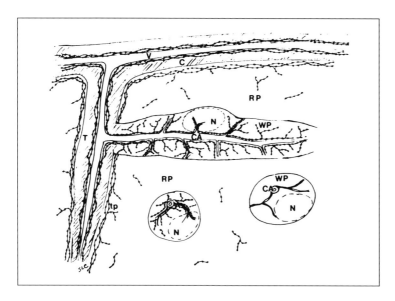

Fig. 2. Schematic drawing of noradrenergic innervation of the spleen. Varicose fibers enter with the splenic artery and its branches (V), continue with those vessels and with the capsule (C) into trabeculae (T), form a subcapsular plexus and associated trabecular-venous plexuses (tp), and follow both the vascular and trabecular plexuses into the white pulp (WP) with the central artery (CA) and its branches. Fibers diverge from this arterial plexus into the white pulp and end among lymphocytes and macrophages in the parenchyma. Only scattered varicosities are found in the red pulp (RP) besides those in trabeculae, and noradrenergic fibers also avoid nodular regions (N) of the white pulp. The white pulp is represented in longitudinal section in the main schematic drawing. Cross sections of the white pulp are included below for distribution of the central arteriolar system (right) and its noradrenergic innervation (left). [From 121, with permission.]

distribution of NE, with which it is usually colocalized [171] SP and CGRP fibers often are very fine (perhaps sometimes below the range of detectable reaction product) and distribute with the vasculature (especially venous and trabecular systems) and among T-cell zones, although other sites of localization such as red pulp of the spleen and the bursa of Fabricius have been described [125, 205]. The SP/CGRP fibers and VIP fibers have been found closely abutting mast cells [46, 108, 148, 155, 189] in various organs, including intestinal mucosa and thymus. However complex the pattern of distribution is in each lymphoid organ, it is clear that neuropeptide-containing nerves distribute among the cells of the immune system; that these cells express receptors for these neuropeptides; and that the nerve terminals are anatomically positioned to provide direct signaling from nerve to lymphoid cell.

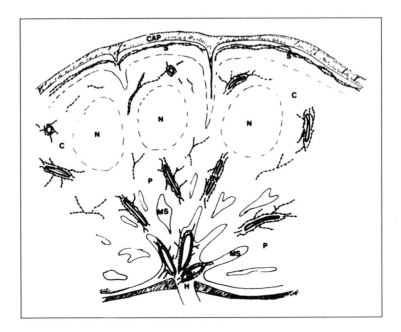

Fig. 3. Schematic drawing of noradrenergic innervation of a lymph node. Varicose fibers enter the node in the hilar region (H), travel with the vasculature (BV) in the medullary cords alongside the medullary sinuses (MS), and branch into the paracortical regions (P) adjacent to the nodules (N). Some varicosities form a subcapsular (S) plexus and give rise to fibers that travel into cortical (C) regions with blood vessels and as free profiles. Noradrenergic fibers are not found in nodular regions. CAP = capsule. [From 121, with permission.]

The presence of neurotransmitters in nerve fibers adjacent to cells of the immune system establishes an anatomical link that may provide a major route for translating central nervous system (CNS) activity into signals that can influence immune function. A large body of evidence has accumulated documenting environmental and psychosocial factors that can influence immune functions through the CNS [6, 7, 10, 16, 17, 109, 115, 150, 171]. Immune responses can be enhanced or suppressed by classical conditioning [8]. Numerous stressors, including bereavement from loss of a spouse, depression, confinement to a nursing home, or examination pressures in medical students, can lead to both altered measures of immune responses and altered health status, presumably as a consequence of the altered immune status, although definitive evidence for such a causal link is not yet available. Stressors in animals also can alter immune responses. Brain lesions in specific autonomic sites of the CNS can result in altered immune responses in either direction, depending

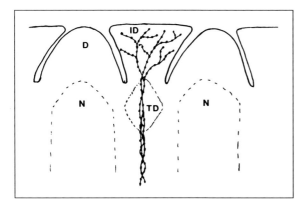

Fig. 4. Schematic drawing of noradrenergic innervation of GALT, represented by rabbit appendix. Noradrenergic fibers enter with the vasculature at the serosal surface, travel with Auerbach's plexus and along the muscularis interna, turn radially and travel in a tortuous internodular plexus between the large nodules (N), plunge through the T-dependent zone (TD) and arborize profusely in the interdomal region (ID) in the lamina propria. Here, the varicosities end among lymphocytes, enterochromaffin cells, and the subepithelial immuno-globulin-secreting plasma cells. The interdomal regions are separated from the adjacent domes (D) by a moat in continuity with the lumen of the gut. [From 121, with permission.]

upon the specific site [151]. Thus, it appears that the CNS is capable of sending signals to the immune system that result in altered responses. The two available routes by which the CNS could signal the immune system include the neuro-endocrine route and the autonomic nerves. Much attention has been focused on the neuroendocrine route in light of the immunological effects (largely immunosuppression) of glucocorticoid administration [146, 188]. However, not all CNS effects on the immune system can be explained by these steroids. Studies of both conditioned immunosuppression [9] and stress-induced lymphocyte hyporesponsiveness [111] have shown the continued presence of these responses in adrenalectomized animals. Many other hormones also have been shown to influence immune responses [34, 91, 95, 112, 137, 139, 146, 147, for review see Torres and Johnson, this vol.]. Central effects of intracerebroventricular CRF [105] and IL-1 [175] administration, and detailed mechanistic evaluation of stress-related changes in cellular immune responses [104, 163], suggest that neural pathways mediate functional effects of CNS outflow. This evidence, coupled with the abundant presence of noradrenergic and peptidergic innerva-tion of lymphoid organs, and appropriate adrenergic or peptidergic receptors on cells of the immune system, has focused our attention on these nerve fibers as a major communication link between the CNS and the immune system.

Innervation of Lymphoid Organs

General Patterns of Innervation of Lymphoid Organs

Noradrenergic postganglionic sympathetic nerve fibers innervate both primary (bone marrow, thymus) (fig. 1) and secondary (spleen, lymph nodes, mucosal-associated lymphoid tissue (MALT)) (fig. 2–4) lymphoid organs. The anatomical connections appear to follow classical patterns from the spinal cord through autonomic sympathetic ganglia. The preganglionic cell bodies are found in the intermediolateral cell column of the spinal cord (e.g. T6-T12 level in rats for the splenic preganglionics), while the ganglion cells are found either in the sympathetic chain or in collateral ganglia (e.g. superior mesenteric-celiac ganglion for splenic postganglionics, superior cervical ganglion and other upper chain ganglia for thymic postganglionics, mesenteric ganglia for gut-associated lymphoid tissue (GALT) postganglionics), thus maintaining the classical two neuron connection from the CNS to the target tissue. The small, unmyelinated noradrenergic fibers generally enter the lymphoid organs with the vasculature, continue into the organ with the vasculature and the capsular/trabecular or septal system, and then arborize into the parenchyma (fig. 5–24) where they form close contacts with lymphocytes and macrophages (fig. 25–29) [79]. Our observations on the ontogeny of splenic noradrenergic fibers in the rat suggest that the directionality of branching is not necessarily from the vasuclar nerve plexuses into the parenchyma; indeed, it may be the other way around [2, 5, 24, 119]. Tyrosine hydroxylase + fibers are present in the spleen at the presumptive border of the marginal sinus before the sinuses and blood vessels are mature; before macrophages and lymphocytes distribute into specific compartments of the splenic white pulp, before smooth muscle cells are present along the arterioles, and before the vascular nerve plexuses have begun to form. It is only as the arterioles mature and become surrounded with smooth muscle cells that innervation along the adventitia develops. These studies further suggest an important relationship between the parenchymal elements that are associated with these nerve fibers.

The specific patterns of fiber distribution differ for each lymphoid organ, but some generalizations can be made. For example, noradrenergic fibers arborize into T-lymphocyte zones, including developing T lymphocytes in the thymus, and macrophage zones of the adult organs, and avoid the follicles or nodules, suggesting that developing, but not necessarily mature, B lymphocytes have much less direct association with noradrenergic innervation. However, this generalization may require modification in ontogeny; since studies of noradrenergic fibers in the developing rat spleen show a close association of B lymphocytes with noradrenergic fibers prior to the development of follicles.

It has become clear that each lymphoid organ must be studied individually for the patterns of distribution of nerve fibers and the possible functions of those fibers, and that the stage of development or maturation can influence the pattern and the extent of this innervation. As further evidence of this individuality of distribution, in the F344 rat, noradrenergic nerve fibers that innervate the spleen and lymph nodes [2, 20, 22, 64, 70, 73, 76] but not the thymus [23], diminish with age, in parallel with the diminution of T-dependent immune function. Similar diminution of peptidergic innervation, other than colocalized NPY in the spleen, has not been seen.

Innervation of Primary Lymphoid Organs

Bone Marrow. Varicose noradrenergic nerve fibers enter the bone marrow of the rat as arteriolar plexuses, follow those vessels into the marrow, and then further distribute into the parenchyma [72, 88, 203], in agreement with the earlier light and electron-microscopic observations of Calvo [42] and Calvo and Forteza-Vila [43]. Nerve terminals end among hematopoietic and lymphopoietic cells of the marrow, and provide the anatomical substrate for delivering neurotransmitter into the extracellular environment of these mobile cells. Of course, for this hypothesis to be substantiated, adrenergic receptors and appropriate second messenger links in the target cells need to be identified.

Peptidergic innervation is also present in bone marrow, but is less well documented. NPY positive fibers have a distribution similar to that of noradrenergic fibers. In addition, megakaryocytes also show NPY immunoreactivity. Substance P [37, 102] and VIP [11] innervation have also been reported, and suggestions have been made that Substance P may influence stem cell development [138, 164].

Thymus. Noradrenergic fibers enter the thymus with the vasculature in both mice and rats as a tangled nerve plexus (fig. 1). Some fibers continue with the vasculature through the interlobular septa into the corticomedullary junction of the thymus, while others form a capsular/subcapsular plexus. The innervation also distributes into the cortex (fig. 5) [23, 66, 72, 79, 121, 200, 201], in general agreement with other studies [41, 129, 178]. Although the noradrenergic fibers are distributed throughout the cortex, a more dense pattern is seen in the outermost cortex, where the immature thymocytes are located, and in association with blood vessels at the corticomedullary junction (fig. 6). As the thymus involutes with age, this pattern becomes even more dense [2, 23, 207]. The noradrenergic varicosities are not only present along vasculature in the thymic cortex, but also branch abundantly into the parenchyma. The possibility that NE from these varicosities can influence thymocytes is strengthened by the demonstration of β-adrenergic receptors on developing thymocytes [182] and the ability of catecholamines to influence the responsiveness of the expression of T alloantigens on these cells [182]. Although noradrenergic innervation is present in the thymus [113, 114, 119, 192, 201, 207], it is not known to what extent it is available as a paracrine secretion, as a neurotransmitter in direct neuroeffector junctions, or both. It also is possible that other cells may be targets of NE in the thymus, including mast cells, eosinophils, or large granular autofluorescent cells [41, 148, 201].

There is also peptidergic innervation of the thymus [50, 52, 118, 148, 172]. NPY generally follows the distribution of noradrenergic fibers, with which it is colocalized [32]. SP and CGRP nerve fibers distribute in the rat thymus along the capsule (fig. 7) and intralobular septa (fig. 8), generally free of vascular association, and enter the thymic cortex from the septa [126]. Along the larger blood vessels of the corticomedullary junction, SP fibers are often among mast cells. VIP fibers distribute mainly along the capsule and intralobular septa and distribute in zones where mast cells are abundant [11, 21, 94, 113], and is also present in thymic cells [93].

The degree of cholinergic innervation of the thymus still remains controversial, largely because techniques for demonstrating peripheral cholinergic nerve fibers are either highly non-specific (AChE histochemistry) or highly variable (ChAT immunoreactivity). Nonetheless, there are several reports in the literature describing cholinergic innervation [54, 60, 141, 142, 181]. However, we have not been able to substantiate any significant degree of cholinergic innervation [30]. Recent studies suggest that there may be vagal components to thymic innervation [13, 14, 152].

Innervation of Secondary Lymphoid Organs
Spleen. Numerous studies, some dating back several decades [165, 191], have shown the presence of nerve fibers in the spleen of all species studied (fig. 9–11). Fluorescence histochemical observations have revealed the abundant

---

Fig. 5. Noradrenergic fibers (small arrowheads) in the thymic cortex. Varicose fibers distribute throughout the cortex, with dense profiles present in the subcapsular region and deep cortical region near the junction with the medulla. The capsular surface is denoted with large arrowheads. Adult rat. Fluorescence histochemistry. × 120.

Fig. 6. Vascular plexuses of noradrenergic fibers in the thymic cortex (denoted by arrowheads). Some nerve fibers distribute into the cortex adjacent to these plexuses. Adult rat. Fluorescence histochemistry. × 240.

Fig. 7. SP nerve fiber (arrowheads) running in a subcapsular location. This long linear profile runs adjacent to mast cells (small arrows). The capsular surface (C) is denoted by large arrowheads. Adult rat. Immunohistochemistry. × 120.

Fig. 8. SP nerve fibers running along a septal (S) region in the thymic cortex, and extending into cortical regions (arrowheads) among thymocytes. Adult rat. Immunohistochemistry. × 120.

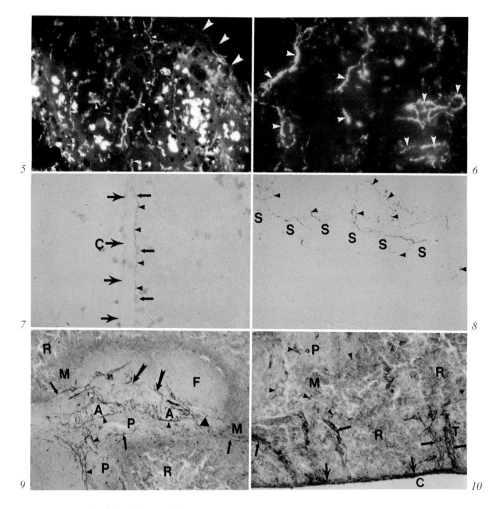

Fig. 9. Peripheral nerve fibers, immunostained by the general nerve marker PGP 9.5, in the white pulp of the spleen. Nerve fibers are present along the vasculature (small arrowheads) of the central arteriolar system (A), in parafollicular sites (large arrowhead) adjacent to the follicles (F), along the marginal sinus and in the marginal zone (M) (small arrows), and within the parenchyma of the PALS (P) (large arrows). R = Red pulp. Adult rat. Immunohistochemistry. × 24.

Fig. 10. Peripheral nerve fibers, immunostained by the general nerve marker PGP 9.5, in the capsular/trabecular system and the white pulp of the speen. Nerve fibers are present along the capsule (C), denoted by large arrows, and within the trabeculae (small arrows) coursing through the red pulp (R). Fibers also are present in the marginal zone (M) and PALS (P) of the white pulp (arrowheads). Adult rat. Immunohistochemistry. × 24.

presence of noradrenergic fibers as a major component of this innervation [48, 49, 72, 82, 89, 121, 168, 169, 200, 201, 206]. Many of these studies focused on the innervation of smooth muscle of the vasculature or the trabecular/capsular system, consistent with physiological evidence that splenic nerve stimulation [176] or application of NE [51] result in splenic capsular/trabecular contraction, and that NE can regulate splenic vascular resistance and blood flow [15, 166]. In addition to these possible smooth muscle targets of noradrenergic innervation, cells of the splenic white pulp also may be targets of these fibers, as suggested by fluorescence histochemical studies [72, 121, 201] and immunocytochemical studies [3, 5, 63, 65, 68, 70, 71, 73, 79, 126].

In the rat, noradrenergic fibers that innervate the spleen originate from cell bodies in the superior mesenteric-celiac ganglion [25, 149], from the splenic nerve, and follow the splenic arterial system into the hilar region of the spleen. Upon entering the spleen, the noradrenergic fibers continue with the vasculature into the trabeculae, contributing to the trabecular system of innervation. In addition, the capsule may be innervated, as it is in the rat, but not the mouse. This pattern is consistent among species that contain an abundance of trabecular smooth muscle as well as species that contain very little trabecular smooth muscle. In rodents, most of the noradrenergic (and tyrosine hydroxylase (TH)-positive) fibers are found in the white pulp and marginal; zone, with only occasional (< 1%) profiles found in the red pulp. The TH-positive fibers form plexuses around the central artery and its branches in the white pulp; additional fibers radiate into the parenchyma of the PALS, often running in parallel with the vasculature several cell layers away from the smooth muscle

Fig. 11. Peripheral nerve fibers, immunostained by the general nerve marker PGP 9.5, in large trabeculae (arrows) coursing through the red pulp (R) of the spleen. These trabeculae converge along large venous sinuses. Adult rat. Immunohistochemistry. × 24.

Fig. 12. TH-positive nerve fibers in the splenic white pulp. These fibers are present in a plexus around the central artery (A), along the marginal sinus (large arrowheads), and in the marginal zone (M) (arrow). Additional nerve fibers course through the parenchyma (small arrowheads) in the PALS (P), among T lymphocytes. R = Red pulp. 14-day-old rat. Immunohistrochemistry. × 120.

Fig. 13. TH-positive nerve fibers in the splenic white pulp. The fibers form a tangled nerve plexus around the central artery (A) and its branches. Fine varicose profiles (arrowheads) course through the parenchyma among T lymphocytes in the PALS (P). A large vein (V) also is innervated abundantly. 14-day-old rat. Immunohistochemistry. × 120.

Fig. 14. TH-positive nerve fibers ending among T lymphocytes in the white pulp of the spleen. The nerve fibers, nickel-enhanced to appear black, travel with the central arteriolar system (A), distribute along the marginal sinus (arrows), and course through the parenchyma (arrowheads) in the PALS (P) among T lymphocytes, immunostained with brown for the general T cell marker OX-19. M = Marginal zone. Adult rat. Double label immunohistochemistry. × 120.

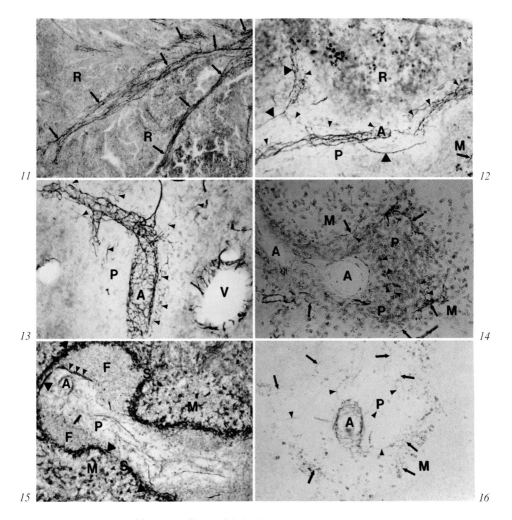

Fig. 15. TH-positive nerve fibers, nickel-enhanced to appear black, in the splenic white pulp along the marginal sinus (S) (large arrowheads), where ED-3-positive macrophages, immunostained brown, are clustered. An additional small nerve fiber bundle (small arrowheads) is found in a parafollicular region. F = Follicle; A = central artery; M = marginal zone. Yong adult rat. Double label immunohistochemistry. × 120.

Fig. 16. NPY nerve fibers in the white pulp of the spleen. NPY fibers form a plexus around the central artery (A), distribute through the parenchyma (arrowheads) in the PALS, and travel among IL-1-beta-positive cells along the marginal sinus and in the marginal zone (M) (arrows). Adult rat. Double label immunohistochemistry (nerve fibers – black; IL-1-β cells – brown). × 120.

(fig. 12, 13). Observations with double-labelled immunocytochemistry for TH and specific markers for cells of the immune system (OX-19 for pan T cells; OX-8 for T suppressor cells; W3/25 for T helper cells) have shown the nerve fibers and terminals directly adjacent to T cells, both helper and suppressor subsets, in the PALS (fig. 14) [3, 5, 63]. Similar dual staining procedures using the ED-3 antibody for antigen-presenting macrophages has shown the close association of TH-positive nerve fibers with these macrophages at the marginal sinus (fig. 15). Additional TH-positive fibers are distributed farther out into the marginal zone, and in a smooth parafollicular location around all margins of the follicles. Only occasionally are nerve fibers present within a follicle. The general lack of association of noradrenergic fibers with developing B lymphocytes may be a feature of adult innervation only; during ontogeny of the spleen during the first 2 weeks of life, before the formation of follicles, the periarteriolar regions are populated by B lymphocytes, and are innervated abundantly by noradrenergic nerve fibers.

The apparent close asociation of TH-positive nerve fibers and terminals with T lymphocytes and macrophages at the light-microscopic level led us to examine these relationships at the electron-microscopic (EM) level [71, 77–81]. Nerve terminals were identified with EM immunocytochemistry by their DAB reaction product, their size and appearance, and their contacts with target

Fig. 17. SP nerve fibers (arrows) traveling along the venous sinuses (V) and in the red pulp (R) of the spleen. Adult rat. Immnohistochemisty. × 24.

Fig. 18. SP nerve fibers (arrows) traveling along the trabeculae and in the red pulp (R) of the spleen. Adult rat. Immunohistochemistry. × 60.

Fig. 19. A long linear SP nerve fiber (arrows) coursing through the white pulp (W) close to the boundary between the PALS and the marginal zone. The border between the white pulp and the red pulp (R) is denoted with arrowheads. Adult rat. Immunohistochemistry. × 60.

Fig. 20. Noradrenergic nerve fibers coursing through the medullary cords (MC) of a popliteal lymph node (large arrowheads), and distributing into the paracortical zone (P) (small arrowheads), where T lymphocytes are found. S = Sinuses. Adult C3H mouse. Fluorescence histochemistry. × 60.

Fig. 21. Noradrenergic nerve fibers (arrowheads) scattered among lymphoid cells in the cortex (C) of a lymph node. Adult NZW mouse. Fluorescence histochemistry. × 120.

Fig. 22. NPY nerve fibers associated with the vascular system (arrows) and parenchymal regions (small arrowheads) of the medullary cords (MC) of a lymph node. S = Sinuses. Adult rat. Immunohistochemistry. × 120.

Fig. 23. SP nerve fibers (arrows) traveling in the medullary cords (MC) along a sinus (S) and among T cytotoxic/suppressor lymphocytes. Adult rat. Double label immunohisto-chemistry (SP nerve fibers – black; OX-8-positive lymphocytes– brown). × 120.

Fig. 24. Noradrenergic nerve fibers (arrowheads) coursing through the lamina propria (LP) of the rabbit appendix. Yellow fluorescent enterochromaffin cells (arrows) are clustered in regions where these nerve fibers abound. Adut New Zealand white rabbit. Fluorescence histochemistry. × 120.

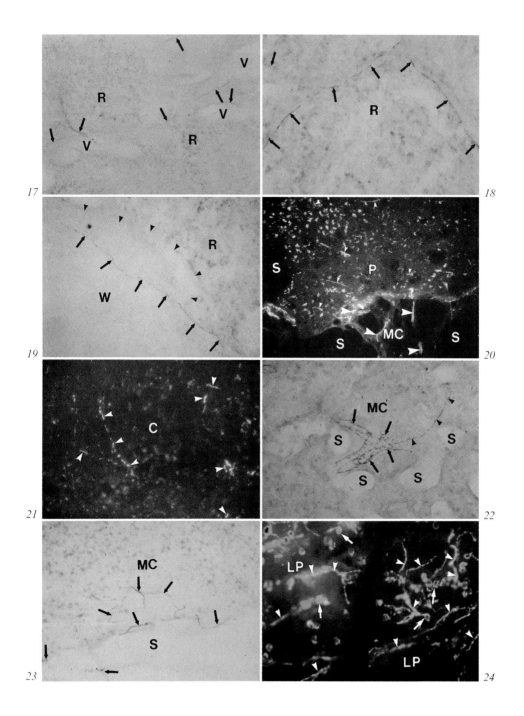

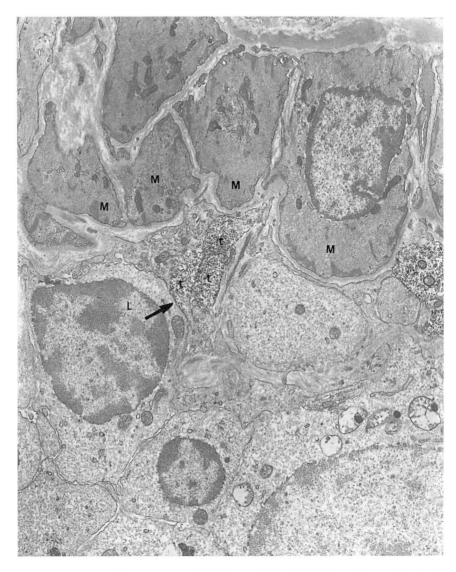

Fig. 25. TH-positive nerve terminals (t) containing the DAB reaction product in the adventitia of a central arteriole of the splenic white pulp. All of these terminals are separated from their adjacent smooth muscle cells (M) by a basement membrane and sometimes additional cell processes. However, a direct apposition is seen (arrow) between one TH-positive nerve terminal and a lymphocyte (L) in the PALS. Fischer 344 rat. EM immunohisto-chemistry. × 15,300.

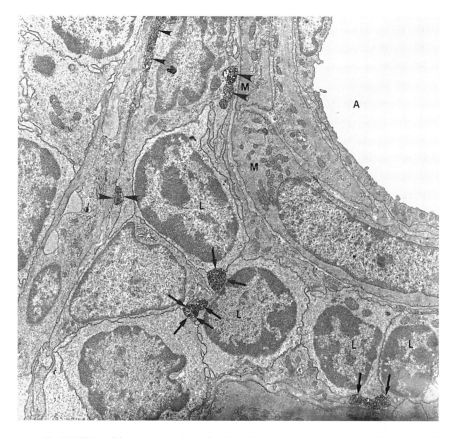

Fig. 26. TH-positive nerve terminals forming direct appositions (arrows and arrowheads) with lymphocytes (L) and other cells in the PALS of the white pulp. The three terminals in the upper center of the micrograph are located in the adventitia, separated from the smooth muscle cells (M) by a basement membrane, but directly abutting a cell on the distal side. The other TH-positive nerve terminals are found within the parenchyma, distant from the adventitia. A = Lumen of the central arteriole. Fischer 344 rat. EM immunohisto-chemistry. × 15,300.

cells. The central arterioles were selected as the first region for these observations due to the clear compartmentation and identification of cells. TH-positive terminals are present in the adventitia of the central arterioles, always separated from the smooth muscle cells by at least the basement membrane, and sometimes by additional cell processes. Therefore, these classical 'neuro-effector junctions' with smooth muscle, by necessity, must exert their influence by a paracrine-like diffusion of NE rather than a close synaptic contact. Some of these same TH-positive terminals in the adventitia directly contact lympho-

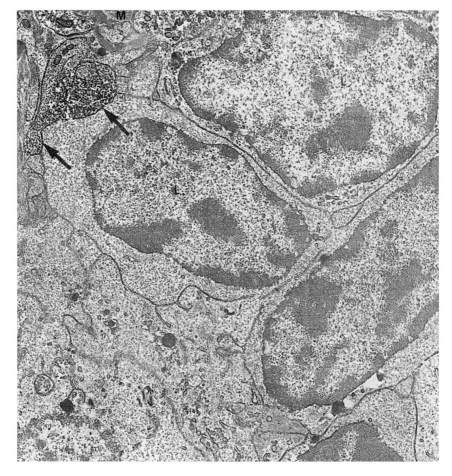

Fig. 27. TH-positive nerve terminals directly abutting (arrows) a lymphocyte (L) in the PALS of the white pulp. The larger terminal forms a smooth apposition, indented in the membrane of the lymphocyte. M = Smooth muscle cell. Fischer 344 rat. EM immunohisto-chemistry. × 21,200.

cytes facing away from the vascular smooth muscle (fig. 25, 26). These contacts form smooth membrane appositions with approximately 6 nm separation, frequently with slightly thickened membranes on both sides. Some of these terminals form indentations in the lymphocyte surface (fig. 27). These synaptic-like contacts are found not only at the junction of the PALS with the arteriolar smooth muscle, but also are present abundantly within the deeper regions of the PALS and at the marginal sinus (fig. 26). Within the PALS, bundles of TH-positive nerve fibers and terminals travel for long distances forming numerous contacts with lymphocytes throughout their course (fig. 28). Thus,

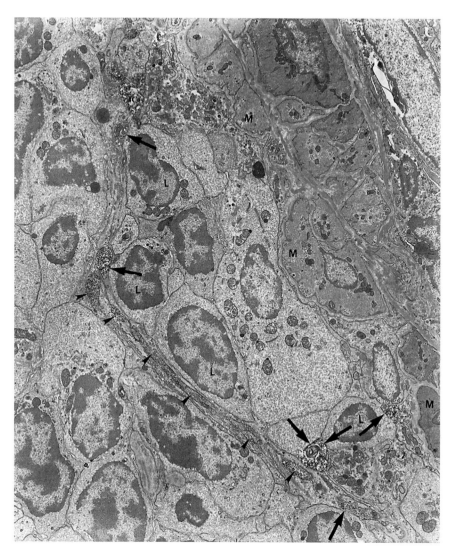

Fig. 28. A bundle of TH-positive nerve terminals is present in the PALS, among lymphocytes, several cell layers deep to the smooth muscle cells (M) of a central arteriole in the white pulp. some of the TH-positive nerve terminals directly contact (arrows) lymphocytes (L) along this nerve bundle, while other terminals show no such direct contacts (arrowheads). The lymphocyte in the lower right has two TH-positive terminals contacting it. Fischer 344 rat. EM immunohistochemistry. × 8,700.

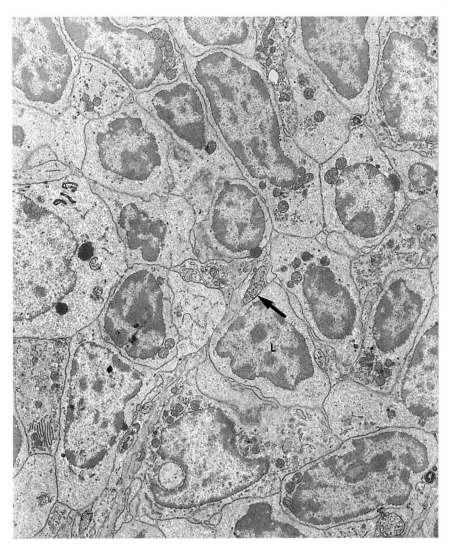

Fig. 29. A TH-positive nerve terminal contacting (arrow) a lymphocyte (L) deep within the PALS of the splenic white pulp. This terminal is part of a nerve bundle that is distant from the vasculature. Fischer 344 rat. EM immunohistochemistry. × 8,700.

it appears that lymphocytes are subject not only to possible influences by the paracrine-like secretion and diffusion of NE, but some, at least, are in direct contact with noradrenergic nerve terminals.

Earlier studies at the EM level reported some nerve fibers adjacent to lymphocytes, reticular cells, or erythrocytes [38, 87, 143, 167, 206]; these observations were viewed either with considerable caution [38], or were dismissed as mistaken identification of platelets rather than nerve terminals [96]. The identification of the TH-positive profiles as nerve terminals is clear at the EM level, and is further substantiated by the loss of TH-positive profiles following denervation either by ganglionectomy or administration of 6-hydroxydopamine. These nerve terminals are adjacent to cells of the immune system, and are often at some distance from vascular smooth muscle cells. These findings suggest that these nerve fibers may influence lymphocytes and macrophages directly in addition to possible regulation of vascular flow or initiation of capsular/trabecular contraction. This nontraditional form of innervation of lymphoid cells that probably are mobile may represent a major link between the CNS and the immune system.

NPY distribution in the spleen follows the same general pattern as that of the noradrenergic, TH-positive fibers, and is generally colocalized with NE (fig. 16) [85, 127, 128, 170, 171]. Because NPY is also found in megakaryocytes and platelets, sympathetic denervation produces little decrease in the NPY content, but depletes NPY immunoreactive nerve fibers.

SP and CGRP nerve fibers enter the spleen with the splenic artery in the hilar region, travel along the venous sinuses and trabecular (fig. 17), and branch into the red pulp (fig. 18) [27, 32, 123, 125]. Additional nerve fibers also were found in the marginal zone and as long linear profiles in the outer PALS of the white pulp (fig. 19). VIP innervation is also present, often associated with vascular elements [21, 26, 129]. In addition, VIP message is present in the spleen, suggesting its presence in lymphoid cells [94].

Splenic innervation has been reported to change with age in F344 rats [2, 18, 28, 29, 132]. In general, noradrenergic innervation decreases, especially after 18 months, in parallel with decreases in T-cell compartments. Similar decreases occur in NPY immunoreactive nerve fibers, but not in Substance P or VIP fibers.

Lymph Nodes. Noradrenergic TH-positive nerve fibers enter cervical, mesenteric, and popliteal lymph nodes with the vasculature at the hilar region in rats and mice (fig. 20) [3, 19, 74, 200, 201]; this innervation is less extensive than noradrenergic innervation of the spleen. The fibers either continue with the vasculature into the medullary cords, or contribute to a capsular/subcapsular plexus. Within the medullary cords, the fibers run adjacent to the vasculature and freely through cellular regions. These fibers continue past the corticomedullary junction and distribute into the paracortical and cortical regions, where T lymphocytes are found (fig. 21). Additional noradrenergic fibers contribute to this innervation from the subcapsular region. The noradrenergic innervation therefore distributes to the medullary cords, the paracortical and cortical regions, the parafollicular areas, the subcapsular sinus, and the capsule, but generally avoids the follicles themselves.

The patterns of noradrenergic innervation of the lymph nodes and spleen show similarities that may reflect a common role. The innervation distributes to sites of entry of T and B lymphocytes, sites of antigen capture, sites of antigen presentation and T-lymphocyte activation, and sites of egress of lymphocytes. The possibility that NE may influence some of these functions is strengthened by functional studies [136] showing a marked diminution of primary and secondary immune responses following denervation of spleen and lymph nodes, and studies showing an influence of catecholamines on egress of activated lymphocytes from the spleen [58, 59] and lymph nodes [144]. It is unlikely that we can identify 'the' role of NE in the spleen or lymph nodes; it is likely that this neurotransmitter can act on numerous cell types in many compartments of secondary lymphoid organs, probably in the presence of differing concentrations of other neurotransmitters and cytokines, to act upon adrenergic receptors found in varying densities on the target cells that may be differentially responsive under varying states of activation. We suggest that at the very least, NE may represent another immunomodulatory substance with considerable functional complexity.

Neuropeptide nerve fibers also are present in lymph nodes. NPY fibers follow the same general course and localization (fig. 22) as noradrenergic nerve fibers, although they may not always be colocalized with NE. VIP fibers were noted along the vasculature in nodal regions of the cortex, with sparse innervation elsewhere [83, 87, 161]. Dynorphin A and CCK nerves were observed in the medulla of guinea pig lymph nodes [117]. SP and CGRP nerve fibers appear to be colocalized and are present in the hilus, beneath the capsule, at the corticomedullary junction, in medullary cords, and in internodal regions (fig. 23) [32, 83, 117, 161]. These nerves are found along the vasculature and among cells of the immune system in the parenchyma. More recently, Romeo et al. [173] reported tyrosine hydroxylase + superior cervical ganglion cells retrogradely labelled from the submaxillary lymph node, containing colocalized NPY or met-enkephalin, suggesting that met-ENK may also be colocalized in noradrenergic fibers innervating lymph nodes.

Mucosal-Associated Lymphoid Tissue. Mucosal-associated lymphoid tissue comprises both organized accumulations of lymphoid cells and follicles, such as Peyer's patches and tonsils, and the more diffuse collections of lymphoid cells found in the loose connective tissue of various mucosae, such as the lamina propria of the gut or the bronchial system. These areas are innervated by autonomic postganglionics from both sympathetic and parasympathetic nervous system, and by the intrinsic neurons of the enteric nervous system. Thus, these areas contain a large number of nerve fibers with an array of different neurotransmitters [185].

Noradrenergic and peptidergic nerve fibers innervate GALT including Peyer's patches [61, 101, 159, 160], tonsils [190, 197, 202], and specialized immune structures such as the rabbit appendix and sacculus rotundus [75, 107]. Even salivary glands have been suggested to have a role in neural-immune modulation [174]. Noradrenergic fibers arise from ganglion cells in the mesenteric ganglia, and enter the gut at the serosal surface in association with large vascular nerve plexuses. These fibers distribute inside the muscularis interna, travel in association with smooth muscle of the gut and blood vessels, and then turn radially to run in internodular septa between the lymph nodules. The nerve plexuses travel towards the lumen of the gut, course directly through the T-dependent area at the base of the lamina propria (fig. 24), and then enter the lamina propria itself. The nerve fibers arborize abundantly in the lamina propria, forming a dense terminal network in the subepithelial region among plasma cells. Noradrenergic terminals appear to form additional associations with lymphocytes and enterochromaffin cells (some which appear to be serotonin-containing) in the lamina propria. No innervation appeared to be present in the nodules or in the crowns of the domes, where B lymphocytes are abundant. Some acetylcholinesterase (AChE)-positive profiles are present, but because this histochemical method is not specific for cholinergic nerves, they are difficult to interpret and may be noradrenergic fibers or even nonneural.

SP, CGRP, VIP and somatostatin nerves are present in the lamina propria of Peyer's patches, where most of the immunological effector cells are found [47, 56, 162, 187, 199]. The SP and CGRP fibers appear closely associated with mast cells in the jejunal intestinal mucosa [184–187]. Ottaway et al. [159] have identified a plexus of VIP nerve fibers coursing with small caliber blood vessels of Peyer's patches.

The innervation of mucosal connective tissue of the lung and bronchial tree (BALT) has also been studied, though in much less detail than that of the gut. Most attention has been paid to VIP innervation [103, 157] and to the relationship between VIP or Substance P fibers and mast cells [92, 155].

Functional Significance of Innervation

In order for NE, or any other putative neurotransmitter, to be accepted as a bona fide neurotransmitter by classical evaluation, it must meet several criteria. The first criterion is the presence and localization of nerve fibers that synthesize the compound in the region where the target cells reside. The sections above document the presence of noradrenergic and peptidergic nerve fibers localized in precise compartments of both primary and secondary lymphoid organs. The second criterion for neurotransmission is release, a criterion for which there is increasing evidence [12, 40, 86, 99, 100, 130, 145, 153, 179, 180, 193] for NE but little for neuropeptides. The third criterion for neurotransmission is the presence of receptors on the target cells, for which an abundance of evidence is available for both adrenergic and peptidergic receptors on lymphocytes, macrophages, and other cells of the immune system [for a detailed review, see ref. 2, 32]. The fourth criterion for neurotransmission is a functional role for the innervation, involving the specific neurotransmitter, that can be revealed by pharmacological or physiological manipulation. In the case of noradrenergic innervation, we have accumulated evidence that NE may inhibit neutrophil oxidative burst activity, inhibit thymocyte proliferation, enhance T-dependent immune responses, enhance cytotoxic T-cell activity and delayed hypersensitivity responses, and exert an inhibitory effect (in lymph nodes) on the severity of expression of adjuvant induced arthritis. We have been unable to reliably demonstrate an inhibitory role for NE in T-cell proliferation. These functional studies are highly complex, reveal possible multiple effects depending on the timing of denervation or stimulation, and may involve simultaneous actions of several mediators on multiple cell types. Detailed reviews of the extensive actions of catecholamines [10, 53, 64, 68, 69, 98, 116, 120–122, 131, 133–135, 183] and neuropeptides [32, 44, 69, 91, 92, 140, 158, 186] on immune functions are available. An assessment of how well these putative neurotransmitters fulfill the criteria for neurotransmission recently has been provided [62].

Feedback

In the above paragraphs, interactions between nerves and lymphoid cells have been examined as a problem of neurotransmission. However, not only do neurotransmitters affect immune function and cytokine production, it is likely that some cytokines also regulate transmitter release both via central nervous system responses by circulating cytokines and by interactions with local nerve terminals innervating lymphoid organs and other peripheral target sites where inflammation or immune responses take place.

Immune System Feedback to the Central Nervous System
Early studies by Besedovsky and colleagues provided evidence that cytokines produced during immune responses could alter hypothalamic activity and neurochemistry [33, 35, 36]. Since then, a number of laboratories have produced

evidence that cytokines feedback to the central nervous system [55]. The initial assumption was that these soluble molecules produced by lymphoid cells were acting on the CNS through the circulation. Findings by Watkins et al. [196], since verified by a number of laboratories indicate that much of this feedback is mediated by the vagus nerve [39, 84, 106, 110, 195]. Furthermore these cytokine-induced CNS changes alter splenic nerve activity, norepinephrine release and turnover, which, in turn, alter immune responses [40, 97, 100, 153, 154, 179, 193, 204]. These studies provide evidence for a complete central feedback loop between the sympathetic nervous system and the immune system.

Local Feedback from Immune System to Nervous System

The presence of direct contacts between nerve terminals and lymphoid cells also suggests the possibility of local feedback. Recent preliminary evidence from our laboratories [Bellinger, unpubl.] suggests that i.p. injections of IL-2 (50 μg/rat) into 3-month-old F344 rats decrease splenic NE content. Immuno-cytochemical staining using an antibody to IL-2 receptor reveals little evidence for IL-2 receptor protein in sympathetic ganglia innervating the spleen. However, within 4 h of IL-2 injection (50 μg), an increase in staining is seen. By 24 h after injection, staining for IL-2R is robust in sympathetic cell bodies in the celiac-superior mesenteric plexus. The superior cervical ganglion from the same rats showed no evidence of IL-2R staining, suggesting that there may be some specificity of the response for sympathetics innervating in spleen. However, the route of administration (i.p.) of IL-2 may account for this difference.

Summary and Conclusions

It now is evident that extensive neural-immune anatomical connections exist between the nervous and immune systems, with close contacts of nerves with lymphocytes and macrophages. The presence of receptors for catecholamines and neuropeptides on these cells, coupled with functional evidence that these neural signals can modulate immune responses, brings these putative neurotransmitters to the forefront as a class of immunomodulatory molecules that can be investigated for possible benefit of disorders resulting from enhanced or suppressed activity of specific aspects of immune function. Furthermore, feedback from the immune system (cytokines) can act locally on lymphoid organ innervation to modulate transmitter release, and can act on the central nervous system via the vagus nerve to alter central pathways relevant to the immune system. It certainly is very clear that extensive bidirectional interactions occur between the nervous and immune systems, and that one system cannot be considered functionally without taking into account the state of activity of the other system.

Acknowledgement

Supported by grant MH42076, NS24761, MH40381, MH47783, MH45681, MH18822, and the Markey Charitable Trust.

References

1   Special issue on peptidergic localization and innervation of lymphoid tissue. Brain Behav Immun 1991;5:1–47.
2   Ackerman KD, Bellinger DL, Felten SY, Felten DL: Ontogeny and senescence of noradrenergic innervation of the rodent thymus and spleen; in Ader R, Felten DL, Cohen N (eds): Psychoneuroimmunology, ed 2. New York, Academic Press, 1991, pp 72–125.
3   Ackerman KD, Felten SY, Bellinger DL, Felten DL: Noradrenergic sympathetic innervation of the spleen. III. Development of innervation in the rat spleen. J Neurosci Res 1987;18:49–54.
4   Ackerman KD, Felten SY, Bellinger DL, Livnat S, Felten DL: Noradrenergic sympathetic innervation of spleen and lymph nodes in relation to specific cellular compartments. Prog Immunol 1987; 6:588–600.
5   Ackerman KD, Felten SY, Dijkstra CD, Livnat S, Felten DL: Parallel development of noradrenergic innervation and cellular compartmentation in the rat spleen. Exp Neurol 1989;103:239–255.
6   Adams DO: Molecular biology of macrophage activation: A pathway whereby psychosocial factors can potentially affect health (review). Psychosom Med 1994;56:316–327.
7   Ader R, Cohen N: The influence of conditioning on immune responses; in Ader R, Cohen N, Felten DL (eds): Psychoneuroimmunology, ed 2. New York, Academic Press, 1991, pp 609–646.
8   Ader R, Cohen N: Psychoneuroimmunology: Conditioning and stress. Ann Rev Psychol 1993;44: 53–85.
9   Ader R, Cohen N, Grota LJ: Adrenal involvement in conditioned immunosuppression. Int J Pharm 1979;1:141–145.
10 Ader R, Felten DL, Cohen N: Interactions between the brain and the immune system. Ann Rev Pharmacol Toxicol 1990;30:561–602.
11 Ahmed M, Bjurholm A, Kreicbergs A, Schultzberg M: Neuropeptide Y, tyrosine hydroxylase and vasoactive intestinal polypeptide-immunoreactive nerve fibers in the vertebral bodies, discs, dura mater, and spinal ligaments of the rat lumbar spine. Spine 1993;18:268–273.
12 Ando T, Ichijo T, Katafuchi T, Hori T: Intracerebroventricular injection of prostaglandin E_2 increases splenic sympathetic nerve activity in rats. Am J Physiol 1995;269:R662–R668.
13 Antonica A, Ayroldi E, Magni F, Paolocci N: Lymphocyte traffic changes induced by monolateral vagal denervation in mouse thymus and peripheral lymphoid organs. J Neuroimmunol 1996;64: 115–122.
14 Antonica A, Magni F, Mearini L, Paolocci N: Vagal control of lymphocyte release from rat thymus. J Autonom Nerv System 1994;48:187–197.
15 Ayers AB, Davies BN, Withrington PG: Responses of the isolated, perfused human spleen to sympathetic nerve stimulation, catecholamines and polypeptides. Br J Pharmacol 1972;44:17–30.
16 Ballieux RE: The mind and the immune system (review). Theoret Med 1994;15:387–395.
17 Bauer SM: Psychoneuroimmunology and cancer: An integrated review (review). J Adv Nurs 1994; 19:1114–1120.
18 Bellinger DL, Ackerman KD, Felten SY, Felten DL: A longitudinal study of age-related loss of noradrenergic nerves and lymphoid cells in the aged rat spleen. Exp Neurol 1992;116: 295–311.
19 Bellinger DL, Ackerman KD, Felten SY, Lorton D, Felten DL: Noradrenergic sympathetic innervation of thymus, spleen and lymph nodes: Aspects of development, aging and plasticity in neural-immune interactions; in Nistico G (ed): Proceedings of a Symposium on Interactions between the Neuroendocrine and Immune Systems. Rome, Pythagora Press, 1989, pp 35–66.

20   Bellinger DL, Ackerman KD, Felten SY, Lorton D, Felten DL: Noradrenergic sympathetic innerva-
     tion of thymus, spleen, and lymph nodes: Aspects of development, aging and plasticity in neural
     immune interaction; in Hadden JW, Masek K, Nistico G (eds): Interactions Among Central Nervous
     System, Neuroendocrine and Immune Systems. Roma, Pythagora Press, 1989, pp 35–66.

21   Bellinger DL, Earnest DJ, Gallagher M, Felten DL: Presence and availability of VIP in primary
     and secondary lymphoid organs (abstract). Soc Neurosci Abstr 1992;18:1009.

22   Bellinger DL, Felten SY, Collier TJ, Felten DL: Noradrenergic sympathetic innervation of
     the spleen. IV. Morphometric analysis in adult and aged F344 rats. J Neurosci Res 1987;18:
     55–63.

23   Bellinger DL, Felten SY, Felten DL: Maintenance of noradrenergic sympathetic innervation in the
     involuted thymus of the aged Fischer 344 rat. Brain Behav Immun 1988;2:133–150.

24   Bellinger DL, Felten SY, Felten DL: Noradrenergic sympathetic innervation of lymphoid organs
     during development, aging, and autoimmunity; in Amenta F (ed): Aging of the Autonomic Nervous
     System. Boca Rato, CRC Press, 1993, pp 243–284.

25   Bellinger DL, Felten SY, Lorton D, Felten DL: Origin of noradrenergic innervation of the spleen
     in rats. Brain Behav Immun 1989;3:291–311.

26   Bellinger DL, Lorton D, Brouxhon S, Felten SY, Felten DL: The significance of vasoactive intestinal
     polypeptide (VIP) in immunomodulation. Adv Neuroimmunol 1996;6:5–27.

27   Bellinger DL, Lorton D, Felten SY, Felten DL: Effects of age on substance P (SP)+nerve fibers
     in the spleen of Fischer 344 rats (abstract). Soc Neurosci Abstr 1989;15:714.

28   Bellinger DL, Lorton D, Felten SY, Felten DL: Age-related alteration in norepinephrine uptake in
     the rat spleen. Soc Neurosci Abstr 1990;16:1210.

29   Bellinger DL, Lorton D, Felten SY, Felten DL: Age-related alterations in norepinephrine uptake
     in the rat spleen (abstract). Soc Neurosci Abstr 1990;16:1210.

30   Bellinger DL, Lorton D, Hamill R, Felten SY, Felten DL: Acetylcholinesterase staining and choline
     acetyltransferase activity in the young adult rat spleen: Lack of evidence for cholinergic innervation.
     Brain Behav Immun 1993;7:191–204.

31   Bellinger DL, Lorton D, Horn L, Felten SY, Felten DL: VIP-immunoreactivity in primary and
     secondary lymphoid organs of the rat. Peptides 1995;submitted.

32   Bellinger DL, Lorton D, Romano T, Olschowka JA, Felten SY, Felten DL: Neuropeptide innervation
     of lymphoid organs. Ann NY Acad Sci 1990;594:17–33.

33   Berkenbosch J, van Oers J, del Rey A, Tilders F, Besedovsky H: Corticotropin-releasing factor-
     producing neurons in the rat activated by interleukin-1. Science 1987;238:524–526.

34   Bernton EW, Bryant HU, Holaday JW: Prolactin and immune function; in Ader R, Cohen N,
     Felten DL (eds): Psychoneuroimmunology, ed 2. New York, Academic Press, 1991, pp 403–428.

35   Besedovsky H, del Rey AE, Sorkin E, Dinarello CA: Immunoregulatory feedback between interleu-
     kin-1 and glucocorticoid hormones. Science 1986;233:652–654.

36   Besedovsky H, Sorkin E, Felix D, Haas H: Hypothalamic changes during the immune response.
     Eur J Immunol 1977;7:323–325.

37   Bjurholm A, Kreicbergs A, Broden E, Schultzberg M: Substance P- and CGRP-immunoreactive
     nerves in bone. Peptides 1989;9:165–171.

38   Blue J, Weiss L: Electron microscopy of the red pulp of the dog spleen including vascular arrange-
     ments, periarterial macrophage sheaths (ellipsoids), and the contractile, innervated reticular mesh-
     work. Am J Anat 1981;161:189–218.

39   Bret-Dibat JL, Bluthe RM, Kent S, Kelley KW, Dantzer R: Lipopolysaccharide and interleukin-
     1 depress food-motivated behavior in mice by a vagal-mediated mechanism. Brain Behav Immun
     1995;9:242–246.

40   Brown R, Li Z, Vriend C, Nirula R, Janz L, Falk J, Nance DM, Dyck DG, Greenberg AH:
     Suppression of splenic macrophage interleukin-1 secretion following intracerebroventricular injec-
     tion of interleukin-1b: Evidence for pituitary-adrenal and sympathetic control. Cell Immunol 1991;
     132:84–93.

41   Bulloch K, Pomerantz W: Autonomic nervous system innervation of thymic related lymphoid tissue
     in wild-type and nude mice. J Comp Neurol 1984;228:57–68.

42   Calvo W: The innervation of the bone marrow in laboratory animals. Am J Anat 1968;123:315–328.

43   Calvo W, Forteza-Vila J: On the development of bone marrow innervation in new-born rats as studied with silver impregnation and electron microscopy. Am J Anat 1969;126:355–359.

44   Carr DJJ, Blalock JE: Neuropeptide hormones and receptors common to the immune and neuroendocrine systems: Bidirectional pathway of intersystem communication; in Ader R, Felten DL, Cohen N (eds): Psychoneuroimmunology, ed 2. New York, Academic Press, 1991, pp 573–588.

45   Chevendra V, Weaver LC: Distribution of neuropeptide Y, vasoactive intestinal peptide and somato-statin in populations of postganglionic neurons innervating the rat kidney, spleen and intestine. Neuroscience 1992;50:727–743.

46   Church MK, El-Lati S, Caulfied JP: Neuropeptide-induced secretion from human skin mast cells. Int Arch Allergy Appl Immunol 1991;94:310–318.

47   Cooke HJ: Neurobiology of the intestinal mucosa. Gastroenterology 1986;90:1057–1081.

48   Dahlström AB, Häggendal J, Hökfelt T: The noradrenaline content of the varicosities of sympathetic adrenergic nerve terminals in the rat. Acta Physiol Scand 1966;67:289–294.

49   Dahlström AB, Zetterström BEM: Noradrenaline stores in nerve terminals of the spleen: Changes during hemorrhagic shock. Science 1965;147:1583–1585.

50   Dardenne M, Savino W: Control of thymus physiology by peptidic hormones and neuropeptides (review). Immunol Today 1994;15:518–523.

51   Davies BN, Withrington PG: The actions of drugs on the smooth muscle and the capsule and blood vessels of the spleen. Pharmacol Rev 1973;25:373–413.

52   de Leeuw FE, Jansen GH, Batanero E, van Wichen DF, Huber J, Schuurman HJ: The neural and neuro-endocrine component of the human thymus. I. Nerve-like structures. Brain Behav Immun 1992;6:234–248.

53   Delrue-Perollet C, Li KS, Vitiello S, Neveu PJ: Peripheral catecholamines are involved in the neuroendocrine and immune effects of LPS. Brain Behav Immunity 1995;9:149–162.

54   Dorko F, Kocisova M, Gregor A, Schmidtova K, Banovska E: Acetylcholinesterase-positive innerva-tion of the thymus in old rats after ovariectomy (Slovak). Bratislavske Lekarske Listy 1996;97: 298–300.

55   Dunn Aj, Wang J: Cytokine effects on CNS biogenic amines (review). Neuroimmunomodulation 1995;2:319–328.

56   Ekblad E, Winther C, Ekman R, Hakanson R, Sundler F: Projections of peptide-containing neurons in rat small intestine. Neuroscience 1987;20:169–188.

57   Elfvin LG, Aldskogius H, Johansson J: Primary sensory afferents in the thymus of the guinea pig demonstrated with anterogradely transported horseradish peroxidase conjugates. Neurosci Lett 1993;150:35–38.

58   Ernström U, Sandberg G: Effects of adrenergic alpha- and beta-receptor stimulation on the release of lymphocytes and granulocytes from the spleen. Scand J Haematol 1973;11:275–286.

59   Ernström U, Söder O: Influence of adrenaline on the dissemination of antibody-producing cells from the spleen. Clin Exp Immunol 1975;21:131–140.

60   Esquifino AI, Cardinali DP: Local regulation of the immune response by the autonomic nervous system (review). Neuroimmunomodulaton 1994;1:265–273.

61   Feher E, Fodor M, Burnstock G: Distribution of somatostatin-immunoreactive nerve fibers in Peyer's patches. Gut 1992;33:1195–1198.

62   Felten DL: Neurotransmitter signaling of cells of the immune system: Important progress, major gaps. Brain Behav Immun 1991;5:2–8.

63   Felten DL, Ackerman KD, Wiegand SJ, Felten SY: Noradrenergic sympathetic innervation of the spleen. I. Nerve fibers associate with lymphocytes and macrophages in specific compartments of the splenic white pulp. J Neurosci Res 1987;18:28–36.

64   Felten DL, Bellinger DL, Felten SY: Autonomic signaling of the immune system: Implications for neural-immune interactions in aging; in Hendrie H, Mendelsohn LG, Readhead C (eds): Brain Aging: Molecular Biology, the Aging Process and Neurodegenerative Disease. Toronto, Hogrefe & Huber, 1990, pp 239–258.

65   Felten DL, Felten SY: Sympathetic noradrenergic innervation of immune organs. Brain Behav Immun 1988;2:293–300.

66   Felten DL, Felten SY: Innervation of the thymus; in Kendall MD, Ritter MA (eds): Thymus Update. London, Harwood Academic Publishers, 1989, pp 73–88.

67   Felten DL, Felten SY: Brain-immune signaling: Substrate for reciprocal immunological signaling of the nervous system; in Frederickson RCA, McGaugh JL, Felten DL (eds): Peripheral Signaling of the Brain: Role in Neural-Immune Interactions, Learning and Memory. Toronto, Hogrefe & Huber, 1991, pp 3–17.

68   Felten DL, Felten SY, Bellinger DL, Carlson SL, Ackerman KD, Madden KS, Olschowka JA, Livnat S: Noradrenergic sympathetic neural interactions with the immune system: Structure and function. Immunol Rev 1987;100:225–260.

69   Felten DL, Felten SY, Bellinger DL, Madden KS: Fundamental aspects of neural-immune signaling (review). Psychother Psychosom 1993;60:46–56.

70   Felten DL, Felten SY, Carlson SL, Bellinger DL, Ackerman KD, Romano TA, Livnat S: Development, aging, and plasticity of noradrenergic sympathetic innervation of secondary lymphoid organs: Implications for neural-immune interactions; in Dahlstrom A, Belmaker RM, Sandler M (eds): Progress in Catecholamine Research. A. Basic Aspects and Peripheral Mechanisms. New York, Liss, 1988, pp 517–524.

71   Felten DL, Felten SY, Carlson SL, Bellinger DL, Ackerman KD, Romano TA, Livnat S: Peripheral innervation of lymphoid tissue; in Freier S (ed): The Neuroendocrine Immune Network. Boca Raton, CRC Press, 1990, pp 9–18.

72   Felten DL, Felten SY, Carlson SL, Olschowka JA, Livnat S: Noradrenergic and peptidergic innervation of lymphoid tissue. J Immunol 1985;135:755s–765s.

73   Felten DL, Felten SY, Madden KS, Ackerman DK, Bellinger DL: Development, maturation, and senescence of sympathetic innervation of secondary immune organs; in Schreibman MP, Scanes CG (eds): Development, Maturation, and Senescence of Neuroendocrine Systems. San Diego, Academic Press, 1989, pp 381–396.

74   Felten DL, Livnat S, Felten SY, Carlson SL, Bellinger DL, Yeh P: Sympathetic innervation of lymph nodes in mice. Brain Res Bull 1984;13:693–699.

75   Felten DL, Overhage JM, Felten SY, Schmedtje JF: Noradrenergic sympathetic innervation of lymphoid tissue in the rabbit appendix: Further evidence for a link between the nervous and immune systems. Brain Res Bull 1981;7:595–612.

76   Felten SY, Bellinger DL, Collier TJ, Coleman PD, Felten DL: Decreased sympathetic innervation of spleen in aged Fischer 344 rats. Neurobiol Aging 1987;8:159–165.

77   Felten SY, Felten DL: Are lymphocytes targets of noradrenergic innervation? In Weiner H, Helhammer D, Murison R, Florin I (eds): Fronteirs of Stress Research. Toronto, Huber, 1989, pp 56–71.

78   Felten SY, Felten DL: Sympathetic noradrenergic neural contacts with lymphocytes and macrophages in the splenic white pulp of the rat: Site of possible bidirectional communication and local regulation between the nervous and immune system; in Bunney WE Jr, Hippius H, Laakman G, Schmauss M (eds): Neuropsychopharmacology. Berlin, Springer, 1990, pp 442–456.

79   Felten SY, Felten DL: The innervation of lymphoid organs; in Ader R, Felten DL, Cohen N (eds): Psychoneuroimmunology, ed 2. New York, Academic Press, 1991, pp 27–69.

80   Felten SY, Olschowka JA: Noradrenergic sympathetic innervation of the spleen. II. Tyrosine hydroxylase (TH)-positive nerve terminals form synaptic-like contacts on lymphocytes in the splenic white pulp. J Neurosci Res 1987;18:37–48.

81   Felten SY, Olschowka JA, Ackerman KD, Felten DL: Catecholaminergic innervation of the spleen: Are lymphocytes targets of noradrenergic nerves? In Dahlström A, Belmaker RH, Sandler M (eds): Progress in Catecholamine Research. A. Basic Aspects and Peripheral Mechanisms. New York, Liss, 1988, pp 525–531.

82   Fillenz M: The innervation of the cat spleen. Proc Roy Soc (Lond) 1970;174:459–468.

83   Fink T, Weihe E: Multiple neuropeptides in nerves supplying mammalian lymph nodes: Messenger candidates for sensory and autonomic neuroimmunomodulation? Neurosci Lett 1988;90:39–44.

84   Fleshner M, Goehler LE, Hermann J, Relton JK, Maier SF, Watkins LR: Interleukin-1 beta induced corticosterone elevation and hypothalamic NE depletion is vagally mediated. Brain Research Bulletin 1995;37:605–610.

85 Fried G, Terenius L, Brodin E, Efendic S, Dockray G, Fahrenkrug J, Goldstein M, Hökfelt T: Neuropeptide Y, enkephalin and noradrenaline coexist in sympathetic neurons innervating the bovine spleen. Biochemical and immunohistochemical evidence. Call Tissue Res 1986;243:495–508.

86 Gaddis RR, Dixon WR: Presynaptic opiate receptors-mediated inhibition of endogenous norepinephrine and dopamine-b-hydroxylase release in the cat spleen, independent of the presynaptic alpha adrenoceptors. J Pharmacol Exp Ther 1982;233:77–83.

87 Galindo B, Imaeda T: Electron microscopic study of the white pulp of the mouse spleen. Anat Rec 1962;143:399–415.

88 Gibson-Berry KL, Richardson C, Felten SY, Felten DL: Immunocytochemical and neurochemical analyses of sympathetic nerves in rat bone marrow. Soc Neurosci Abstr 1993;19:944.

89 Gillespie JS, Kirpekar SM: The localization of endogenous and infused noradrenaline in the spleen. J Physiol 1965;179:46P–47P.

90 Giron LT, Crutcher KA, Davis JN: Lymph nodes: A possible site for sympathetic neuronal regulation of immune responses. Ann Neurol 1980;8:520–525.

91 Goetzl EJ, Turck C, Sreedharan S: Production and recognition of neuropeptides by cells of the immune system; in Ader R, Cohen N, Felten DL (eds): Psychoneuroimmunology, ed 2. New York, Academic Press, 1991, pp 263–282.

92 Goetzl EJ, Xia M, Ingram DA, Kishiyama JL, Kaltreider HB, Byrd PK, Ichikawa S, Sreedharan SP: Neuropeptide signaling of lymphocytes in immunological responses. Int Arch Allergy Immunol 1995;107:202–204.

93 Gomariz RP, De La Fuente M, Hernanz A, Leceta J: Occurrence of vasoactive intestinal peptide (VIP) in lymphoid organs. Ann NY Acad Sci 1992;650:13–18.

94 Gomariz RP, Delgado M, Naranjo JR, Mellstrom B, Tormo A, Mata F, Leceta J: VIP gene expression in rat thymus and spleen. Brain Behav Immun 1993;7:271–278.

95 Heijnen CJ, Kavelaars A, Ballieux RE: Corticotropin-releasing hormone and proopiomelanocortin-derived peptides in the modulation of immune function; in Ader R, Felten DL, Cohen N (eds): Psychoneuroimmunology, ed 2. New York, Academic Press, 1991, pp 429–446.

96 Heusermann U, Stutte HJ: Electron microscopic studies of the innervation of the human spleen. Cell Tiss Res 1977;184:225–236.

97 Hori T, Katafuchi T, Take S, Kaizuka Y, Ichijo T, Shimizu N: The hypothalamo-sympathetic nervous system modulates peripheral cellular immunity (review). Neurobiology 1995;3:309–317.

98 Hori T, Katafuchi T, Take S, Shimizu N, Niijima A: The autonomic nervous system as a communication channel between the brain and the immune system (review). Neuroimmunomodulation 1995; 2:203–215.

99 Hurst S, Collins SM: Interleukin-1b modulation of norepinephrine release from rat myenteric nerves. Am J Physiol 1993;264:G30–G35.

100 Ichijo T, Katafuchi T, Hori T: Central interleukin-1 beta enhances splenic sympathetic nerve activity in rats. Brain Res Bull 1994;34:547–553.

101 Ichikawa S, Sreedharan SP, Goetzl EJ, Owen RL: Immunohistochemical localization of peptidergic nerve fibers and neuropeptide receptors in Peyer's patches of the cat ileum. Regul Pept 1994;54: 385–395.

102 Imai S, Hukuda S, Maeda T: Substance P-immunoreactive and protein gene product 9.5-immunoreactive nerve fibers in bone marrow of rat coccygeal vertebrae. J Orthopaed Res 1994;12:853–859.

103 Inoue N, Magari S, Sakanaka M: Distribution of peptidergic nerve fibers in rat bronchus-associated lymphoid tisse: Light microscopic observations. Lymphology 1990;23:155–160.

104 Irwin M: Stress-induced immune suppression: Role of brain corticotropin releasing hormone and autonomic nervous system mechanisms (review). Adv Neuroimmunol 1994;4:29–47.

105 Irwin M, Vale W, Britton KT: Central corticotropin-releasing factor suppresses natural killer cytotoxicity. Brain Behav Immun 1987;1:81–87.

106 Jansen AH, Liu P, Weisman H, Chernick V, Nance DM: Effect of sinus denervation and vagotomy on c-fos expression in the nucleus tractus solitarius after exposure to CO_2. Pflügers Arch Eur J Physiol 1996;431:876–881.

107 Jesseph JM, Felten DL: Noradrenergic innervation of the gut-associated lymphoid tissues (GALT) in the rabbit. Anat Rec 1984;208:81A–810.

108   Johnson AR, Erdos EG: Release of histamine from mast cells by vasoactive peptides. Proc Soc Exp Biol Med 1973;142:1252–1256.

109   Justice B: Critical life events and the onset of illness (review). Compreh Ther 1994;20:232–238.

110   Kapcala LP, He JR, Gao Y, Pieper JO, DeTolla LJ: Subdiaphragmatic vagotomy inhibits intra-abdominal inerleukin-1 beta stimulation of adrenocorticotropin secretion. Brain Res 1996;728:247–254.

111   Keller SE, Weiss JM, Scheiffer SJ, Miller NE, Stein M: Stress-induced suppression of immunity in adrenalectomized rats. Science 1983;221:1301–1304.

112   Kelley KW: Growth hormone in immunobiology; in Ader R, Cohen N, Felten DL (eds): Psychoneuroimmunology, ed 2. New York, Academic Press, 1991, pp 337–402.

113   Kendall MD, Al-Shawaf AA: Innervation of the rat thymus gland. Brain Behav Immunol 1991;5:9–28.

114   Kendall MD, Atkinson BA, Munoz FJ, de la Riva C, Clarke AG, von Gaudecker B: The noradrenergic innervation of the rat thymus during pregnancy and in the post-partum period. J Anat 1994;185:617–625.

115   Kiecolt-Glaser R: Psychoneuroimmunology and health consequences: Data and shared mechanisms (review). Psychosom Med 1995;57:269–274.

116   Kruszewska B, Felten SY, Moynihan J: Alterations in cytokine and antibody production following chemical sympathectomy in two strains of mice. J Immunol 1995;155:4613–4620.

117   Kurkowski R, Kummer W, Heym C: Substance P-immunoreactive nerve fibers in tracheobronchial lymph nodes of the guinea pig: Origin, ultrastructure and coexistence with other peptides. Peptides 1990;11:13–20.

118   Lacey CB, Elde RP, Seybold VS: Localization of vasoactive intestinal peptide binding sites in the thymus and bursa of Fabricius of the chick. Peptides 1991;12:383–391.

119   Leposavic G, Micic M, Ugresic N, Bogojevic M, Isakovic K: Components of sympathetic innervation of the rat thymus during late fetal and postnatal development: Histofluorescence and biochemical study. Sympathetic innervation of the rat thymus. Thymus 1992;19:77–87.

120   Livnat S, Eisen J, Felten DL, Felten SY, Irwin J, Madden KS, Sundaresan PJ: Behavioral and sympathetic neural modulation of immune function; in Dahlstrom A, Belmaker RM, Sandler M (eds): Progress in Catecholamine Research. A. Basic Aspects and Peripheral Mechanisms, New York, Liss, 1988, pp 539–546.

121   Livnat S, Felten SY, Carlson SL, Bellinger DL, Felten DL: Involvement of peripheral and central catecholamine systems in neural-immune interactions. J Neuroimmunol 1985;10:5–30.

122   Livnat S, Madden KS, Felten DL, Felten SY: Regulation of the immune system by sympathetic neural mechanisms. Prog Neuro-psychopharmacol Biol Psychiatry 1987;11:145–152.

123   Lorton D, Bellinger DL, Felten SY, Felten DL: Substance P (SP) and calcitonin gene-related peptide (CGRP) innervation of the rat spleen. Soc Neurosci Abstr 1989;15:714.

124   Lorton D, Bellinger DL, Felten SY, Felten DL: Substance P innervation of the rat thymus. Peptides 1990;11:1269–1275.

125   Lorton D, Bellinger DL, Felten SY, Felten DL: Substance P Innervation of spleen in rats: Nerve fibers associate with lymphocytes and macrophages in specific compartments of the spleen. Brain Behav Immun 1991;5:29–40.

126   Lorton D, Hewitt D, Bellinger DL, Felten SY, Felten DL: Noradrenergic reinnervation of the rat spleen following chemical sympathectomy with 6-hydroxydopamine: Pattern and time course of reinnervation. Brain Behav Immun 1990;4:198–222.

127   Lundberg JM, Rudehill A, Sollevi A, Fried G, Wallin G: Co-release of neuropeptide Y and noradrenaline from pig spleen in vivo: Importance of subcellular storage, nerve impulse frequency and pattern, feedback regulation and resupply by axonal transport. Neuroscience 1989;28:475–486.

128   Lundberg JM, Rudehill A, Sollevi A, Hamberger B: Evidence for co-transmitter role of neuropeptide Y in the pig spleen. Br J Pharmacol 1989;96:675–687.

129   Lundberg JM, Änggård A, Pernow J, Hökfelt T: Neuropeptide Y-, substance P- and VIP-immunoreactive nerves in cat spleen in relation to autonomic vascular and volume control. Cell Tissue Res 1985;239:9–18.

130   MacNeil BJ, Jansen AH, Greenberg AH, Nance DM: Activation and selectivity of splenic sympathetic nerve electrical activity response to bacterial endotoxin. Am J Physiol 1996;270:R264–R270.

131 Madden KS, Ackerman KD, Livnat S, Felten SY, Felten DL: Patterns of noradrenergic innervation of lymphoid organs and immunological consequences of denervation; in Goetzl E, Spector NH (eds): Neuroimmune Networks: Physiology and Diseases. New York, Liss, 1989, pp 1–8.

132 Madden KS, Bellinger DL, Snyder E, Maida M, Felten DL: Alterations in sympathetic innervation of thymus and spleen in aged mice (abstract). 1st Int Conf Immunol Aging 1996, June 16–19.

133 Madden KS, Felten SY, Felten DL, Bellinger DL: Sympathetic nervous system–immune system interactions in young and old Fischer 344 (F344) rats. Ann NY Acad Sci 1995;771:523–534.

134 Madden KS, Felten SY, Felten DL, Sundaresan PR, Livnat S: Sympathetic neural modulation of the immune system. I. Depression of T cell immunity in vivo and in vitro following chemical sympathectomy. Brain Behav Immun 1989;3:72–89.

135 Madden KS, Livnat S: Catecholaminergic action on immunologic reactivity; in Ader R, Felten DL, Cohen N (eds): Psychoneuroimmunology, ed 2. New York, Academic Press, 1991, pp 283–310.

136 Madden KS, Sanders VM, Felten DL: Catecholamine influences and sympathetic neural modulation of immune responsiveness (review). Ann Rev Pharmacol Toxicol 1995;35:417–448.

137 Maestroni GJM, Conti A: Role of the pineal neurohormone melatonin in the psychoneuroendocrine-immune network; in Ader R, Cohen N, Felten DL (eds): Psychoneuroimmunology, ed 2. New York, Academic Press, 1991, pp 465–513.

138 Manske JM, Sullivan EL, Andersen SM: Substance P mediated stimulation of cytokine levels in cultured murine bone marrow stromal cells. Adv Exp Med Biol 1995;383:53–64.

139 McCruden AB, Stimson WH: Sex hormones and immune function; in Ader R, Felten DL, Cohen N (eds): Psychoneuroimmunology, ed 2. New York, Academic Press, 1991, pp 475–493.

140 McGillis JP, Mitsuhaski M, Payan DG: Immunologic properties of substance P; in Ader R, Felten DL, Cohen N (eds): Psychoneuroimmunology, ed 2. San Diego, Academic Press, 1991, pp 209–223.

141 Micic M, Leposavic G, Ugresic N: Relationships between monoaminergic and cholinergic innervation of the rat thymus during aging. J Neuroimmunol 1994;49:205–212.

142 Micic M, Leposavic G, Ugresic N, Bogojevic M, Isakovic K: Parasympathetic innervation of the rat thymus during first life period: Histochemical and biochemical study. Thymus 1992;19:173–182.

143 Moore RD, Mumaw VR, Schoenberg MC: The structure of the spleen and its functional implications. Exp Molec Path 1964;3:31–50.

144 Moore TC: Modification of lymphocyte traffic by vasoactive neurotransmitter substances. Immunology 1984;52:511–518.

145 Mughal S, Cuschieri A, Kharbat BA: Histochemical localization of adenosine triphosphatase activity in thymus: A light microscopical and ultrastructural study. Histochem J 1986;18:341–350.

146 Munck A, Guyre PM: Glucocorticoids and immune function; in Ader R, Felten DL, Cohen N (eds): Psychoneuroimmunology, ed 2. San Diego, Academic Press, 1991, pp 447–474.

147 Murphy WJ, Durnum SK, Longo DL: Differential effects of growth hormone and prolactin on murine T cell development and function. J Exp Med 1993;178:231–236.

148 Müller S, Weihe E: Interrelation of peptidergic innervation with mast cells and ED1-positive cells in rat thymus. Brain Behav Immun 1991;5:55–72.

149 Nance DM, Burns J: Innervation of the spleen in the rat: Evidence for absence of afferent innervation. Brain Behav Immun 1989;3:281–290.

150 Nee LE: Effects of psychosocial interactions at a cellular level (review). Social Work 1995;40:259–262.

151 Neveu PJ: Asymmetrical brain modulation of immune reactivity in mice: A model for studying interindividual differences and physiological population heterogeneity? [published erratum appears in Life Sci 1992;50:1469] (review). Life Sci 1992;50:1–6.

152 Niijima A: An electrophysiological study on the vagal innervation of the thymus in the rat. Brain Res Bul 1995;38:319–323.

153 Niijima A, Hori T, Aou S, Oomura Y: The effects of interleukin-1β on the activity of adrenal, splenic and renal sympathetic nerves in the rat. J Autonom Nerv Syst 1991;36:183–192.

154 Niijima A, Hori T, Katafuchi T, Ichijo T: The effect of interleukin-1 beta on the efferent activity of the vagus nerve to the thymus. J Autonom Nerv Syst 1995;54:137–144.

155 Nilsson G, Alving K, Ahlstedt S, Hokfelt T, Lundberg JM: Peptidergic innervation of rat lymphoid tissue and lung: relation to mast cells and sensitivity to capsaicin and immunization. Cell Tissue Res 1990;262:125–133.

156 Nio DA, Moylan RN, Roche JK: Modulation of T lymphocyte function by neuropeptides: Evidence for their role as local immunoregulatory elements. J Immunol 1993;150:5281–5288.

157 Nohr D, Weihe E: The neuroimmune link in the bronchus-associated lymphoid tissue (BALT) of cat and rat: Peptides and neural markers. Brain Behav Immun 1991;5:84–101.

158 Ottaway C: Vasoactive intestinal peptide and immune function; in Ader R, Felten DL, Cohen N (eds): Psychoneuroimmunology, ed 2. San Diego, Academic Press, 1991, pp 225–262.

159 Ottaway CA, Lewis DL, Asa SL: Vasoactive intestinal peptide-containing nerves in Peyer's patches. Brain Behav Immun 1987;1:148–158.

160 Pfoch M, Unsicker K: Electron microscopic study on the innervation of Peyer's patches of Syrian hamster. Z Zellforsch 1972;123:425–429.

161 Popper P, Mantyh CR, Vigna SR, Magioos JE, Mantyh PW: The localization of sensory nerve fibers and receptor binding sites for sensory neuropeptides in canine mesenteric lymph nodes. Peptides 1988;9:257–267.

162 Probert L, de Mey J, Polak JM: Distinct subpopulations of enteric p-type neurones contain substance P and vasoactive intestinal polypeptide. Nature 1981;294:470–471.

163 Rabin BS, Cunnick JE, Lysle DT: Stress-induced alteration of immune function. Prog NeuroEndocrinImmunol 1990;3:116–124.

164 Rameshwar P, Gascon P: Substance P (SP) mediates production of stem cell factor and interleukin-1 in bone marrow stroma: Potential autoregulatory role for these cytokines in SP receptor expression and induction. Blood 1995;86:482–490.

165 Reigele L: Uber die mikroscopische innervation der milz. Z Zellforschmikrosk Anat 1929;9:511–533.

166 Reilly FD: Innervation and vascular pharmacodynamics of the mammalian spleen. Experientia 1985;41:187–192.

167 Reilly FD, McCuskey PA, Miller ML, McCuskey RS, Meineke HA: Innervation of the periarteriolar lymphatic sheath of the spleen. Tissue Cell 1979;11:121–126.

168 Reilly FD, McCuskey RS: Studies of the hemopoietic microenvironment. VII. Neural mechanisms in splenic microvascular regulation in mice. Microvasc Res 1977;14:293–302.

169 Reilly FD, McCuskey RS, Meineke HA: Studies of the hemopoietic microenvironment. VIII. Adrenergic and cholinergic innervation of the murine spleen. Anat Rec 1976;185:109–118.

170 Romano T, Olschowka JA, Felten SY, Felten DL: Tyrosine hydroxylase and neuropeptide Y positive nerve fibers in the spleen of the beluga whale (abstract). Assoc Aquatic Anim Res 1989.

171 Romano TA, Felten SY, Felten DL, Olschowka JA: Neuropeptide-Y innervation of the rat spleen: Another potential immunomodulatory neuropeptide. Brain Behav Immun 1991;5:116–131.

172 Romano TA, Felten SY, Olschowka JA, Felten DL: Noradrenergic and peptidergic innervation of lymphoid organs in the beluga, *Delphinapterus leucas:* An anatomical link between the nervous and immune systems. J Morphol 1994;221:243–259.

173 Romeo HE, Fink T, Yanaihara N, Weihe E: Distribution and relative proportions of neuropeptide Y- and proenkephalin-containing noradrenergic neurones in rat superior cervical ganglion: Separate projections to submaxillary lymph nodes. Peptides 1997;15:1479–1487.

174 Sabbadini E, Berczi I: The submandibular gland: A key organ in the neuro-immuno-regulatory network? (review). Neuroimmunomodulation 1995;2:184–202.

175 Sanders SK, Becker KJ, Cierpial MA, Carpenter DM, Rankin LA, Fleener SL, Ritchie JC, Simpson PE, Weiss JM: Intracerebroventricular infusion of interleukin-I rapidly decreases peripheral cellular immune responses. J Neuroimmunol 1989;86:6398–6402.

176 Schiff JM: Leçons sur la physiologie de la digestion, 1867, vol 2, p 416.

177 Schultzberg M, Svenson SB, Unden A, Bartfai T: Interleukin-1-like immunoreactivity in peripheral tissues. J Neurosci Res 1987;18:184–189.

178 Sergeeva VE: Histotopography of catecholamines in the mammalian thymus. Bull Exp Biol Med 1974;77:456–458.

179 Shimizu N, Hori T, Nakane H: An interleukin-1 beta-induced noradrenaline release in the spleen is mediated by brain corticotropin-releasing factor: An in vivo microdialysis study in conscious rats. Brain Behav Immun 1994;8:14–23.

180 Shimizu N, Kaizuka Y, Hori T, Nakane H: Immobilization increases norepinephrine release and reduces NK cytotoxicity in spleen of conscious rat. am J Physiol 1996;271:R537–R544.

---

181 Singh U, Fatani JA, Mohajir AM: Ontogeny of cholinergic innervation of thymus in mouse. Dev Comp Immunol 1987;11:627–635.

182 Singh U, Owen JJT: Studies on the maturation of thymus stem cells: The effects of catecholamines, histamine, and peptide hormones on the expression of T alloantigens. Eur J Immunol 1976;6: 59–62.

183 Spengler RN, Chensue SW, Giacherio DA, Blenk N, Kunkel SL: Endogenous norepinephrine regulates tumor necrosis factor-a production from macrophages in vitro. J Immunol 1994;152: 3024–3031.

184 Stead RH: Innervation of mucosal immune cells in the gastrointestinal tract (review). Regional Immunol 1992;4:91–99.

185 Stead RH, Bienenstock J, Stanisz AM: Neuropeptide regulation of mucosal immunity. Immunol Rev 1987;100:333–359.

186 Stead RH, Tomioka M, Pezzati P, Marshall J, Croitoru K, Perdue M, Stanisz A, Bienenstock J: Interaction of the mucosal immune and peripheral nervous systems; in Ader R, Felten DL, Cohen N (eds): Psychoneuroimmunology, ed 2. San Diego, Academic Press, 1991, pp 177–208.

187 Stead RH, Tomioka M, Quinonez G, Simon G, Felten SY, Bienenstock J: Intestinal mucosal mast cells in normal and nematode-infected rat intestines are in intimate contact with peptidergic nerves. Proc Natl Acad Sci USA 1987;84:2975–2979.

188 Sternberg EM, Chrousos GP, Wilder RL, Gold PW: The stress response and the regulation of inflammatory disease (review). Ann Intern Med 1992;117:854–866.

189 Theoharides TC, Douglas WW: Mast cell histamine secretion in response to somatostatin analogues: Structural considerations. Eur J Pharmacol 1981;73:131–136.

190 Ueyama T, Kozuki K, Houtani T, Ikeda M, Kitajiri M, Tamashita T, Kumazawa T, Nagatsu I, Sugimoto T: Immunolocalization of tyrosine hydroxylase and vasoactive intestinal polypeptide in nerve fibers innervating human palatine tonsil and paratonsillar glands. Neurosci Lett 1990;116: 70–74.

191 Utterback RA: The innervation of the spleen. J Comp Neurol 1944;81:55–68.

192 Vizi ES, Orso E, Osipenko ON, Hasko G, Elenkov IJ: Neurochemical, electrophysiological and immunocytochemical evidence for a noradrenergic link between the sympathetic nervous system and thymocytes. Neuroscience 1995;68:1263–1276.

193 Vriend CY, Zuo L, Dyck DG, Nance DM, Greenberg AH: Central administration of interleukin-1 beta increases norepinephrine turnover in the spleen. Brain Res Bull 1993;31:39–42.

194 Walcott B, McLean JR: Catecholamine-containing neurons and lymphoid cells in a lacrimal gland of the pigeon. Brain Res 1985;328:129–137.

195 Watkins LR, Goehler LE, Relton JK, Tartaglia N, Silbert L, Martin D, Maier SF: Blockade of interleukin-1 induced hyperthermia by subdiaphragmatic vagotomy: Evidence for vagal mediation of immune-brain communication. Neurosci Lett 1995;183:27–31.

196 Watkins LR, Maier SF, Goehler LE: Cytokine-to-brain communication: A review & analysis of alternative mechanisms. Life Sci 1995;57:1011–1026.

197 Weihe E, Krekel J: The neuroimmune connection in human tonsils. Brain Behav Immun 1991;5: 41–54.

198 Weihe E, Muller S, Fink T, Zentel HJ: Tachykinins, calcitonin gene-related peptide and neuropeptide Y in nerves of the mammalian thymus: Interactions with mast cells in autonomic and sensory neuroimmunomodulation. Neurosci Lett 1989;100:77–82.

199 Weisz-Carrington P, Nagomoto N, Farraj M, Buschmann R, Rypins EB, Stanisz A: Analysis of SP/VIP fiber association with T4 and T8 lymphocytes in normal human colon; in Mestechky J (ed): Advances in Mucosal Immunology. New York, Plenum Press, 1995, pp 559–561.

200 Williams JM, Felten DL: Sympathetic innervation of murine thymus and spleen: A comparative histofluorescence study. Anat Rec 1981;199:531–542.

201 Williams JM, Peterson RG, Shea PA, Schmedtje JF, Bauer DC, Felten DL: Sympathetic innervation of murine thymus and spleen: Evidence for a functional link between the nervous and immune systems. Brain Res Bull 1981;6:83–94.

202 Yamashita T, Kumazawa H, Kozuki K, Amano H, Tomoda K, Kumazawa T: Autonomic nervous system in human palatine tonsil. Acta Otolaryngol 1984;416:63–71.

203 Yamazaki K, Allen TD: Ultrastructural morphometric study of efferent nerve terminals on murine bone marrow stromal cells, and the recognition of a novel anatomical unit: The 'neuro-reticular complex'. Am J Anat 1990;187:261–276.

204 Zalcman S, Green-Johnson JM, Murray L, Wan W, Nance DM, Greenberg AH: Interleukin-2-induced enhancement of an antigen-specific IgM plaque-forming cell response is mediated by the sympathetic nervous system. J Pharmacol Exp Therapeut 1994;271:977–982.

205 Zentel HJ, Weihe E: The neuro-B cell link of peptidergic innervation in the bursa Fabricii. Brain Behav Immun 1991;5:132–147.

206 Zetterström BEM, Hökfelt T, Norberg K-A, Olsson P: Possibilities of a direct adrenergic influence on blood elements in the dog spleen. Acta Chir Scand 1973;139:117–122.

207 Zirbes T, Novotny GE: Quantification of thymic innervation in juvenile and aged rats. Acta Anat 1992;145:283–288.

Dr. Suzanne Stevens-Felten, University of Rochester School of Medicine,
Department of Neurobiology and Anatomy, Box 603, 601 Elmwood Avenue,
Rochester, NY 14642 (USA)
Tel. (716) 275 2030, Fax (716) 442 8766, E-Mail: felten@medinfo.rochester.edu

Blalock JE (ed): Neuroimmunoendocrinology, 3rd rev ed.
Chem Immunol. Basel, Karger, 1997, vol 69, pp 132–154

....

Neuroendocrine Peptide Receptors on Cells of the Immune System

Hildegardo H. Garza, Jr.[a], *Daniel J.J. Carr*[b]

[a] Department of Ophthalmology, Louisiana State University Eye Center;
[b] Departments of Microbiology, Immunology, and Parasitology and Pharmacology,
Louisiana State University Medical Center, New Orleans, La., USA

Introduction

Over the course of the past 3–4 years, a tremendous effort has been made in the further characterization of neuropeptide receptors on cells of the immune system. The previous review [1] focused on the biochemical, pharmacological, and biological evidence for the existence of these receptors on lymphocytes, monocytes/macrophages, granulocytes, and hematopoietic-derived cell lines. However, with the advent of molecular biological techniques, it has been possible to definitively identify neuropeptide receptors at the molecular level and in some systems, identify receptor-linked signaling cascades as summarized in table 1. As an example, the adrenoceptor-immune system interaction illustrates the intimate relationship between receptor ligation and intracellular signaling events ultimately influencing the humoral and cellular immune responses [2]. In addition, the review discusses receptors for molecules and neurotransmitters that have not previously been covered but for which evidence would indicate such receptors exist on cells of the immune system and play a role in immunophysiology. A summary of the distribution of neuroendocrine peptide receptors on cells of the immune system is given in table 2.

Cannabinoid Receptor

Whereas the active constituent of cannabis Δ^9-tetrahydrocannabinol (THC) is not a neuropeptide, there is a growing body of literature suggesting that it has significant immunosuppressive properties and may aid the progres-

Table 1. Summary of receptor properties

Receptor class	General immunomodulatory effect	Mechanism in immunocytes
Cannabinoid	suppressive	Ca^{2+}, adenylate cyclase
Corticotropin	stimulatory	Ca^{2+}, adenylate cyclase
Dopamine	unknown	unknown
Serotonin	stimulatory	unknown
Opioid	suppressive – in vivo stimulatory – in vitro	7 transmembrane spanning region, G protein
Sigma	suppressive	unknown
Arginine vasopressin	stimulatory	unknown
Prolactin	stimulatory	Raf-1 phosphorylation, MAP kinase activation
Somatostatin	suppressive	unknown
Substance P	stimulatory	G protein activation, Ca^{2+}, MAP kinase activation
Vasoactive intestinal peptide	suppressive	adenylate cyclase
Insulin-like growth factor	stimulatory	p56 Lck tyrosine kinase, IRS-I activation, PPI-3 kinase activation
Calcitonin gene-related peptide	suppressive	adenylate cyclase

sion of infectious diseases [3–5]. Moreover, reports suggest that THC acts directly on lymphocytes and monocytes/macrophages through the suppression of intracellular Ca^{2+} mobilization and adenylate cyclase activity [6–8]. These findings are consistent with the notion that cells of the immune system express binding sites for THC.

The existence of cannabinoid receptors was originally demonstrated in the brain by stereoselective radioreceptor assays [9]. These results were confirmed by the cloning of the receptor from a rat [10] and human [11] cDNA library. A second cannabinoid receptor was identified from a human promyelocytic cell line, HL-60 [12]. Ligand-binding studies and RT-PCR have confirmed the existence of cannabinoid binding sites on cells of the immune system

Table 2. Neuroendocrine peptide receptors on cells of the immune system

Receptor	Cell/tissue	$K_d(K_i)$, nM	B_{max}	References
Cannabinoid	spleen cell	0.910	87 fmol/10^6 cells	13
Cannabinoid	spleen	7.2		14
Cannabinoid	lymph node	3.8		14
Cannabinoid	Peyer's patches	4.0		14
Dopamine D_5	human PBMCs	0.58	2.2 fmol/10^6 cells	40
Serotonin				
5HT1A	activated T cell	1.2		53
5HT2	activated T cell	128		53
μ opioid	splenocytes	960	27 nmol/10^7 cells	1
$μ_3$ opioid	granulocyte	44	1630 fmol/mg	83
κ opioid	EL-4 murine thymoma	60	2.7 pmol/10^6 cells	1
κ opioid	P388d$_1$ murine macrophage line	17	54 fmol/10^6 cells	1
ACTH	rat splenic T cells	0.087	1,100 sites/cell	1
ACTH		4	30,000 sites/cell	1
ACTH	rat splenic B cells	0.090	3,600 sites/cell	1
ACTH		4.3	38,000 sites/cell	1
β-Endorphin	EL-4 murine thymoma	65		1
β-Endorphin	murine splenocytes	4.1	0.1–0.3 fmol/10^6 cells	1
β-Endorphin	U937 human promonocyte line	12	40 fmol/10^6 cells	1
Sigma	PBMCs	26.4		93
Sigma	PBMCs	26.4	752 fmol/mg	93
Sigma	T lymphocytes	401	382 fmol/10^6 cells	95
Sigma	B lymphocytes	302	1,145 fmol/10^6 cells	95
Sigma	thymocytes (high)	277	161 fmol/10^6 cells	95
Sigma	thymocytes (low affinity)	2,500	31 fmol/10^6 cells	95
Sigma	splenocytes	40.8	2,320 fmol/mg	97
Sigma	spleen	0.66	5,646 fmol/mg	98
Sigma	PBMCs	2.4	219,483 sites/cell	98
AVP	PBMCs	0.47		1
AVP	PBMCs	0.5	7.6 fmol/8 × 10^6 cells	106
Prolactin	lymphocytes	1.7	360 sites/cell	1
Prolactin	LGLs	0.300	660 sites/cell	1

Table 2 (continued)

Receptor	Cell/tissue	$K_d(K_i)$, nM	B_{max}	References
Somatostatin	gut-associated lymphoid tissue	1.3		127
Somatostatin	PBMCs	700	300–500 sites/cell	1
Somatostatin	activated lymphocytes	11	7×10^5 sites/cell	1
Somatostatin	Jurkat T cell line	0.003	100 sites/cell	1
Substance P	IM-9 B lympho-blastoid line	0.21	4,838 sites/cell	133
Substance P	T cells	0.400	7,000 sites/cell	1
Substance P	splenic T cells	0.620	195 sites/cell	1
Substance P	Peyer's patch T cells	0.500	647 sites/cell	1
Substance P	splenic B cells	0.640	190 sites/cell	1
Substance P	Peyer's patch B cells	0.920	975 sites/cell	1
VIP	lamina propria T cells	9.08		142
VIP	monocytes	0.250	9,600 sites/cell	1
VIP	T-enriched cells	0.470	1,700 sites/cell	1
VIP	B-enriched cells	0.430	1,400 sites/cell	1
VIP	LGLs	0.390	2,400 sites/cell	1
VIP	splenocytes	0.100	1,600 sites/cell	1
VIP	splenocytes	0.220	900 sites/cell	1
VIP	Peyer's patch lymphocytes	0.240	500 sites/cell	1
IGF	Jurkat T	1.77	230 sites/cell	156

[13, 14]. One hypothesis that has arisen suggests that the brain-derived THC receptor (termed CB1) is primarily found within the nervous system and testis while the peripheral THC receptor (termed CB2) primarily resides within immune cells [15]. Future studies will reveal whether this idea holds true. However, a recent investigation has detected CB1 mRNA by RT-PCR and CB1 protein expression by Western blot analysis that is upregulated following mitogen (phytohemagglutinin) stimulation in the human T-cell leukemia cell line, Jurkat [16]. Another study found little if any CB1 mRNA or protein expressed in primary spleen cells using mutational RT-PCR and immunocyto-chemical techniques [17]. However, this same study did find CB1 mRNA in the human T-lymphoblast Molt-4 cells and rat thymus cells [17]. Future studies are required to elucidate the apparent dichotomy of receptor expression between primary and immortalized cells as well as how the distribution of THC binding sites on leukocyte subpopulations influences immune homeostasis and disease processes. In addition, the finding of an endogenous ligand for the

cannabinoid receptor [18] that is active on cells of the immune system [19, 20] points to a need to fully characterize the CB1 and CB2 types of cannabinoid receptors within the immune system.

Corticotropin Receptor

The expression of the corticotropin (ACTH) receptor on lymphocytes has important implications relative to autocrine and paracrine function of an immune response. Within the confines of an inflammatory response, cortico-tropin-releasing hormone (CRF) and ACTH are reportedly elevated in tissues including the spleen and thymus [21, 22]. In addition, it has recently been shown that lymphocyte-derived ACTH is biologically active using the Y-1 adrenal cell line as an indicator [23]. The consequences of ACTH on the physiology of cells of the immune system have previously centered on antibody production [1]. Recent studies have shown that the stress-related polypeptide enhances IL-4 and anti-CD40-induced IgE production through CD14 + monocytes [24]. Whereas ACTH pretreatment of peripheral blood mononuclear cells elicited IL-6 and TNF-α production, neither cytokine corresponded to the elevated IgE synthesis in the presence of IL-4 [24]. Other studies suggest that ACTH may play a role in the activation of T cells [25] but it has no measurable direct effect on natural killer (NK) cell activity [26, 27] indicating some degree of selective receptor expression.

ACTH has been shown to upregulate ACTH binding sites and 2- and 4-kb ACTH receptor mRNA transcripts (2 to 6-fold) through the activation of a cAMP pathway in murine Y–1 and human H295 adrenocortical cells [28]. However, the type 2 cytokine TGF-β has previously been reported to downregulate ACTH binding and block ACTH-mediated upregulation of ACTH binding sites on bovine adrenocortical cells [29]. Within the immune system, this observation would suggest that TGF-β acts as a feedback inhibitor of ACTH receptors on lymphocytes during a type 2-elicited humoral immune response.

Recently, the ACTH receptor (designated MC5-R) was cloned from primary rat splenic lymphocytes [Clarke, pers. commun.]. Subsequent work has shown that the receptor could be amplified from rat splenocyte library and splenic lymphocytes stimulated with or without concanavalin A over 72 h but not from rat thymocytes. These results are consistent with the observation showing that ACTH receptors could be detected from B and T lymphocytes but not from thymocytes [30]. Although the mitogen-stimulated spleen cells display elevated (2 to 3-fold) levels of ACTH binding sites [30], there is no evidence of an increase at the transcriptional level as determined by competitive RT-PCR, suggesting that the receptor is controlled post-transcriptionally

[Clarke, pers. commun.]. Polyclonal antibody generated to the amino-terminal domain of the MCR-5 receptor reacts with a protein from quiescent lymphocytes or adrenal cells with an apparent molecular weight of 57–60 kD whereas the antibody recognizes proteins that have apparent molecular weights of 33–35 and 57–60 kD from concanavalin A-stimulated lymphocytes. Considering that the amino acid sequence of the lymphocyte MCR-5 ACTH receptor predicts a protein of 32 kD suggests that the 57 to 60-kD protein recognized by the polyclonal antibody may be the mature glycosylated form of the MCR-5 receptor. Recent studies have investigated signaling cascades coupled to the lymphocyte ACTH receptor. The addition of corticotropin (1–39 or 1–25) was found to increase Ca^{2+} uptake and cAMP synthesis in a dose- and time-dependent manner [31]. However, ACTH (11–24) or α-MSH (ACTH 1–13) had no effect. The transient nature of Ca^{2+} uptake is predicted to involve microdomains on the plasma membrane of the receptor expressing cell that coordinates signal transduction processes [32]. This explanation would suggest that ACTH signaling acts as an ancillary stimulant that would modify cell activation.

Neurotransmitter Receptors

Dopamine is a neurotransmitter that may have an important role in human disease including Parkinson's disease, neuropsychiatric, and hypertensive disorders. Early work suggested that dopamine, either through direct or indirect action on lymphocytes, could modify both humoral and cell-mediated immune parameters [33]. The potential direct action of dopamine on lymphocytes was supported by radioligand binding studies that showed [^{3}H]spiroperidol binding to lymphocytes [34]. The binding capacity for spiroperidol was found to be elevated on lymphocytes obtained from schizophrenic patients [35, 36] but reduced on lymphocytes from patients with idiopathic Parkinson's [37]. Whereas there has been some controversy on this latter point [38], recent studies [39, 40] support and expand upon the original observation suggesting the existence of specific dopamine receptors on lymphocytes.

The molecular characterization of dopamine receptors indicates the existence of at least 5 subtypes, D_1-D_5, that can be classified into two receptor families; dopamine D_1-like receptors (includes D_1 and D_5) and dopamine D_2-like receptors (includes D_2-D_4) [41, 42].

Both D_3 and D_5 dopamine receptor transcripts have been identified in human peripheral blood lymphocytes [43, 44] and a high-affinity dopamine transport system has recently been identified in lymphocytes as well [45]. The latter observation has important implications regarding cocaine modification of immune function [46, 47] and human immunodeficiency virus (HIV) replication in peripheral blood mononuclear cells [48] through the action of cocaine in the inhibition of dopamine uptake by the lymphocytes [45].

Another neurotransmitter serotonin has also been shown to modify immune function. Specifically, serotonin ($10^{-4} - 10^{-6}$ M) has been shown to augment natural killer activity through a monocyte-dependent pathway [49]. Serotonin uptake pathways in peripheral blood mononuclear cells have also been identifed [50] and such pathways may directly or indirectly influence natural killer activity [51]. Serotonin receptors ($5HT1_A$) have been described on monocytes [52] as well as activated T lymphocytes [53] supporting the potential direct effect of this neurotransmitter on immunocompetence [54–56].

Opioid and Nonopioid Receptors

There is continuing precedence of an immunomodulatory role for endogenous opioids during acute and chronic inflammatory processes in situ [57–60]. However, these endogenous opioid peptides (including endorphins, enkephalins, and dynorphins) bind to opioid and nonopioid β-endorphin receptors on leukocytes as defined by the sensitivity to naloxone. Relative to the β-endorphin-specific receptor, there has been some progress in the last 5–6 years in the biochemical characterization and regulation of the receptor. In the A20 B-cell lymphoma line, a high-affinity ($K_d = 9 \times 10^{-11} M$) and a low-affinity ($2 \times 10^{-8}$ M) binding site have been identified [61]. Stimulation of these cells with concanavalin A results in a loss of the high-affinity site whereas treatment of cells with the glucocorticoid agonist dexamethasone results in an increase in the number of low-affinity sites. Using an antibody generated to the complementary portion of the carboxyl-terminus of β-endorphin, the putative biochemical profile of the monocytic U937 β-endorphin-specific receptor has been described [62]. Two distinct bands of 56–58 and 64 kD were identified by immunoblotting while chemical crosslinking in the presence of the antibody showed specific labeling of components with apparent molecular weights of 44 and 59 kD. While the investigators suggest that the 56 to 58-kD species in the Western blot analysis is consistent with the 59-kD protein observed during chemical crosslinking, there is no explanation for the discrepancy in the size of the other labeled proteins. It is possible that the 64-kD protein is albumin as this is a typical carrier protein when using ^{125}I-labeled β-endorphin and has been previously suspect in opioid receptor labeling experiments [63]. The 44-kD protein moiety may represent a nonglycosylated version of the binding site or a tightly coupled G protein although additional studies are required to address this issue. The size of the immunogenic and predicted binding site of the β-endorphin-specific receptor parallels the reported size of the opioid receptors (i.e. δ and μ) as previously reviewed [1]. It is possible that the β-endorphin-specific receptor is a splice variant of one of the opioid receptors found on cells of the immune system.

Significant progress has been made in the characterization of opioid receptors on cells of the immune system by a number of different investigative teams primarily as a result of the cloning of brain δ [64, 65], κ [66], and μ [67, 68] opioid receptors. These studies indicate that the receptors belong to the rhodopsin superfamily characterized by multiple (7) hydrophobic membrane-spanning regions. In addition, deletion and site-directed mutagenesis studies have identified potential regions important for agonist/antagonist activity [69–71]. Opioid receptor transcripts isolated from cells of the immune system were initially described by Kieffer's group [72] and substantiated by additional studies by these and several other teams using primary and immortalized hematopoietic-derived cells [72–77]. However, these studies only determined partial sequences of the open reading frame for each of the opioid receptor types that were found to be 98–99% homologous to the brain opioid receptor sequences. The first report of a full-length opioid receptor expressed by cells of the immune system was a κ opioid reeptor found on the T-cell lymphoma R1.1 [78]. These results confirmed previous pharmacological studies showing a κ opioid receptor on the R1.1 cells that was coupled to guanine nucleotide-binding protein [79, 80]. A second full-length opioid receptor (δ) constitutively expressed in thymocytes has also been identified and sequenced [81]. Whereas no full-length μ receptor has been cloned from lymphoid tissue, there is precedence for novel binding traits for μ alkaloid selectivity on immune cells [82–83]. These receptors have clearly been shown to have functional significance within the immune system by numerous laboratories [84]. A nonopioid 'orphan' receptor having sequence homology (60%) with the cloned opioid receptors has also recently been cloned and sequenced in murine lymphocytes [85]. The receptor is upregulated following cell activation with mitogens. Likewise, the receptor reportedly has functional significance with mitogen-induced lymphocyte proliferation and polyclonal antibody production but not IL-6 production on the generation of cytotoxic T lymphocytes as determined by antisense experiments [84, 85]. A similar 'orphan' opioid receptor has been confirmed in activated human lymphocytes as well [86]. Whereas the endogenous ligand for this receptor has been isolated from brain tissue [87, 88], preliminary results using RT-PCR assays and specific oligonucleotide primers for the orphanin ligand suggest that it is either absent or below the limits of detection in lymphocytes treated with or without mitogen (fig. 1). These results suggest that opioids are 'fine-tuners' within the immune system considering both the association of opioids with infectious pathogens [89] or opioid command of neurotransmitter release [90] for dissemination of chemical syntax.

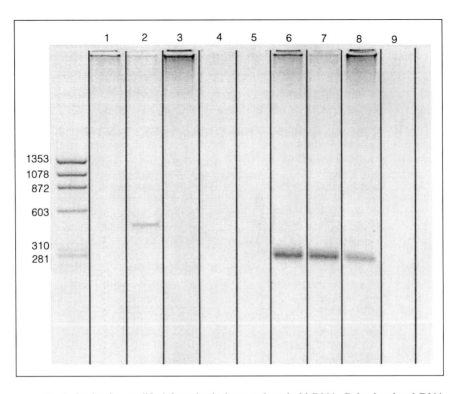

Fig. 1. Orphanin amplified from brain but not lymphoid RNA. Polyadenylated RNA was prepared from brain tissue or splenic lymphocytes (stimulated 48–72 h with or without concanavalin A). First strand cDNA synthesis was performed on equivalent amounts of RNA with a cDNA synthesis kit (Promega, Madison, Wisc., USA). PCR was performed on equivalent amounts of cDNA used as template per sample. Orphanin oligonucleotide primers were: sense, 5′CTTCTCCAGTGTGTTCAGCAGTT–3′ and antisense, 5′-GTCAT-GAGCCCTTCCACGATGC-3′ for a predicted amplified product of 239 bp. The far left lane represents the HaeIII digest of OX174 RF DNA molecular weight marker. Lanes 1 and 6, amplified product from unstimulated splenic lymphocytes; lanes 2 and 7, amplified product from brain; lanes 3 and 8, amplified product from stimulated splenic lymphocytes; lanes 4 and 9, primer control; lane 5, water blank. Lanes 1–4 represent RT-PCR product using orphanin-specific oligonucleotide primers and lanes 6–9 represent RT-PCR product using GAPDH-specific oligonucleotide primers.

Sigma Receptors

Although somewhat controversial, there is a growing body of literature suggesting the existence of sigma binding sites on cells of the immune system. Sigma compounds were originally described as novel opioids that elicit psycho-tomimetic actions and included such ligands as phencyclidine or PCP [91].

However, the current dogma places sigma receptors as enantioselective but nondopaminergic, nonopioid, nonphencyclidine, saturable sites located both in the central nervous system as well as peripherally [92]. Conventional radiore-ceptor assays have identified sigma-type receptors on both human and mouse leukocytes [93–96]. Photoaffinity labeling experiments suggest that the site has an apparent molecular weight of 57 kD electrophoresed under reducing or nonreducing conditions [97]. Activation of the receptor with sigma ligands has been shown to suppress proinflammatory cytokine synthesis [98], suppress natural killer activity [99], and alter B-cell proliferation [100]. Suppression of graft-vs.-host disease and delayed-type hypersensitivity granuloma formation in mice has also been noted [101]. However, definitive proof of the existence of a sigma receptor has not been forthcoming using molecular techniques. The idea that a sigma receptor may be related to novel opioid-binding sites on immune cells [96] is interesting but presently untested.

Arginine Vasopressin Receptor

Arginine vasopressin (AVP) receptors present on the surface of immune cells appear to be of the V_1 subtype similar to those classified on hepatic cells that mediate calcium mobilization [102]. Functionally, AVP ($10^{-9} - 10^{-10}$ M) has been shown to facilitate the production of γ-interferon (γ-IFN) by substi-tuting for interleukin-2 (IL-2) as a helper signal in murine splenocytes [103]. This response is blocked by the V_1 antagonist [d(CH$_2$)1/5 Tyr-(Me)]AVP but not by another V_1 antagonist, [d(CH$_2$)1/5D Tyr(Et^{2}Val^4)]AVP or V_2 antagonists [104]. This suggests the presence of a novel V_1 subtype on immunocytes.

Two independent studies have reported the presence of AVP receptors on peripheral blood mononuclear cells (PBMCs). These receptors were saturable, selective, and of high affinity ($K_d = 0.47 \pm 0.17$ nM [105]) or ($K_d = 0.5$ nM, $B_{max} = 7.6$ fmol/8 $\times$ 10^6 cells [106]). The authors of the latter study had previ-ously described the enhancing effect of a single-dose AVP on the autologous mixed lymphocyte assay [107] which was augmented further by the daily addition of AVP. This augmentation appeared to be influenced by the presence of arginine in position 8 of this nine amino acid polypeptide.

Prolactin Receptor

The receptor for prolactin (PRL) is a member of the hematopoietic recep-tor family that includes the receptors for interleukins 2–7. This receptor has been cloned and sequenced from both rat liver [108] and Nb2, a PRL-dependent T-lymphocyte cell line [109]. PCR analysis had been used to detect the presence of PRL receptor gene expression in B cells, T cells, and monocytes [110] and this finding was later confirmed by the demonstration of a heterogenous population of PRL-receptor-positive splenocytes by flow cytometry [111]. This study reported that 20% of primary splenic lymphocytes express PRL receptor and of this subset, 33% were kappa light chain positive and the remainder were CD4 or CD8 positive. Gagnerault et al. [112] later expanded these findings to the primary lymphoid tissues (thymus and bone marrow) and discovered that greater than 90% of lymphocytes in these tissues expressed PRL receptor, but that thymocytes expressed PRL receptor at a lower density than bone marrow lymphocytes [112]. In addition, this study revealed that in primary lymphoid organs, all four subsets of T lymphocytes frequently expressed PRL receptor ($>85\%$), in contrast to a lower frequency of expression in the periphery (~50–65%). Subsequently, closer investigation of hematopoietic tissues revealed that while thymocytes were frequently positive, receptor densities were low with the exception of a minority of double-negative (CD4–/CD8–) and single-positive CD4+ T cells which were strongly labeled with fluorescently labeled anti-PRL receptor antibody [113]. In peripheral blood, all B cells, all monocytes, and 75% of T lymphocytes, expressed PRL receptor [113].

Several studies have shown that density of lymphocytic PRL receptor expression can be modulated in response to various stimuli. In vivo and in vitro administration of the T-cell mitogen, concanavalin A, has been shown to increase the density of lymphocyte PRL receptor expression [112, 114]. Increases in PRL receptor expression may also play a role in development of autoimmune disease as suggested by the NZB murine model of autoimmunity where the percentage of T lymphocytes bearing PRL receptors as well as receptor density increases with age [112]. Similarly, it has been demonstrated that PRL receptor expression, as determined by radioreceptor assay, varies with the menstrual cycle in females and appears to be mediated at the transcriptional level by PRL receptor mRNA availability [115].

Some data has been obtained on the potential pathway by which PRL-receptors mediate their effects in lymphocytes. In NB2 cells, PRL induced the phosphorylation of the p72–74 serine/threonine kinase, c-Raf-1. This phosphorylated form was capable of autokinase and substrate kinase activities. In contrast, Raf-1 phosphorylation was constitutive in Sp, which is a PRL-independent T lymphocyte line derived from NB2. In NB2 cells, Raf-1 coprecipitated with the PRL receptor [116]. It has also been shown that activation of the PRL receptor leads to rapid tyrosyl phosphorylation of MAP kinase and the subsequent translocation of MAP kinase to the nucleus with kinetics identical to that for nuclear accumulation of PRL itself [117]. Studies have been done to elucidate the role of PRL as a second signal necessary but not sufficient for T lymphocyte proliferation, specifically, escape from cell cycle phase G1 [118, 119]. These studies have shown that administration of IL-2 and PRL to the T lymphocyte-derived cell line L2 resulted in the sequential expression of interferon regulatory factor-1, c-myc, proliferating cell nuclear antigen, thymidine kinase, cyclin B, and histone H3 followed by subsequent entry of the cell into the S phase. In summary, it would appear that PRL receptors can play a role in the activation of lymphocytes, although no studies to date have addressed the consequence of a lack of PRL receptors on 25% of the T-lymphocyte population. It is tempting to speculate that PRL receptor-negative T lymphocytes reflect an anergic status.

Somatostatin Receptor

Somatostatin (SOM) suppresses or inhibits many of the functional responses of lymphocytes. It has been shown to inhibit in vivo primary antibody response to sheep red blood cells in a dose-dependent fashion and that the inhibition was abrogated by co-adminstsration of neurokinin A but not substance P [120]. Similarly, in lymphocytes from atopic patients, SOM has been shown to decrease spontaneous IgE production by a mechanism that requires the presence of T cells and monocytes in addition to B cells [121]. SOM also inhibited IgE production by modulating switching induced by IL-4 plus anti-CD 40 mAb in a T-cell- and monocyte-dependent fashion [121]. In a dose-dependent fashion, SOM inhibits nataural killer activity in vitro without affecting the cytolytic potential of these cells as defined by anti-CD16-mediated target redirection [122].

The SOM analog angiopeptin has been shown to decrease the adhesiveness of rat leukocytes to unstimulated and IL-1β-activated rat heart endothelial cells [123]. Another analog of SOM, SMS 201–995, inhibits CD2/phytohemagglutinin-mediated proliferation, but not anti-CD3-mediated T-cell proliferation [124]. The importance of SOM as a paracrine/autocrine inhibitor of lymphocyte proliferation was demonstrated by experiments wherein endogenous SOM production was blocked by the addition of SOM-specific antisense oligonucleotide resulting in enhanced proliferation [125]. In one instance, SOM was shown to increase the IL-2 secretion, but not the proliferation, of a T-cell-derived antigen-specific cell line, A040.1 [126].

SOM receptors were evaluated in four human gut-associated lymphoid tissues (palatine tonsils, ileal Peyer patches, vermiform appendix, and colonic solitary lymphatic follicles) by receptor autoradiography. All four tissues were somatostatin receptor positive ($K_d = 1.3 \pm 0.6$ nM); the receptors were preferentially located in the germinal centers, with the luminal part of the center more strongly labeled than the basal part. The corona of the follicles and the primary follicles without germinal centers did not have SOM receptors [127].

Inflammatory lymphocytes obtained from murine hepatic granulomas induced by schistosomiasis express only SOM receptor subtype II mRNA but not subtypes I or III [128]. SOM (at nanomolar concentrations) has been shown to increase the release of cytotoxic factors such as H_2O_2, nitric oxide, and TNF by rat peritoneal macrophages, although micromolar concentrations were inhibitory [129].

Substance P Receptors

Substance P (SP), which is known to regulate blood pressure, peristalsis of the gut, and salivation, is thought to modulate certain B lymphocyte responses [130]. However, the presence of SP receptors on human lymphocytes may be in question. Prior studies have demonstrated high affinity ($K_d = 400–800$ pM) SP receptors on circulating and mucosal T and B cells of human and murine origin [1] and the presence of SP receptor-specific mRNA and protein in LPS-stimulated macrophages [131, 132]. However, one study has failed to find SP receptors on either human peripheral blood lymphocytes or jejunal intraepithelial lymphocytes by radioreceptor assay [133]. This finding was supported by experiments which show that SP-mediated mobilization of intracellular calcium cannot be blocked by an SP receptor antagonist and furthermore that an amphiphilic SP receptor antagonist could mimic SP in this system [134]. It has been proposed that SP can mediate its effects by means of three distinct mechanisms: (1) a neurokinin-1 receptor-dependent pathway; (2) a receptor-independent pathway, which leads to activation of heterotrimeric G proteins and calcium influx, and (3) a non-neurokinin-receptor-dependent pathway which is present in monocytes and B cells and leads to the activation of MAP kinase [135].

Vasoactive Intestinal Peptide Receptor

High-affinity vasoactive intestinal peptide (VIP) receptors have been characterized on monocytes, T-enriched lymphocytes, T-depleted lymphocytes, B-enriched lymphocytes, and large granular lymphocytes (LGLs) [1]. VIP administration has varied immunological outcomes which range from lymphocyte development (adhesion and trafficking) to lymphoproliferative effects to lymphocyte and macrophage function. VIP receptors have been localized to the margins of follicles present in the Peyer's patches [136] and in macrophages in the lung [137]. Two types of VIP receptors (VIPR1 and VIPR2) have been found to localize to different nonlymphoid tissues of the central nervous system. This differential expression is mirrored by T lymphocytes which express VIPR1 constitutively but can be induced (by activation or by VIP alone) to express VIPR2 [138]. While VIPR1 mRNA has been detected in murine T lymphocytes [139] and the human VIPR1 gene has been localized to the short arm of chromosome 3 (3p22) [140], it has been suggested that VIPR2 predominates over VIPR1 in the mediation of intracellular Ca^{2+} mobilization and cAMP responses in the T lymphocyte [141].

T cells of the lamina propria have been shown to express high-affinity VIP receptors ($K_d = 9.08$ nM) which respond to VIP by producing IL-5 [142]. In mesenteric lymph node lymphocytes, VIP receptors have been observed to maintain rapid turnover of surface receptor [143] and can be triggered to increase cellular cAMP levels [144].

It has been suggested that VIP may exert its immunomodulatory effects indirectly by regulating cytokine production. In Con A-stimulated splenic lymphocytes, VIP downregulated IL-2 mRNA and protein expression (but not interferon-γ) by increasing cellular cAMP [145]. Anti-CD3-elicited lymphocyte proliferation was indirectly reduced following the inhibition of IL-2 and IL-4 secretion [146]. While IL-2 inhibition was again reduced by a transcriptional mechanism, IL-4 inhibition was modulated at a posttranscriptional level [146].

VIP may influence immune function by modulating lymphocyte cell-surface adhesion molecules. The B-lymphoblast cell line Raji has been shown to increase surface expression of lymphocyte-function-associated (LFA-1) adhesin and intercellular adhesion molecule-1 (ICAM-1) in response to VIP administration [147]. These results were supported and extended by the observation that VIP can increase ICAM and VCAM integrins on both resting and activated T cells, although more effectively on quiescent T cells [148]. This study also suggested that VIP is strongly chemotactic for unstimulated lymphocytes but less so for activated ones [148]. This suggests that VIP preferentially affects resting lymphocytes in contrast to other chemokines such as RANTES which targets activated lymphocytes. A contradictory observation has been made which suggests that VIP significantly inhibits lymphocyte chemotaxis through a cAMP-mediated pathway in both resting and activated splenic and thymic lymphocytes [149].

In the microenvironment of the granuloma, VIP may play a role as a paracrine regulator of the immune response. Murine Schistosomiasis granuloma-derived T cells spontaneously secrete IL-5 that is increased by the addition of VIP, while splenic T cells did not secrete IL-5, nor was IL-5 secretion induced by the addition of VIP [150]. These experiments also showed that during activation of splenic T cells, VIP had no effect on IL-5 production; however, 24 h after removal of the proliferative stimulus, these same cells would secrete IL-5 in response to VIP [150]. VIP was also observed to suppress proliferation of granuloma-derived T cells in response to mitogen or specific antigen by decreasing IL-2 secretion [151]. Thus, in the granuloma, a feedback regulatory cycle can be demonstrated: (1) eosinophils secrete VIP; (2) VIP reduces T lymphocyte proliferation but increases IL-5 secretion, and (3) IL-5 enhances the growth and differentiation of eosinophils.

Insulin-Like Growth Factor Receptor

Insulin-like growth factor (IGF) receptor has been shown to mediate a proliferative effect on human peripheral blood T cells [152]. Both receptor types (IGFR-I and IGFR-II) have been found on CD4 + and CD8 + T cells, B cells, and monocytes [153], but IGFR-I appears to be responsible for increased proliferation [152]. Other studies have shown the presence of IGFR-I and II mRNA in unstimulated peripheral blood lymphocytes that begin production of IGF-I and II following stimulation with phytohemagglutinin [154]. Production of IGF-I by TNF-α-stimulated macrophages [155] would suggest the potential for paracrine regulation of the immune system.

High-affinity IGFR-I has been demonstrated by radioreceptor assay on the Jurkat T cell line ($K_d = 1.77$ nM, $B_{max} = 230$ receptors/cell) and that ligand binding induces the phosphorylation of a 95-kD tyrosine kinase [156]. Other studies indicate that IGF-I may induce another tyrosine kinase, p56 Ick, which is associated with T lymphocyte receptors [157]. One potential substrate for this tyrosine kinase may be insulin receptor substrate I (IRS-I) which is activated by phosphorylation of tyrosines within YMXM or YXXM motifs. Differential expression of IRS-I in immunocytes may initiate divergent signaling pathways in human thymocytes and peripheral blood T lymphocytes. In thymocytes, IGFR-I ligand binding induces the phosphorylation of a 160- to 180-kD protein (pp170) which becomes associated with phosphatidylinositol-3 kinase. This complex could be immunoprecipitated by anti-IRS-I. In circulating T cells, IRS-I appears to be less abundantly expressed, and, as a result, this pathway does not appear to be activated in these cells [158].

One study suggests that IGFR-II may be associated with naive peripheral T cells because CD45RA-expressing CD4 + and CD8 + T cells were 2.3- and 1.7-fold more likely to express IGFR-II than their CD45RO + counterparts [159].

Calcitonin Gene-Related Peptide Receptors

Two forms of calcitonin gene-related peptide (CGRP) have been discovered: CGRP I and CGRP II. Although the gene products are highly conserved, they arise from separate genes, probably resulting from gene duplication. Functional high-affinity CGRP receptors have been characterized on T and B lymphocytes and have been linked to adenylate cyclase activity [160]. Experiments performed on the murine pre-B cell line 70Z/3 have confirmed these findings and have also identified a prospective 103-kD receptor that can be superinduced by LPS administration [161]. In this cell line, CGRP activated adenylate cyclase resulting in a rise in intracellular cAMP [162]. This rise in cAMP significantly inhibited surface immunoglobulin expression by lowering the steady state levels of μ and κ immunoglobulin mRNA [162].

Acknowledgments

The authors would like to thank Drs. Hans-Peter Nothacker and Olivier Civelli of Hoffmann-La Roche AG for their collaboration concerning the orphanin studies. This work was supported by NIH grants from the National Eye Institute EY06789 (H.H.G.) and the National Institute of Neurological Disorders and Stroke NS35470 (D.J.J.C.).

References

1   Carr DJJ: Neuroendocrine peptide receptors on cells of the immune system; in Blalock JE (ed): Neuroendocrinimmunology. Chem Immunol. Basel, Karger, 1991, vol 52, pp 84–105.

2   Sanders VM: The role of adrenoceptor-mediated signals in the modulation of lymphocyte function. Adv Neuroimmunol 1995;5:283–298.

3   Morahan PS, Klykken PC, Smith SH, Harris LS, Munson AE: Effects of cannabinoids on host resistance to *Listeria monocytogenes* and herpes simplex virus. Infect Immun 1979;23:670–674.

4   Klein TW, Newton C, Widen R, Friedman H: Δ^9-Tetrahydrocannabinol injection induces cytokine-mediated mortality of mice infected with *Legionella pneumophila*. J Pharmacol Exp Ther 1993;267: 635–640.

5   Specter S, Lancz G, Westrich G, Friedman H: Delta-9-tetrahydrocannabinol augments murine retroviral induced immunosuppression and opportunistic infection. Int J Immunopharmacol 1991; 13:411–417.

6   Yebra M, Klein TW, Friedman H: Δ^9-Tetrahydrocannabinol suppresses concanavalin A induced increase in cytoplasmic free calcium in mouse thymocytes. Life Sci 1992;51:151–156.

7   Kaminski NE, Koh WS, Yang KH, Lee M, Kessler FK: Suppression of the humoral immune response by cannabinoids is partially mediated through inhibition of adenylate cyclase by a pertussis toxin-sensitive G-protein coupled mechanism. Biochem Pharmacol 1994;48:1899–1908.

8   Zhu W, Newton C, Kaaka Y, Friedman H, Klein TW: Δ^9-Tetrahydrocannabinol enhances the secretion of interleukin 1 from endotoxin-stimulated macrophagaes. J Pharmacol Exp Ther 1994; 270:1334–1339.

9   Devane WA, Dysarz FA III, Johnson MR, Melvin LS, Howlett A: Determination and characterization of a cannabinoid receptor in rat brain. Mol Pharmacol 1988;34:605–613.

10   Matsuda LA, Lolait SJ, Brownstein MJ, Young AC, Bonner TI: Structure of a cannabinoid receptor and functional expression of the cloned cDNA. Nature 1990;346:561–564.

11   Gerard CM, Molleraeau C, Vassart G, Parmentier M: Molecular cloning of a human cannabinoid receptor which is also expressed in testis. Biochem J 1991;279:129–134.

12   Munro S, Thomas KL, Abu-Shaar M: Molecular characterization of a peripheral receptor for cannabinoids. Nature 1993;365:61–65.

13   Kaminski NE, Abood ME, Kessler FK, Martin BR, Schatz AR: Identification of a functionally relevant cannabinoid receptor on mouse spleen cells that is involved in cannabinoid-mediated immune modulation. Mol Pharmacol 1992;42:736–742.

14   Lynn AB, Herkenham M: Localization of cannabinoid receptors and nonsaturable high-density cannabinoid binding sites in peripheral tissues of the rat: Implications for receptor-mediated immune modulation by cannabinoids. J Pharmacol Exp Ther 1994;268:1612–1623.

15   Galiegue S, Mary S, Marchand J, Dussosoy D, Carriere D, Crayon P, Bouaboula M, Shire D, Le Fur G, Cassellas P: Expression of central and peripheral cannabinoid receptors in human immune tissues and leukocyte subpopulations. Eur J Biochem 1995;232:54–61.

16   Daaka Y, Friedman H, Klein TW: Cannabinoid receptor proteins are increased in Jurkat, human T cell line after mitogen activation. J Pharmacol Exp Ther 1996;276:776–783.

17   Pettit DAD, Anders DL, Harrison MP, Cabral GA: Cannabinoid receptor expression in immune cells. Adv Exp Med Biol 1996;402:119–129.

18   Devane WA, Hanus L, Breuer A, Petwee RG, Stevenson LA, Griffin G, Gibson D, Mandelbaum A, Etinger A, Mechoulam R: Isolation and structure of a brain constituent that binds to the cannabinoid receptor. Science 1992;258:1946–1949.

19   Schwarz H, Blanco FJ, Lotz M: Anandamide, an endogenous cannabinoid receptor agonist inhibits lymphocyte proliferation and induces apoptosis. J Neuroimmunol 1994;55:107–115.

20   Lee M, Yang KD, Kaminski NE: Effects of putative cannabinoid receptor ligands, anandamide and 2-arachidonyl-glycerol, on immune function in B6C3F1 mouse splenocytes. J Pharmacol Exp Ther 1995;275:529–536.

21   Jessop DS, Lightman SL, Chowdrey HS: Effects of a chronic inflammatory stress on levels of pro-opiomelanocortin-derived peptides in the rat spleen and thymus. J Neuroimmunol 1994;49:197–203.

22   Chowdrey HS, Lightman SL, Harbuz MS, Larsen PJ, Jessop DS: Contents of corticotropin-releasing hormone and arginine vasopressin immunoreactivity in the spleen and thymus during a chronic inflammatory stress. J Neuroimmunol 1994;53:17–21.

23   Clarke BL, Gebhardt BM, Blalock JE: Mitogen-stimulated lymphocytes release biologically active corticotropin. Endocrinology 1993;132:983–988.

24   Aebischer I, Stampfli MR, Zurcher A, Miescher S, Urwyler A, Frey B, Luger T, White RR, Stadler BM: Neuropeptides are potent modulators of human in vitro immunoglobulin E synthesis. Eur J Immunol 1994;24:1908–1913.

25   Kavellars A, Ballieux R, Heijnen C: Modulation of the immune response by proopiomelanocortin derived peptides. II. Influence of adrenocorticotropin hormone on the rise of intracellular free calcium concentration after T cell activation. Brain Behavior Immun 1988;2:57–66.

26   McGlone J, Lumpkin E, Norman R: Adrenocorticotropin stimulates natural killer cell activity. Endocrinology 1991;129:1653–1658.

27   van Ierssel GJHM, Mieremet-Ooms MAC, van der Zon AM, van Hogezand RA, Wagtmans MJ, van der Sluys Veer A, Lamers CBHW, Verspaget HW: Effect of cortisol and ACTH on corticosteroid-suppressed peripheral blood natural killer cells from healthy volunteers and patients with Crohn's disease. Immunopharmacology 1996;34:97–104.

28   Mountjoy KG, Bird IM, Rainey WE, Cone RD: ACTH induces up-regulation of ACTH receptor mRNA in mouse and human adrenocortical cell lines. Mol Cell Endocrinol 1994;99:R17–R20.

29   Rainey WE, Viard I, Saez JM: Transforming growth factor β treatment decreases ACTH receptors on ovine adrenocortical cells. J Biol Chem 1989;264:21474–21477.

30   Clarke BL, Bost KL: Differential expression of functional adrenocorticotropic hormone receptors by subpopulations of lymphocytes. J Immunol 1989;143:464–469.

31   Clarke BL, Moore DR, Blalock JE: Adrenocorticotropic hormone stimulates a transient calcium uptake in rat lymphocytes. Endocrinology 1994;135:1780–1786.

32   Clarke BL: Calcium uptake by ACTH-stimulated lymphocytes: what is the physiological significance? Adv Neuroimmunol 1995;5:271–281.

33   Nagy E, Berczi I, Wren GE, Asa SL, Kowacs K: Immunomodulation by bromocriptine. Immunopharmacology 1983;6:231–235.

34   Le Fur G, Phan T, Uzan A: Identification of stereospecific [³H]spiroperidol binding sites in mammalian lymphocytes. Life Sci 1980;26:1139–1148.

35   Bondy G, Ackenheil M: ³H-Spiperone binding sistes in lymphocytes as possible vulnerability marker in schizophrenia. J Psychiatr Res 1987;21:521–529.

36   Grodzicki J, Pardo M, Schved G, Schlosberg A, Fuchs S, Kanety H: Differences in [³H]-spiperone binding to peripheral blood lymphocytes from neuroleptic responsive and nonresponsive schizophrenic patients. Biol Psychiatry 1990;27:1327–1330.

37   Le Fur G, Meininger V, Phan T, Gerard A, Baulac M, Uzan A: Decrease in lymphocyte [³H]spiroperidol binding sites in Parkinsonism. Life Sci 1980;27:1587–1591.

38   Arnold G, Bondy B, Bandmann O, Gasser TH, Schwarz J, Trenkwalder C, Wagner M, Poewe W, Oertel WH: ³H-spiperone binding to lymphocytes fails in the differential diagnosis of de novo Parkinson syndromes. J Neural Transm 1993;5:107–116.

39   Santambrogio L, Lipartiti M, Bruni A, Dal Toso R: Dopamine receptors on human T- and B-lymphocytes. J Neuroimmunol 1993;45:113–120.

40   Ricci A, Amenta F: Dopamine D_5 receptors on human peripheral blood lymphocytes: A radioligand binding study. J Neuroimmunol 1994;53:1–7.

41   Sibley DR, Monsma FJ Jr: Molecular biology of dopamine receptors. Trends Pharmacol Sci 1992; 13:61–69.

42   Gingrich JA, Caron MG: Recent advances in the molecular biology of dopamine receptors. Annu Rev Neurosci 1993;16:299–321.

43   Takahashi N, Nagai Y, Ueno S, Saeki Y, Yanagihara T: Human peripheral blood lymphocytes express D5 dopamine receptor gene and transcribe the two pseudo genes. FEBS Lett 1992;314: 23–25.

44   Nagai Y, Ueno S, Saeki Y, Soga F, Yanagihara T: Expression of the D3 dopamine receptor gene and a novel variant transcript generated by alternative splicing in human peripheral blood lymphocytes. Biochem Biophys Res Commun 1993;194:386–374.

45   Faraj BA, Olkowski L, Jackson RT: A cocaine-sensitive active dopamine transport in human lymphocytes. Biochem Pharmacol 1995;50:1007–1014.

46   Ou DW, Shen ML, Luo YD: Effects of cocaine on the immune system in Balb/C mice. Clin Immunol Immunopathol 1989;52:305–312.

47   Bagasra O, Forman L: Functional analysis of lymphocyte subpopulations in experimental cocaine abuse. I. Dose-dependent activation of lymphocyte subsets. Clin Exp Immunol 1989;77:289–293.

48   Peterson PK, Gekker G, Chao CC, Schut R, Molitor TW, Balfour HH Jr: Cocaine potentiates HIV-1 replication in human peripheral blood mononuclear cell cultures. J Immunol 1991;146:81–84.

49   Hellstrand K, Hermodsson S: Role of serotonin in the regulation of human natural killer cell cytotoxicity. J Immunol 1987;139:869–875.

50   Laplanche JL, Beaudry P, Launay JM, Dreux C, Goussault Y: Initial evidence for serotonin uptake by human peripheral blood lymphocytes. Biog Amines 1985;193:200.

51   Gabrilovac J, Cicin-Sain L, Osmak M, Jernej B: Alteration of NK- and ADCC-activities in rats genetically selected for low or high platelet serotonin level. J Neuroimmunol 1992;37:213–222.

52   Hellstrand K, Hermodsson S: Monocyte-mediated suppression of IL-2-induced NK-cell activation. Scand J Immunol 1990;32:183–192.

53   Aune TM, McGrath KM, Sarr T, Bombara MP, Kelley KA: Expression of 5HT1a receptors on activated human T cells: Regulation of cyclic AMP levels and T cell proliferation by 5-hydroxytryptamine. J Immunol 1993;151:1175–1183.

54   Sternberg EM, Trial J, Parker CW: Effect of serotonin on murine macrophages: Suppression of Ia expression by serotonin and its reversal by 5-HT₂ serotonergic receptor antagonists. J Immunol 1986;137:276–282.

55   Choquet D, Korn H: Dual effects of serotonin on a voltage-gated conductance in lymphocytes. Proc Natl Acad Sci USA 1988;85:4557–4561.

56   Nordlind K, Sundstrom E: Different modulating effects of the monoamines, adrenaline, noradrena-line and serotonin on the DNA synthesis response of human peripheral blood T lymphocytes activated by mercuric chloride and nickel sulfate. Int Arch Allergy Appl Immunol 1988;87:317–320.

57   Przewlocki R, Hassan AHS, Lason W, Epplen C, Herz A, Stein C: Gene expression and localization of opioid peptides in immune cells of inflamed tissue: Functional role in antinociception. Neuro-science 1992;48:491–500.

58   Cepeda MS, Lipkowski AW, Langlade A, Osgood PF, Ehrlich HP, Gargreaves K, Szyfelbein SK, Carr DB: Local increases of subcutaneous β-endorphin immunoactivity at the site of thermal injury. Immunopharmacology 1993;25:205–213.

59   Panerai AE, Radulovic J, Monastra G, Manfredi B, Locatelli L, Sacerdote P: β-Endorphin concentra-tions in brain areas and peritoneal macrophages in rats susceptible and resistant to experimental allergic encephalomyelitis: A possible relationship between tumor necrosis factor α and opioids in the disease. J Neuroimmunol 1994;51:169–176.

60   Jessop DS, Renshaw D, Lightman SL, Harbuz MS: Changes in ACTH and β-endorphin immunoreac-tivity in immune tissues during a chronic inflammatory stress are not correlated with changes in corticotropin-releasing hormone and arginine vasopressin. J Neuroimmunol 1995;60:29–35.

61   Shaker M, Shahabi NA, Sharp BM: Expression of naloxone-resistant β-endorphin binding sites on A20 cells: Effects of concanavalin A and dexamethasone. Immunopharmacology 1994;28:183–192.

62   Shahabi NA, Bost KL, Madhok TC, Sharp BM: Characterization of antisera to the naloxone-insensitive receptor for β-endorphin on U937 cells generated by using the complementary peptide strategy. J Pharmacol Exp Ther 1992;263:876–883.

63   Scheideler MA, Zukin RS: Reconstitution of solubilized delta-opiate receptor binding sites in lipid vesicles. J Biol Chem 1990;265:15176–15182.

64   Kieffer BL, Befort K, Gaveriaux-Ruff C, Hirth CG: The δ-opioid receptor: Isolation of a cDNA by expression cloning and pharmacological characterization. Proc Natl Acad Sci USA 1992;89: 12048–12052.

65   Evans CJ, Keith D, Magendzo K, Morrison H, Edwards RH: Cloning of a delta opioid receptor by functional expression. Science 1992;258:1952–1955.

66   Yasuda K, Raynor K, Kong H, Breder CD, Takeda J, Reisine T, Bell GI: Cloning and functional comparison of κ and δ opioid receptors from mouse brain. Proc Natl Acad Sci USA 1993;90: 6736–6740.

67   Thompson RC, Mansour A, Akil H, Watson SJ: Cloning and pharmacological characterization of a rat μ opioid receptor. Neuron 1993;11:903–913.

68   Wang JB, Imai Y, Eppler CM, Gregor P, Spivak CE, Uhl GR: μ opiate receptor: cDNA cloning and expression. Proc Natl Acad Sci USA 1993;90:10230–10234.

69   Kong H, Raynor K, Yasuda K, Moe ST, Portoghese PS, Bell GI, Reisine T: A single residue, aspartic acid 95, in the δ opioid receptor specifies selective high affinity agonist binding. J Biol Chem 1993;268:23055–23058.

70   Surratt CK, Johnson PS, Moriwaki A, Seidleck BK, Blaschak CJ, Wang JB, Uhl GR: Charged transmembrane domain amino acids are critical for agonist recognition and intrinsic activity. J Biol Chem 1994;269:20548–20553.

71   Kong H, Raynor K, Yano H, Takeda J, Bell GI, Reisine T: Agonists and antagonists bind to different domains of the cloned κ opioid receptor. Proc Natl Acad Sci USA 1994;91:8042–8046.

72   Gaveriaux-Ruff G, Simonin F, Peluso J, Defort K, Kieffer B: Expression of opioid receptors mRNAs in immune cells. Regul Pept 1994;54:103–104.

73   Chuang LF, Chuang TK, Killam KF Jr, Chuang AJ, Kung H, Yu L, Chuang RY: Delta opioid receptor gene expression in lymphocytes. Biochem Biophys Res Commun 1994;202:1291–1299.

74   Chuang LF, Chuang TK, Killam KF Jr, Qiu Q, Wang XR, Lin J, Kung H, Sheng W, Chao C, Yu L, Chuang RY: Expression of kappa opioid receptors in human and monkey lymphocytes. Biochem Biophys Res Commun 1995;209:1003–1010.

75   Sedqi M, Roy S, Ramakrishnan S, Elde R, Loh HH: Complementary DNA cloning of a μ-opioid receptor from rat peritoneal macrophages. Biochem Biophys Res Commun 1995;209:563–574.

76   Gaveriaux C, Peluso J, Simonin F, Laforet J, Kieffer B: Identification of κ- and δ-opioid receptor transcripts in immune cells. FEBS Lett 1995;369:272–276.

77   Chuang TK, Killam KF Jr, Chuang LF, Kung H, Sheng WS, Chao CC, Yu L, Chuang RY: Mu opioid receptor gene expression in immune cells. Biochem Biophys Res Commun 1995;216:922–930.

78   Belkowski SM, Zhu J, Liu-Chen L-Y, Eisenstein TK, Adler MW, Rogers TJ: Sequence of κ-opioid receptor cDNA in the R1.1 thymoma cell line. J Neuroimmunol 1995;62:113–117.

79   Lawrence DM, Bidlack JM: The kappa opioid receptor expressed on the mouse R1.1 thymoma cell line is coupled to adenylyl cyclase through a pertussis toxin-sensitive guanine nucleotide-binding regulatory protein. J Pharmacol Exp Ther 1993;266:1678–1683.

80   Joseph DB, Bidlack JM: The kappa opioid receptor expressed on the mouse R1.1 thymoma cell line down-regulates without desensitizing during chronic opioid exposure. J Pharmacol Exp Ther 1995;272:970–976.

81   Sedqi M, Roy S, Ramakrishnan S, Loh HH: Expression cloning of a full-length cDNA encoding delta opioid receptor from mouse thymocytes. J Neuroimmunol 1996;65:167–170.

82   Roy S, Ge B-L, Loh HH, Lee NM: Characterization of [³H]morphine binding to interleukin-1-activated thymocytes. J Pharmacol Exp Ther 1992;263:451–456.

83   Makman MH, Bilinger TV, Stefano GB: Human granulocytes contain an opiate alkaloid-selective receptor mediating inhibition of cytokine-induced activation and chemotaxis. J Immunol 1995;154:1323–1330.

84   Carr DJJ, Rogers TJ, Weber RJ: The relevance of opioids and opioid receptors on immunocompetence and immune homeostasis. Proc Soc Exp Biol Med 1996;213:248–257.

85   Halford WP, Gebhardt BM, Carr DJJ: Functional role and sequence analysis of a lymphocyte orphan opioid receptor. J Neuroimmunol 1995;59:91–101.

86   Wick MJ, Minnerath SR, Roy S, Ramakrishnan S, Loh HH: Expression of alternate forms of brain opioid 'orphan' receptor mRNA in activated human peripheral blood lymphocytes and llymphocytic cell lines. Mol Brain Res 1995;32:342–347.

87   Meunier J-C, Mollereau C, Toll L, Suaudeau C, Moisand C, Alvinerie P, Butour J-L, Guillemot J-C, Ferrara P, Monsarrat B, Mazargull H, Vassart G, Parmentier M, Costentin J: Isolation and structure of the endogenous agonist of opioid receptor-like ORL₁ receptor. Nature 1995;377:532–535.

88   Reinscheid RK, Nothacker H-P, Bourson A, Ardati A, Henningsen RA, Bunzow JR, Grandy DK, Langen H, Monsma FJ Jr, Civelli O: Orphanin FQ: A neuropeptide that activates an opiodlike G protein-coupled receptor. Science 1995;270:792–794.

89   Chao CC, Gekker G, Hu S, Sheng WS, Shark KB, Bu D-F, Archer S, Bidlack JM, Peterson PK: κ opioid receptors in human microglia downregulate human immunodeficiency virus 1 expression. Proc Natl Acad Sci USA 1996;93:8051–8056.

90   Ovadia H, Magenheim Y, Behar O, Rosen H: Molecular characterization of immune derived proenkephalin mRNA and the involvement of the adrenergic system in its expression in rat lymphoid cells. J Neuroimmunol 1996;68:77–83.

91   Martin WR, Eades CE, Thompson JA, Huppler RE: The effects of morphine- and nalorphine-like drugs in the nondependent and morphine-dependent chronic spinal dog. J Pharmacol 1976;197:517–532.

92   Walker JM, Bowen WD, Walker FO, Matsumoto RR, DeCosta B, Rice KC: Sigma receptor: Biology and function. Pharmacol Rev 1990;42:355–402.

93   Wolfe SA Jr, Kulsakdinum C, Battaglia G, Jaffe JJ, De Souza EB: Initial identification and characterization of sigma receptors on human peripheral blood leukocytes. J Pharmacol Exp Ther 1988;247:1114–1119.

94   Su T-P, London ED, Jaffe JH: Steroid binding at sigma receptors suggests a link between endocrine, nervous, and immune systems. Science 1988;240:219–221.

95   Carr DJJ, De Costa BR, Radesca L, Blalock JE: Functional assessment and partial characterization of [³H](+)-pentazocine binding sites on cells of the immune system. J Neuroimmunol 1991;35:153–166.

96   Whitlock BB, Liu Y, Chang S, Saini P, Ha BK, Barrett TW, Wolfe SA Jr: Initial characterization and autoradiographic localization of a novel sigma/opioid binding site in immune tissues. J Neuroimmunol 1996;67:83–96.

97   Garza HH Jr, Mayo S, Bowen WD, DeCosta BR, Carr DJJ: Characterization of a (+)-azidophenazocine-sensitive sigma receptor on splenic lymphocytes. J Immunol 1993;151:4672–4680.

98 Derocq J-M, Bourrie B, Segui M, LeFur G, Casellas P: In vivo inhibition of endotoxin-induced pro-inflammatory cytokine production by the sigma ligand SR 31747. J Pharmacol Exp Ther 1995; 272:224–230.

99 Carr DJJ, Mayo S, Woolley TW, DeCosta BR: Immunoregulatory properties of (+)-pentazocine and sigma ligands. Immunology 1992;77:527–531.

100 Liu Y, Wolfe SA Jr: Haloperidol and spiperone potentiate murine splenic B cell proliferation. Immunopharmacology 1996;34:147–159.

101 Cassellas P, Bourrie B, Canat X, Carayon P, Buisson I, Paul R, Breliere J-C, LeFur G: Immunopharmacological profile of SR 31747: In vitro and in vivo studies on humoral and cellular responses. J Neuroimmunol 1994;52:193–203.

102 Fishman JB, Dickey BF, Fine RE: Purification and characterization of the rat liver vasopressin (V1) receptor. J Biol Chem 1987;262:14049–14055.

103 Johnson HM, Torres BA: Regulation of lymphokine production by arginine vasopressin and oxytocin: Modulation of lymphocyte function by neurohypophyseal hormones. J Immunol 1985;135:773s–775s.

104 Johnson HM, Torres BA: Immunoregulatory properties of neuroendocrine peptide hormones; in Blalock JE, Bost KL (eds): Neuroimmunoendocrinology. Prog Allergy. Basel, Karger, 1988, vol 43, pp 37–67.

105 Elands J, Van Woundenberg A, Resink A, de Kloet ER: Vasopressin receptor capacity of human blood peripheral mononuclear cells is sex dependent. Brain Behav Immun 1990;4:30–38.

106 Bell J, Adler MW, Greenstein JI, Liu-Chen LY: Identification and characterization of ^{125}I arginine vasopressin binding sites on human peripheral blood mononuclear cells. Life Sci 1993;52:95–105.

107 Bell J, Adler MW, Greenstein JI: The effect of arginine vasopressin on the autologous mixed lymphocyte reaction. Int J Immunopharmacol 1992;14:93–103.

108 Boutin J, Jolicoeur C, Okamura H, Gagnon J, Edery M, Shirota M, Banuille D, Dusanter-Fourt I, Dijiane J, Kelly P: Cloning and expression of the rat prolactin receptor, a member of the growth hormone/PRL receptor gene family. Cell 1988;53:69–77.

109 Ali S, Edery M, Pellegrini I, Lesueur L, Paly J, Djiane J, Kelly PA: The Nb2 form of prolactin receptor is able to activate a milk protein gene promoter. Mol Endocrinol 1992;6:1242-1248.

110 Pellegrini I, Lebrun JJ, Ali S, Kelly PA: Expression of prolactin and its receptor in human lymphoid cells. Mol Endocrinol 1992;6:1023–1031.

111 Viselli SM, Mastro AM: Prolactin reeptors are found on heterogeneous subpopulations of rat splenocytes. Endocrinology 1993;132:571–576.

112 Gagnerault MC, Touraine P, Savino W, Kelly PA, Dardenne M: Expression of prolactin receptors in murine lymphoid cells in normal and autoimmune situations. J Immunol 1993;150:5673–5681.

113 Dardenne M, de Moraes MdC, Kelly PA, Gagnerault MC: Prolactin receptor expression in human hematopoietic tissues analyzed by flow cytofluorometry. Endocrinology 1994;134:2108–2114.

114 Gala RR, Shevach EM: Identification by analytical flow cytometry of prolactin receptors on immunocompetent cell populations in the mouse. Endocrinology 1993;133:1617–1623.

115 Athreya BA, Zulian F, Godillot AP, Weiner DB, Williams WV: Prolactin receptor levels on lymphocytes vary with menstrual cycle in women. Pathobiology 1994;62:34–42.

116 Clevenger CV, Torigoe T, Reed JC: Prolactin induces rapid phosphorylation and activation of prolactin receptor-associated RAF-1 kinase in a T-cell line. J Biol Chem 1994;269:5559–5565.

117 Buckley AR, Rao YP, Buckley DJ, Gout PW: Prolactin-induced phosphorylation and nuclear translocation of MAP kinase in Nb2 lymphoma cells. Biochem Biophys Res Commun 1994;204: 1158–1164.

118 Clevenger CV, Sillman AL, Hanley-Hyde J, Prystowsky MB: Requirement for prolactin during cell cycle regulated gene expression in cloned T-lymphocytes. Endocrinology 1992;130:3216–3222.

119 Prystowsky MB, Clevenger CV: Prolactin as a second messenger for interleukin 2. Immunomethods 1994;5:49–55.

120 Eglezos A, Andrews PV, Helme RD: In vivo inhibition of the rat primary antibody response to antigenic stimulation by somatostatin. Immunol Cell Biol 1993;71:125–129.

121 Kimata H, Yoshida A, Fujimoto M, Mikawa H: Effect of vasoactive intestinal peptide, somatostatin, and substance P on spontaneous IgE and IgG4 production in atopic patients. J Immunol 1993; 150:4630–4640.

122   Sirianni MC, Annibale B, Fais S, Delle Fave G: Inhibitory effect of somatostatin-14 and some analogues on human natural killer cell activity. Peptides 1994;15:1033–1036.

123   Leszczynski D, Dunsky K, Josephs MD, Zhao Y, Foegh ML: Angiopeptin, a somatostatin-14 analogue, decreases adhesiveness of rat leukocytes to unstimulated and IL-1 beta-activated rat heart endothelial cells. Life Sci 1995;57:L217–L223.

124   Radosevic-Stasic B, Trobonjaca Z, Lucin P, Cuk M, Polic B, Rukavina D: Immunosuppressive and antiproliferative effects of somatostatin analog SMS 201–995. Int J Neurosci 1995;81:283–297.

125   Aguila MC, Rodriguez AM, Aguila-Mansilla HN, Lee WT: Somatostatin antisense oligodeoxynucleotide-mediated stimulation of lymphocyte proliferation in culture. Endocrinology 1996;137:1585–1590.

126   Nio DA, Moylan RN, Roche JK: Modulation of T lymphocyte function by neuropeptides. Evidence for their role as local immunoregulatory elements. J Immunol 1993;150:5281–5288.

127   Reubi JC, Horisberger U, Waser B, Gebbers JO, Laissue J: Preferential location of somatostatin receptors in germinal centers of human gut lymphoid tissue. Gastroenterology 1992;103:1207–1214.

128   Elliott DE, Metwali A, Blum AM, Sandor M, Lynch R, Weinstock JV: T lymphocytes isolated from the hepatic granulomas of schistosome-infected mice express somatostatin receptor subtype II (SSTR2) messenger RNA. J Immunol 1994;153:1180–1186.

129   Chao TC, Cheng HP, Walter RJ: Somatostatin and macrophage function: Modulation of hydrogen peroxide, nitric oxide and tumor necrosis factor release. Regul Pept 1995;58:1–10.

130   Bost KL, Pascual DW: Substance P: A late-acting B lymphocyte differentiation cofactor. Am J Physiol 1992;262:C537–545.

131   Bost KL: Quantification of macrophage-derived substance P receptor mRNA using competitive polymerase chain reaction; in Sharp BM, Eisenstein TK, Madden JJ, Friedman H (eds): The Brain Immune Axis and Substance Abuse. Adv Exp Med Biol. New York, Plenum Press, 1995, vol 373, pp 219-223.

132   Kincy-Cain T, Bost KL: Increased susceptibility of mice to Salmonella infection following in vivo treatment with the substance P antagonist, spantide II. J Immunol 1996;157:255–264.

133   Roberts AI, Taunk J, Ebert EC: Human lymphocytes lack substance P receptors. Cell Immunol 1992;141:457–465.

134   Kavelaars A, Jeurissen F, von Frijtag Drabbe Kunzel J, Herman van Roijen J, Rijkers GT, Heijnen CJ: Substance P induces a rise in intracellular calcium concentration in human T lymphocytes in vitro: Evidence of a receptor-independent mechanism. J Neuroimmunol 1993;42:61–70.

135   Kavelaars A, Jeurissen F, Heijnen CJ: Substance P receptors and signal transduction in leukocytes. Immunomethods 1994;5:41–48.

136   Ichikawa S, Sreedharan SP, Goetzl EJ, Owen RL: Immunohistochemical localization of peptidergic nerve fibers and neuropeptide receptors in Peyer's patches of the cat ileum. Regul pept 1994;54: 385–395.

137   Ichikawa S, Sreedharan SP, Owen RL, Goetzl EJ: Immunochemical localization of type I VIP receptor and NK-1-type substance P receptor in rat lung. Lung Cell Mol Physiol 1995;12:L584–L588.

138   Delgado M, Martinez C, Johnson MC, Gomariz RP, Ganea D: Differential expression of vasoactive intestinal peptide receptors 1 and 2 (VIP-R1 and VIP-R2) mRNA in murine lymphocytes. J Neuroimmunol 1996;68:27–38.

139   Johnson MC, McCormack RJ, Delgado M, Martinez C, Ganea D: Murine T-lymphocytes express vasoactive intestinal peptide receptor 1 (VIP-R1) mRNA. J Neuroimmunol 1996;68:109–119.

140   Sreedharan SP, Huang JX, Cheung MC, Goetzl EJ: Structure, expression, and chromosomal localization of the type I human vasoactive intestinal peptide receptor gene. Proc Natl Acad Sci USA 1995; 92:2939–2943.

141   Xia M, Sreedharan SP, Goetzl EJ: Predominant expression of type II vasoactive intestinal peptide receptors by human T lymphoclastoma cells: Transduction of both Ca^{2+} and cyclic AMP signals. J Clin Immunol 1996;16:21–30.

142   Blum AM, Mathew R, Cook GA, Metwali A, Felman R, Weinstock JV: Murine mucosal T cells have VIP receptors functionally distinct from those on intestinal epithelial cells. J Neuroimmunol 1992;39:101–108.

143   Ottaway CA: Receptors for vasoactive intestinal peptide on murine lymphocytes turn over rapidly. J Neuroimmunol 1992;38:241–253.

144 Ottaway CA: Role of sulfhydryl groups in the binding of vasoactive intestinal peptide to its receptor on murine lymphocytes. J Neuroimmunol 1992;39:49–56.

145 Ganea D, Sun L: Vasoactive intestinal peptide downregulates the expression of IL-2 but not of IFN gamma from stimulated murine T lymphocytes. J Neuroimmunol 1993;47:147–158.

146 Sun L, Ganea D: Vasoactive intestinal peptide inhibits interleukin (IL)-2 and IL-4 production through different molecular mechanisms in T cells activated via the T cell receptor/CD3 complex. J Neuroimmunol 1993;48:59–69.

147 Robichon A, Sreedharan SP, Yang J, Shames RS, Gronroos EC, Cheng PP, Goetzl EJ: Induction of aggregation of Raji human B–lymphoblastic cells by vasoactive intestinal peptide. Immunology 1993;79:574–579.

148 Johnston JA, Taub DD, Lloyd AR, Conlon K, Oppenheim JJ, Kevlin DJ: Human T lymphocyte chemotaxis and adhesion induced by vasoactive intestinal peptide. J Immunol 1994;153:1762–1768.

149 Delgado M, De la Fuente M, Martinez C, Gomariz RP: Pituitary adenylate cyclase-activating polypeptides (PACAP27 and PACAP38) inhibit the mobility of murine thymocytes and splenic lymphocytes: comparison with VIP and implication of cAMP. J Neuroimmunol 1995;62:137–146.

150 Mathew RC, Cook GA, Blum AM, Metwali A, Felman R, Weinstock JV: Vasoactive intestinal peptide stimulates T lymphocytes to release IL-5 in murine schistosomiasis mansoni infection. J Immunol 1992;148:3572–3577.

151 Metwali A, Blum A, Mathew R, Sandor M, Lynch RG, Weinstock JV: Modulation of T lymphocyte proliferation in mice infected with Schistosoma mansoni: VIP suppresses mitogen- and antigen-induced T cell proliferation possibly by inhibiting IL-2 production. Cell Immunol 1993;149:11–23.

152 Johnson EW, Jones LA, Kozak RW: Expression and function of insulin-like growth factor receptors on anti-CD3-activated human T lymphocytes. J Immunol 1992;148:63–71.

153 Xu X, Mardell C, Xian CJ, Zola H, Read LC: Expression of functional insulin-like growth factor-1 receptor on lymphoid cell subsets of rats. Immunology 1995;85:394–399.

154 Nyman T, Pekonen F: The expression of insulin-like growth factors and their binding proteins in normal human lymphocytes. Acta Endocrinol 1993;128:168–172.

155 Noble PW, Lake FR, Henson PM, Riches DW: Hyaluronate activation of CD44 induces insulin-like growth factor-1 expression by a tumor necrosis factor-alpha-dependent mechanism in murine macrophages. J Clin Invest 1993;91:2368–2377.

156 Cross RJ, Elliott LH, Morford LA, Roszman TL, McGillis JP: Functional characterization of the insulin-like growth factor I receptor on Jurkat T cells. Cell Immunol 1995;160:205–210.

157 Aguayo J, Wohlik N, Perez MV, Pineda G: Effect of insulin-like growth factor I on HLA-DR antigen expression in cultured human thyrocytes: A component of the autoimmune process? Rev Med Chil 1994;122:248–252.

158 Kooijman R, Lauf JJ, Kappers AC, Rijkers GT: Insulin-like growth factor induces phosphorylation of immunoreactive insulin receptor substrate and its association with phosphatidylinositol-3 kinase in human thymocytes. J Exp Med 1995;182:593–597.

159 Kooijman RK, Scholtens LE, Rijkers GT, Zegers BJ: Differential expression of type I insulin-like growth factor receptors in different stages of human T cells. Eur J Immunol 1995;25:931–935.

160 McGillis JP, Humphreys S, Reid S: Characterization of functional calcitonin gene-related peptide receptors on rat lymphocytes. J Immunol 1991;147:3482–3489.

161 McGillis JP, Humphreys S, Rangnekar V, Ciallella J: Modulation of B lymphocyte differentiation by calcitonin gene-related peptide (CGRP). I. Characterization of high-affinity CGRP receptors on murine 70Z/3 cells. Cell Immunol 1993;150:391–404.

162 McGillis JP, Humphreys S, Rangnekar V, Ciallella J: Modulationn of B lymphocyte differentiation by calcitonin gene-related peptide (CGRP). II. Inhibition of LPS-induced kappa light chain expression by CGRP. Cell Immunol 1993;150:405–416.

Daniel J.J. Carr, PhD, LSU Medical Center, Department of Microbiology and Immunology, 1901 Perdido Street, New Orleans, LA 70112–1393 (USA)
Tel. (504) 568 4412, Fax (504) 568 2918

Blalock JE (ed): Neuroimmunoendocrinology, 3rd rev ed.
Chem Immunol. Basel, Karger, 1997, vol 69, pp 155–184

....

Neuroendocrine Peptide Hormone Regulation of Immunity

Barbara A. Torres, Howard M. Johnson

Department of Microbiology and Cell Science, University of Florida,
Gainesville, Fla., USA

Introduction

It is now well established that so-called 'non-neuroendocrine' peripheral
tissues such as the gut, pancreas, reproductive organs, lymph nodes, thymus,
and spleen can produce a variety of hormones or hormone-like activities.
An intriguing aspect of hormone production by cells and tissue of the
immune system and by closely associated nonimmune tissues such as the gut
is their possible regulation of immune function. It is of particular interest
that studies carried out over the last few years with lymphocytes stimulated
by specific antigens, microbial superantigens, and mitogens have shown that
cells of the immune system can produce several polypeptide hormones that
are known to be produced also by the pituitary [1]. Perhaps the most notable
observation was the demonstration that lymphocyte-derived corticotropin
(ACTH) is the same as pituitary-derived ACTH as ascertained by amino
acid sequencing [2].

Data presented in this review support the view that neuroendocrine polypeptide hormones can regulate several important immune functions. These
include antibody production, lymphocyte cytotoxicity, lymphokine production, hypersensitivity, and macrophage and neutrophil activation and chemotaxis. We will focus particularly on immunoregulation by: neuropeptides
derived from the polyprotein proopiomelanocortin (POMC), enkephalins, the
posterior pituitary hormones vasopressin and oxytocin, vasoactive intestinal
peptide, substance P, the gonadotropins, growth hormone, prolactin, somatostatin, and thyrotropin. The data provide compelling evidence for a regulatory
circuit between the immune and neuroendocrine systems whereby neuropep-

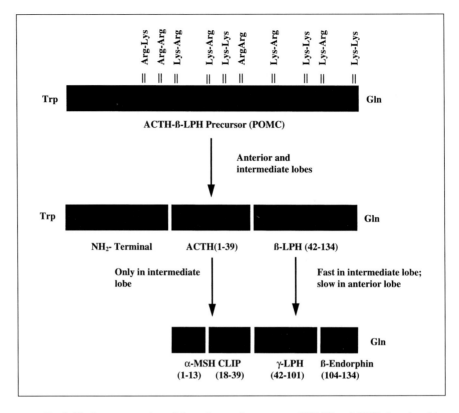

Fig. 1. Pituitary processing of the polyprotein precursor POMC to ACTH, β-endorphin, and other active peptides.

tides have a profound effect on positive and negative regulation of immune function at concentrations similar to those required for mediation of their classical functions.

POMC and Proenkephalin Products

Both ACTH and β-endorphin are classically produced in the pituitary gland from the polyprotein precursor POMC (fig. 1) [3]. ACTH is a single-chain polypeptide comprised of 39 amino acids that regulates the stress response in individuals through release of adrenal steroids. An investigation of the possible immunoregulatory role of neuropeptides that are derived from POMC was prompted by the observation that ACTH and endorphin-like activities were produced by lymphocytes that were infected with Newcastle disease virus [4, 5]. ACTH, either synthetic or natural, was a potent inhibitor of antibody production by lymphocytes [6]. This was illustrated in an in vitro plaque-forming cell (PFC) assay [7], where mouse spleen cells readily produced specific antibodies when stimulated with protein antigens such as sheep red blood cells (SRBC) or with carbohydrate complexes such as dinitrophenyl-Ficoll (DNP-Ficoll). ACTH preferentially suppressed antibody responses to protein antigens as compared to carbohydrate-type antigens. Although B cells are the source of antibodies, helper T cells are also required for an optimal response to protein antigens like SRBC, while antibody production to DNP-Ficoll is less T-cell dependent [8]. Thus, ACTH may suppress the antibody response in part by blocking helper T-cell signals. ACTH also acts at an early stage in the antibody response, where cell-cell interactions such as T cell-B cell collaborations are most likely to occur.

Consistent with ACTH effects on T and B cell function is the demonstration of ACTH receptors on both cell types [9]. The ACTH agonist $(^{125}I\text{-}Tyr^{23})Phe^2\text{-}Nle^4\text{-}ACTH$ was used to identify two types of binding sites on both normal rat T and B lymphocytes. The lymphocyte receptor displayed characteristics similar to the receptor on adrenal cells. One site has an approximate $K_d = 9 \times 10^{-11}$ M with 32,000 sites/cell, and the other had a $K_d = 4 \times 10^{-9}$ M with 38,000 sites/cell. The number of high affinity sites could be substantially increased by lipopolysaccharide (LPS) or concanavalin A (Con A) stimulation of B or T cells, respectively. Modulation of receptor number upon cell stimulation suggests that the ACTH receptors may be important in immunoregulation.

The structural basis of ACTH suppression of the antibody response can be ascertained by comparing the ACTH cleavage peptide α-melanocyte-stimulating hormone (α-MSH; $ACTH_{1-13}$ acetylated and amidated) and corticotropin-like intermediate peptide (CLIP; $ACTH_{18-39}$) with $ACTH_{1-39}$ for suppression of the anti-SRBC response (fig. 1). Neither α-MSH nor CLIP could suppress the antibody response [6]. $ACTH_{1-24}$, like $ACTH_{1-39}$, has full steroidogenic activity yet had no effect on antibody production, which suggests a dissociation of immunoregulatory and steroidogenic properties of $ACTH_{1-39}$.

In contrast to the inhibitory effects of ACTH on antibody production in the murine spleen cell system, others [10] have shown that ACTH enhances the growth and differentiation of enriched cultures of human tonsilar B cells. ACTH at nanomolar concentrations enhanced the proliferation of activated B cells by two- and threefold in the presence of interleukin-4 (IL-4) or recombinant interleukin-2 (IL-2). Furthermore, ACTH enhanced IL-2 and B-cell differentiation factor-induced IgM and IgG immunoglobulin secretion by activated B cells at concentrations similar to those for enhancement of proliferation. ACTH did not affect B-cell function in the absence of the interleukins. In a recent study, ACTH and other POMC-derived peptide hormones were shown to modulate the IL-4-driven class switch to IgE in human B cells in vitro [11]. Additionally, ACTH has been shown to inhibit the in vitro antibody response of primed human peripheral lymphocytes to tetanus toxoid at relatively low concentrations (10^{-13} and 10^{-17} M), while enhancing the response at higher concentrations [12]. ACTH as well as β-endorphin also inhibited the secretory immunoglobulin response to a polyclonal mitogen in the mouse system [13]. Thus, it appears that ACTH may either inhibit or enhance B-cell function, probably depending on factors such as lymphokines and on the presence of accessory T cells.

The production of the immunoregulatory lymphokine gamma-interferon (IFNγ) in a mouse spleen cell system is also suppressed by ACTH in a manner similar to suppression of the antibody response [14]. IFNγ production in humans or mice involves macrophages [15] and helper T cells, in addition to the IFNγ-producing cells [16, 17]. ACTH appears to inhibit IFNγ production by interfering with helper cell function, since the blockage can be reversed by factors that restore helper cell competence [14]. The structural requirements for ACTH suppression of IFNγ production are the same as for the suppression of antibody production, with α-MSH, CLIP, and $ACTH_{1-24}$ having no regulatory effect [14].

The endogenous opiates β-, γ-, and α-endorphin are also contained in POMC, and are composed of amino acids 61–69, 61–77, and 61–76, respectively, of β-lipotropin (β-LPH) (fig. 1). The production of ACTH by lymphocytes is associated with production of endorphin-like activities, which suggests a role for a POMC-like precursor in the formation of these lymphocyte-derived hormones [5]. Direct evidence for receptors on mouse spleen cell membranes for endogenous opiates was established in binding studies with ^{3}H[Met]-enkephalin [6]. At least one type of binding site for [Met]-enkephalin was present with a $K_d = 5.9 \times 10^{-10}$ M. Indirect evidence for [Met]-enkephalin receptors on human lymphocytes was shown by enhancement of rosette formation by naloxone [18]. Naloxone is an antagonist for α-endorphin and other opiates in that it competes for binding to specific receptors in the brain. A nonopiate receptor for β-endorphin on human lymphocytes has also been reported where naloxone does not block binding [19]. Thus, lymphocytes may contain both opiate and nonopiate receptors for endogenous opiates such as β-endorphin.

The endorphins β, γ, and α, were examined for possible regulation of the in vitro antibody response to SRBC in the murine system [6]. α-Endorphin was a potent inhibitor of the anti-SRBC PFC response at concentrations as low as 5×10^{-8} M (table 1). β- and γ-endorphin were minimally inhibitory, in spite of their structural similarity to α-endorphin. The α-endorphin amino

Table 1. Effect of endorphins and enkephalins on the in vitro anti-SRBC PFC response

Hormone	Concentration μM	PFC/culture ± SD	% suppression
α-Endorphin	0.5	637 ± 246	92
	0.05	2,720 ± 302	60
	0.005	6,333 ± 652	7
β-Endorphin	6	5,320 ± 567	22
γ-Endorphin	5	5,133 ± 580	25
[Leu]-Enkephalin	2	2,460 ± 692	64
	0.2	2,520 ± 240	63
	0.02	5,453 ± 670	20
[Met]-Enkephalin	2	1,880 ± 250	73
	0.2	4,040 ± 454	41
Control	–	6,840 ± 697	–

C57Bl/6 mice spleen cells (1.5×10^{-7} in 1 ml) were used for the PFC response. Hormones and SRBC were added to cultures on day 0 and PFC responses were determined on day 5.

acid sequence is contained within the amino acid sequence of both β- and γ-endorphin, which suggests that α-endorphin suppression of antibody production is controlled by a stringent signal at the level of ligand-receptor interaction. As shown in table 2, naloxone was able to block α-endorphin-induced suppression of the PFC response by binding to receptors on the spleen cells that are similar to those of opiate receptors found in the brain.

Although β-endorphin is a poor suppressor of the PFC response relative to α-endorphin, it competed with α-endorphin for an opiate-like receptor and thus blocked the suppression of the antibody response (table 2). The naloxone and β-endorphin competition data indicate the following: (a) endorphin receptors similar to those in the brain are present on spleen cells and probably lymphocytes in general; (b) α- and β-endorphin probably bind to the same receptors; (c) binding of the endorphin receptor does not necessarily activate immunosuppressive events as illustrated by the blocking of α-endorphin effects by the opiate antagonist naloxone and by β-endorphin. In fact, β-endorphin has been shown to enhance T-cell proliferation and IL-2 production [20].

In addition to the murine system, α-endorphin can also suppress the primary in vitro antibody response of human blood lymphocytes to the T-cell-dependent antigen ovalbumin [21]. α-Endorphin inhibited antibody pro-

Table 2. Blockage of α-endorphin suppression of the in vitro anti-SRBC PFC response by naloxone and β-endorphin

α-Endorphin μM	Naloxone μM	β-Endorphin μM	PFC/culture	% suppression	p
Experiment 1					
0.5	0	0	853 ± 234	85	<0.01
0.5	3	0	4,567 ± 1,055	18	NS
0	3	0	4,310 ± 1,259	22	
0	0	0	5,540 ± 658	–	
Experiment 2					
5	0	0	3,220 ± 707	76	<0.05
5	0	12	7,360 ± 905	46	NS
0	0	12	6,140 ± 877	55	
0	0	0	13,680 ± 1,018	–	

C57Bl/6 female mice spleen cells (1.5×10^{-7} in 1 ml) were used for the PFC response. Hormones and SRBC were added to cultures on day 0 and PFC responses were determined by day 5. p values are based on comparison with the naloxone (n = 3) and β-endorphin (n = 2) controls, respectively. NS = Not significant.

duction to ovalbumin by blocking both T- and B-cell function. The suppression probably occurred via binding to the opiate receptor on the lymphocytes, since α-endorphin lacking the N-terminal amino acid tyrosine was not inhibitory. An intact amino-terminus is required for α-endorphin binding to its receptors [22].

[Leu]- and [Met]-enkephalin are also endogenous opiates, but have their own polyprotein precursors [23]. Interestingly, [Met]-enkephalin is contained within the N-terminal sequence of all three endorphins (residues 61–65). Both [Leu]- and [Met]-enkephalin were intermediate in their antibody suppressive properties in the mouse spleen cell system, more suppressive than β-endorphin but less suppressive than α-endorphin (table 1) [6]. This suggests that there are stringent steric requirements for endorphin and enkephalin interaction with receptors on the cell membrane in a manner suitable for induction of immunosuppression, with the amino-terminal end of the endorphins playing an important role. Others have similarly found β-endorphin, [Leu]-enkephalin, and [Met]-enkephalin to suppress the in vitro antibody response [24–28].

Of interest is the observation that rats subjected to opiate-type stress have been reported to show suppressed splenic natural killer (NK) cell activity and lymphocyte proliferation in vitro [29, 30]. This suppression was blocked by the opiate antagonist naltrexone, suggesting that endogenous opiates mediate some forms of stress-induced suppression of the immune response. But this observation was not correlated with similar in vivo reductions in immune function. While elevated circulating corticosterone was observed, it was of insufficient duration to affect the immune response [30]. Other interesting aspects of the immunoregulatory function of POMC-derived peptides are the observations that the opiate peptides α-endorphin, β-endorphin, and/or [Met]-enkephalin can: (a) enhance the natural cytotoxicity of lymphocytes and macrophages toward tumor cells [31–36]; (b) enhance or inhibit T-cell mitogenesis; the enhancement may be due to induction of IL-2 [20, 37–41]; (c) enhance T-cell rosetting [41]; (d) stimulate human peripheral blood mononuclear cell chemotaxis [42, 43]; (e) inhibit T-cell chemotactic factor production [44]; (f) inhibit IFNγ production by cultured human peripheral blood mononuclear cells [45], and (g) inhibit major histocompatibility (MHC) class II antigen expression [46]. Inhibition of MHC class II antigen expression is a possible mechanism for the suppressive effects of these hormones.

Arginine Vasopressin

Arginine vasopressin (AVP) is a neurohypophyseal (posterior pituitary) nonapeptide that is classically produced in the magnocellular neurons of the supraoptic and paraventricular nuclei of the hypothalamus. It is transported to the posterior pituitary where it is released into the circulation [47]. Its effects include: (a) antidiuretic activity on specific receptors in the kidney [48]; (b) vasopressor activity which, in concert with other peptide hormones, regulates systemic arterial pressure [49]; (c) modulation of the stress response by direct stimulation of release of ACTH and by enhancement of ACTH release by corticotropin releasing factor [50]; (d) enhancement of learning and memory, functioning as a neurotransmitter [51]. Recently, a number of peripheral tissues and organs have been shown to also produce AVP or an AVP-related peptide(s). These include the testis, ovary, uterus, adrenal gland, superior cervical ganglion, spleen, and thymus [52–54]. The presence of AVP and related peptides in the thymus has led to speculation of its role in T-cell education and differentiation [55–58]. In addition, various areas of the central nervous system have also been shown to produce AVP [51]. These multiple sources of AVP are consistent with the multiple physiological functions that have recently been shown to be associated with this hormone.

AVP plays an important role in positive regulation of IFNγ production by providing a helper signal [59, 60]. The helper cell signal for IFNγ production is mediated by the helper T-cell lymphokine IL-2 [16]. The experimental

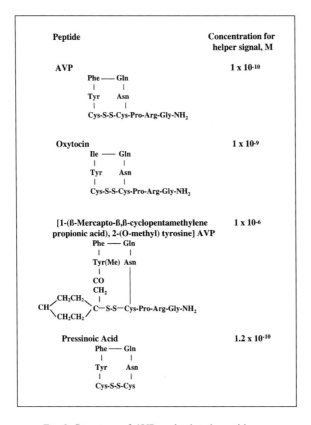

Peptide	Concentration for helper signal, M

AVP 1×10^{-10}

Oxytocin 1×10^{-9}

[1-(ß-Mercapto-ß,ß-cyclopentamethylene propionic acid), 2-(O-methyl) tyrosine] AVP 1×10^{-6}

Pressinoic Acid 1.2×10^{-10}

Fig. 2. Structure of AVP and related peptides.

approach demonstrating AVP replacement of the IL-2 helper signal for IFNγ production in mouse spleen cell cultures was to first remove helper cells or helper cell function by treatment of cultures with appropriate monoclonal antibodies and complement or with the metabolic inhibitor mitomycin C [59]. Competence for IFNγ production was restored by addition of AVP to cultures along with a T-cell mitogen such as staphylococcal enterotoxin A (SEA) [59] (fig. 2). Pressinoic acid, the six amino acid ring structure of AVP, appears to be the critical structure for the AVP helper signal, since it restored competence for IFNγ production at a concentration similar to that of AVP. Oxytocin, which has an isoleucine in place of phenylalanine in position 3 of the ring, had to be added at tenfold greater concentrations for similar help. Isoleucine pressinoic acid, the six amino acid ring of oxytocin, was less effective than oxytocin in providing the helper signal. Thus, the six amino acid ring structure of AVP is important for providing the helper signal to lymphocytes for induction of IFNγ with a possible minor role for the three C-terminal amino acids. The classical functions of AVP such as the antidiuretic and vasopressor activities require the three C-terminal amino acids in addition to an intact pressinoic acid ring [61]. This suggests that the AVP receptor on lymphocytes is novel.

In order to better characterize the AVP lymphocyte receptor, V_1 and V_2 receptor antagonists and agonists were examined for their effects on AVP function and binding to lymphocytes. The V_1 antagonist [1-(β-mercapto-β,β-cyclopentamethylene propionic acid), 2-(O-methyl)tyrosine]AVP was a potent competitor of ^{3}H-AVP binding on both liver and spleen cell membranes [62]. In contrast, pressinoic acid did compete with ^{3}H-AVP for binding to the V_1 receptor on spleen cell membranes, but not liver. This suggests that the lymphocyte AVP receptor was unique, yet related to that on liver cells. Functionally, of the several V_1 and V_2 agonists and antagonists examined, only the V_1 antagonist[1-(β-mercapto-β,β-cyclopentamethylene propionic acid), 2-(O-methyl)tyrosine]AVP blocked the AVP signal for IFNγ production [60]. Importantly, another V_1 antagonist[1-(β-mercapto-β,β-cyclopentamethylene propionic acid), 2-D-(O-ethyl)tyrosine, 4-valine]AVP had no effect on AVP function. IL-2 help was not affected by any AVP antagonists tested. The findings provide direct and functional evidence that lymphocytes possess specific receptors for AVP that are V_1-like but novel. Similarly, human B cells and macrophages have been shown to express V_1-like AVP receptors [63].

Thus, AVP provides a positive signal for induction of IFNγ [59] as compared to the negative signal of ACTH described previously [14]. Whereas ACTH inhibits IFNγ production by blocking a required helper function [14], AVP provides its positive signal by replacing a required helper T-cell function, the production of IL-2. It is not known whether ACTH blocks helper cell function by inhibiting production of IL-2. The current scheme for the cellular interactions that regulate IFNγ production in the murine system and the positive role of AVP in induction, along with the negative role of ACTH, is summarized in figure 3. The model suggests a possible interaction between AVP and ACTH regulation of lymphocyte function that was previously not appreciated.

Thyroid-Stimulating Hormone (Thyrotropin, TSH) and Related Hormones

Structurally, TSH is a 28-kD glycoprotein that is made up of two noncovalently linked subunits designated α and β. The α-subunit resembles that of several other neuropeptides, namely follicle-stimulating hormone

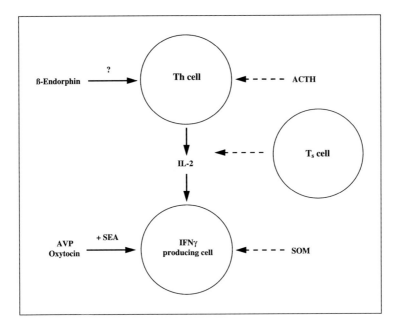

Fig. 3. IFNγ production is regulated by the dynamic interaction between helper (T$_h$), suppressor (T$_s$), and IFNγ-producing cells. Helper cells provide IL-2. ACTH blocks helper cell function. Suppressor cells absorb IL-2. AVP can replace IL-2 helper signal. β-Endorphin may enhance IL-2 production, and SOM may decrease IFNγ production. ⟶ = Positive signal; -----→ = negative signal.

(FSH), human chorionic gonadotropin (hCG), and luteinizing hormone (LH) [64]. The β-subunit is unique for each of these hormones and is responsible for the specificity of their actions. A conformational determinant requiring regions on both subunits constitutes the receptor-binding portion of TSH [65].

Initial observations of hypothyroidism in thymectomized or athymic mice suggested a relationship between the thyroid and the immune system [66]. In fact, human lymphocytes stimulated with the T-cell mitogen SEA were shown to produce immunoreactive TSH [67] and TSH beta subunit mRNA has been detected in such cells as well [68]. Lymphocyte-derived and pituitary TSH were antigenically related and had the same molecular mass and structure. Production of immunoreactive TSH by the T lymphoblast line MOLT-4 could be induced in a dose-dependent fashion by thyrotropin-release hormone (TRH) and its induction inhibited by triiodothyronine (T$_3$) [69].

In addition to TSH being produced by cells of the immune system, some lymphoid cells express TSH receptors. Monocytes, NK cells, and mitogen-stimulated B cells, but not phytohemagglutinin (PHA)-stimulated T cells or resting T and B lymphocytes, have been found to bind TSH [70]. TSH receptor transcripts have been found in normal-nonactivated human lymphocytes and these transcripts are identical to those found in thyroid tissue [71]. It was suggested that aberrant expression of the TSH receptor on lymphoid cells may act as the trigger for anti-TSH receptor autoantibody production observed in the circulation of patients with Graves' disease. Binding of TSH to mitogen-stimulated B cells was associated with an increase in immunoglobulin production. This is consistent with functional studies where both human and bovine TSH enhanced the in vitro antibody response to the T-dependent antigen SRBC in the mouse spleen cell system at concentrations in the range of 0.1 nM [72]. TSH had to be present during the first 24–48 h of 96-hour cultures for enhancement of the antibody response, suggesting that TSH affected an early event in the antibody response. TSH also enhanced the antibody response to the *Brucella abortus*-trinitrophenyl (BA-TNP) antigen, which is a less T-dependent antigen than SRBC, yet TSH enhancement of antibody production still required the presence of T cells [73]. Thus, in the immune system, TSH functions to augment both T-dependent and T-independent antibody production. TSH secretion by, and activity on, immune cells may have profound positive regulatory influences on resultant antibody responses.

In addition to its effects on B cells, TSH modulates T-cell activity. TSH has been shown to increase proliferation of mouse spleen cells in response to T-cell mitogens and IL-2 [74]. Further, IL-2-driven NK cytotoxic activity was augmented, suggesting a regulatory role for TSH in immune function. The ability of TSH to enhance T-cell responses may, in part, explain its effects on T-dependent B-cell responses.

The structural similarity of TSH with FSH, hCG, and LH would suggest that these hormones should also be investigated both as possible products and as potential regulators of lymphocyte function. Immunoreactive hCG is produced by lymphocytes in the mixed lymphocyte reaction, and it has been proposed that since the blastocyst is implanted in a lymphocyte infiltrate, lymphocyte-derived hCG may play an important role in enhancing implantation of the allogeneic fetus [75]. hCG has been shown to inhibit cytotoxic T-cell and NK-cell killing, T-cell mitogenesis and mixed lymphocyte reactions, potentially via the induction of suppressor cell activity [76, 77]. This would indicate that diversity at the major histocompatibility complex and the subsequent production of hCG would suppress the maternal immune response thereby facilitating fetal survival.

Substance P

Substance P is an eleven amino acid peptide that is a member of the tachykinin family of sensory neuropeptides, which cause tachycardia by lowering peripheral blood pressure. As a group the tachykinins are characterized by C-terminal amino acid sequence Phe-X-Gly-Leu-Met-NH$_2$, where X is an aromatic or aliphatic amino acid [78]. Substance P is found in the central nervous system and peripheral sensory nerves that innervate organs and tissues such as the gastrointestinal tract, respiratory tract, visual system, skin, and, relevant to the human system, in lymph nodes and spleen [79]. The wide tissue distribution of substance P is consistent with the central role that it is thought to play in pain [79]. Other effects of substance P on nonneural tissues include contraction of intestinal smooth muscle, arteriolar vasodilatation, increased secretion by salivary glands and nasal epithelium, and alteration of microvascular permeability [79]. The latter effect may facilitate cell traffic to local sites of inflammation.

Three tachykinin receptors have been cloned and classified on the basis of relative potencies of various mammalian tachykinins. Human peripheral T cells and the human lymphoblastoid cell line IM-9 express a substance P receptor similar to the NK-1 prototype receptor [80]. Substance P binds to the lymphocyte receptor with $K_d = 4 - 8.7 \times 10^{-10}$ M, with 7,000 and 25,000 receptors/cell, for T and B cells, respectively [80–82]. Cross-linking of labeled substance P to IM-9 cells and membranes under conditions which minimized proteolysis detected a 58-kD protein [83]. Interaction of substance P with its receptor-stimulated phosphatidylinositol (PI) turnover in IM-9 cells, and the nonhydrolyzable GTP analog GppNHP inhibited substance P binding [82]. The substance P receptor appears to be coupled to a guanine nucleotide-binding (G) protein and belongs to a family of G protein-linked receptors with seven hydrophobic transmembrane domains. Through the use of analogs and truncated peptides, it has been suggested that the C-terminal portion of substance P is required for binding to its receptor and that the N-terminal basic amino acids are required for cell activation [84]. In addition to binding the NK 1-like receptor, substance P has also been found to bind a novel receptor on B cells and monocytes which transduces an intracellular signal via MAP kinases [85].

Substance P has been shown to modulate the activity of cells involved in inflammation. Substance P is a chemoattractant for immune cells and can influence their metabolism and stimulate cell proliferation. On rat tissue mast cells, substance P bound to specific receptors to induce histamine and leukotriene release at micromolar concentrations [86]. The hypersensitivity effects of substance P such as vasodilatation and alteration of microvascular permeability appear to be mediated by substance P-induced factors such as histamine and the leukotrienes. In contrast to the activation of tissue mast cells to release mediators, substance P has no effect on basophils [86]. Thus, the hypersensitivity effects of substance P are cell specific.

Substance P has also been reported to stimulate chemotaxis and lysosomal enzyme secretion by rabbit neutrophils [87]. This function of substance P may be dependent on the C-terminal substituent peptide and operate via the receptor for the synthetic chemotactic peptide N-formylmethionylleucyl-phenylalanine (fMLP). The fact that approximately 1,000 times more substance P than fMLP was requred for competitive binding against fML[^{3}H]P and for chemotaxis may suggest that substance P enhanced neutrophil chemotaxis via cross-reactivity with the fMLP receptor rather than through interaction with a primary substance P receptor. Substance P has been shown to stimulate neutrophil phagocytosis [87–89], as well as increase adhesion of neutrophils to bronchial epithelial cells [90]. The substance P N-terminal peptide is structurally similar to the phagocytosis stimulatory tetrapeptide tufsin [88], and was as effective as intact substance P in activation for phagocytosis. In this case, receptor competition studies suggested that substance P and its N-terminal peptide stimulated phagocytosis by binding to the tufsin receptor.

Substance P has a stimulatory effect on lymphocytes with respect to both T-cell proliferation and immunoglobulin production by B cells [91, 92]. Approximately 10% of CD8+ T cells and 18% of CD4+ T cells express specific substance P receptors [93]. The receptor on the helper/inducer subpopulation may be related to their ability to stimulate immunoglobulin synthesis. In the human and mouse systems, substance P-stimulated and/or enhanced T-cell mitogen-induced proliferation by 60–70% as reflected by incorporation of [^{3}H]thymidine ([^{3}H]TdR) [91]. Unlike neutrophil chemotaxis which does not necessarily involve the NK-1 receptor, the lymphocyte proliferative effects of substance P reside in the C-terminal end of the molecule as the octapeptide substance P$_{4-11}$ was as effective as intact substance P in inducing proliferation. Thus, various functions can apparently involve different parts of the substance P molecule. In addition to T-cell proliferative effects, substance P has also been reported to stimulate immunoglobulin production of the IgA and IgM but not IgG class in an in vitro mouse system [92]. Thus, substance P has a positive regulatory effect on both T-cell and B-cell function.

Monocytes respond chemotactically to substance P and its activity could not be blocked by fMLP antagonists [94]. In the activation of guinea pig macrophages, substance P could stimulate production of the arachidonic acid metabolites, leukotriene C$_4$, and prostaglandin E, as well as O$_2^-$, hydrogen peroxide and the cytokines, IL-1, TNFα, and IL-6 [89, 95]. Tumor necrosis factor-α (TNFα) was induced in human mononuclear cells cultured in the presence of substance P [96]. Further, the truncated peptide, substance P(4–11), also induced significant levels of TNFα. Cytokine production may further affect lymphocyte function. For example, IL-6 production could lead to enhanced immunoglobulin synthesis by B cells. Substance P also augmented macrophage phagocytosis with the release of lysosomal enzymes [89]. Since substance P is widely distributed in nervous tissue, it has been suggested that it may play a role in neurologic disorders such as allergic neuritis, multiple sclerosis, and polyneuritis, which are characterized by extensive macrophage infiltration at focal sites of ongoing tissue damage [89]. Further, substance P may exacerbate rheumatoid arthritis by stimulation of macrophage-like synoviocytes in the joints [97]. Homology has been observed between the amyloid β protein deposited in the brains of patients with Alzheimer's disease and the tachykinins [98]. Substance P could reverse both early neurotrophic and late neurotoxic effects of an amyloid β protein peptide. Therefore, substance P may have neuronal effects opposite to amyloid β protein, but recent reports indicate that amyloid β protein-related peptides do not interact at the substance P receptor itself [99].

Vasoactive Intestinal Peptide

Vasoactive intestinal peptide (VIP) is a 28-amino acid neurotransmitter with partial sequence homology to glucagon, secretin, and growth hormone-releasing hormone [78]. It was initially isolated from porcine intestinal tissue and was found to act as a vasodilator of enteric blood vessels. VIP is found in the autonomic and central nervous system, and in both cholinergic and peptidergic neurons innervating several tissues such as the intestine [100], pituitary [101], heart [102], kidney [103], skin [104], thymus [105], and spleen [106]. A wide range of physiological actions have been ascribed to VIP: (a) stimulation of water secretion by the intestine and pancreatic acinar cells [107]; (b) stimulation of prolactin secretion by the pituitary [108]; (c) stimulation of glycogenolysis by liver [109] and brain [110]; (d) inhibition of somatostatin release by the hypothalamus [111]; (e) relaxation of smooth muscles in the trachea [112], intestines [107] and urogenital tract [113], and (f) dilation of small blood vessels [78].

Human polymorphonuclear leukocytes, eosinophils, and rat mast cells have been demonstrated to contain immunoreactive VIP [114, 115]. Rat thymocytes residing in thymus, spleen, and lymph nodes have been shown to contain VIP [116]. In the past it has not been clear whether such cells actually synthesize VIP or simply store VIP obtained from peptidergic neurons innervating immunologic tissue. Recently, it has been demonstrated that rat T cells (from thymus, spleen and lymph node) and B cells (from spleen and lymph node) express VIP transcripts [117]. On the other hand, rat basophil leukemia cells produce, store, and release upon appropriate stimulation distinct forms of VIP not found in other tissues [118]. These cells do not appear to have pathways necessary to produce intact VIP_{1-28}. Instead, the predominant form produced here is VIP_{10-28} with the C-terminal asparagine as a free acid. Longer forms of N-terminally extended VIP have also been detected; however, their amino acid sequences remain to be determined. It will be interesting to determine the effects of these factors on the immune system.

VIP has been reported to have an inhibitory effect on a number of immune responses. It inhibits mitogen-stimulated proliferation of mouse lymphocytes isolated from spleen, Peyer's patches, and mesenteric lymph nodes [119]. T lymphocytes seem to be the primary target of VIP-mediated inhibition since proliferative responses to T-cell mitogens such as Con A and PHA were affected, but proliferation induced by the B-cell mitogen LPS was not inhibited. The findings are consistent with the observation that T cells, but not B cells, have high-affinity receptors for VIP [120].

In addition to affecting proliferation in response to mitogenic stimulation, VIP has also been demonstrated to modulate cytokine production. For example, VIP has been shown to inhibit the production of IL-2 [121–123] and IFNγ [121] from mitogen-stimulated lymphocytes. VIP has also been found to down-regulate the expression of IL-4 [124] and IL-10 [124, 125] in stimulated mouse T cells.

Immunoglobulin production was also shown to be affected by VIP [92]. IgA production by Con A-stimulated lymphocytes from spleen and mesenteric lymph nodes was slightly increased by VIP (30 and 20%, respectively) whereas IgA production by Peyer's patches-derived lymphocytes was significantly increased (70%). Interestingly, IgM production in Peyer's patches was increased (80%) by VIP but was unaffected in spleen and lymph nodes. However, IgA production by mitogen-stimulated human peripheral blood mononuclear cells was unaffected by VIP [126]. IgA is the predominant immunoglobulin produced in Peyer's patches, and IgA-producing lymphocytes are more abundant in these tissues than in lymph nodes or spleen [127, 128]. The site-specific VIP effects on immunoglobulin production can perhaps be explained by differences in T-cell subpopulations in these organs.

VIP and related peptides have been reported to affect human NK cell activity [129, 130], inhibiting tumoricidal activity at VIP concentrations ranging from 10^{-7} to 10^{-10} M. Although these concentrations are higher than those normally found in peripheral blood (10^{-11} M), concentrations in the vicinity of VIP-secreting neurons have been estimated to be 10^{-9} to 10^{-10} M [131]. VIP effects on macrophage-mediated tumoricidal activity were also investigated, and although VIP alone did not affect tumor cell killing, it potentiated the suppressive effects of noradrenaline [132]. Others have demonstrated that VIP and its related peptides derived from preproVIP, peptide histidine methionine (PHM-27) and peptide histidine valine (PHV-42), inhibited NK activity. The order of potency being VIP > PHV-42 > PHM-27. Interestingly, the VIP antagonist [p-chloro-Phe[6],Leu[17]]-VIP at 10^{-8} M inhibited the effects of VIP but not PHM-27 or PHV-42, thus suggesting the existence of different receptors for prepro-VIP-derived peptides [133].

Evidence also suggests that VIP can modulate lymphocyte traffic. Egress of lymphocytes from popliteal lymph nodes is inhibited by VIP treatment [134]. In another report, mouse T lymphocytes were pretreated with VIP for 18 h, reinjected into syngeneic subjects and their subsequent in vivo localization was monitored [135]. Lymphocytes pretreated with VIP showed a reduced ability to migrate back to mesenteric lymph nodes and Peyer's patches. Lymphocyte distribution in spleen and blood was unaffected. Lymphocytes pretreated with VIP and washed of excess VIP showed decreased specific binding of ^{125}I-VIP with Scatchard analysis indicating a marked reduction in the number of binding sites/cell. The altered expression of VIP receptors was not associated with a concomitant alteration in expression of Thy-1, Lyt-1, or Lyt-2 phenotypic markers. Binding of VIP to its lymphocyte receptor appeared to result in a decreased expression of the VIP receptor. Downregulation of the VIP receptor may, in turn, affect the interaction of lymphocytes with lymphoid tissue, causing decreased infiltration into mesenteric lymph nodes and Peyer's patches.

Receptors for VIP have been shown to exist on a number of immune effector cells, including human peripheral blood lymphocytes [136], mouse T lymphocytes [119], human mononuclear cells [120], rat B and T lymphocytes [137], and the human lymphoblastic cell lines Molt-4B [138], SUP-T1 [139], and SKW6.4 [140]. Human lymphocytes possess both high- and low-affinity VIP receptors, with the high-affinity receptor having a $K_d = 4.7 \times 10^{-10}$ M and the low affinity receptor having a $K_d = 8 \times 10^{-10}$ M. These lymphocyte receptors are similar in specificity and K_d to the high- and low-affinity VIP receptors found in brain, endocrine, and intestinal tissue [141].

There appears to exist a differential expression of receptors on the various lymphocyte phenotypes [142]. For example, human T-cell-enriched PBL preparations demonstrated enhanced binding of ^{125}I-VIP as compared to unseparated or T-cell-depleted preparations. Enriched populations of CD4 and CD8 cells showed even higher binding capacity; however CD4 was greater than CD8 in this regard. Also, ^{125}I-VIP specifically bound to large granular and B lymphocytes, with the latter having the lowest binding capacity.

Cross-linking studies have been performed to characterize the VIP receptor. Through the use of various cross-linkers, a 47-kD protein has been isolated from Molt-4B lymphoblasts and GH$_3$ pituitary cells. Rat frontal cortex and pancreatic acinar cells have also been demonstrated to have a 47- to 48-kD cross-linked protein. Liver and intestinal epithelium, on the other hand, demonstrated two cross-linked species: a high-molecular-weight (73–86 kD), high-affinity protein and a low-molecular-weight (30–36 kD), low-affinity protein.

Further studies were performed on Molt-4B lymphoblasts and GH$_3$ pituitary cells to determine the functionality of the VIP receptor. VIP caused a cascade of intracellular events in these cells: activation of adenylate cyclase, accumulation of cAMP, activation of cAMP protein kinase, and phosphorylation of specific cellular proteins [107, 143].

It has been proposed that G proteins modulate VIP receptor interaction with adenylate cyclase [141]. G proteins act as transmembrane signals and interact with the catalytic subunit of adenylate cyclase to either inhibit (via G$_i$) or stimulate (via G$_s$) enzymatic activity [144]. Interaction of VIP with its high-affinity receptor results in G protein, G$_s$, stimulation of adenylate cyclase. Somatostatin, a known inhibitor of cAMP formation in adenohypophyseal cells, antagonizes VIP effects, perhaps by facilitating the interaction of G protein, G$_i$, with either G$_s$ or adenylate cyclase [141].

An interesting model emerges from the reported data on VIP and its immunomodulatory effects. VIP synthesized and secreted by either immune effector cells or neurons innervating lymphoid tissue can act on VIP receptor-bearing cells (such as T lymphocytes), resulting in inhibition of proliferative responses, IgA production, and migration of lymphocytes to lymphoid tissues such as mesenteric lymph nodes and Peyer's patches. These inhibitory effects may be the result of activation of adenylate cyclase. The stimulation of adenylate cyclase may be the result of activation of adenylate cyclase. The stimulation of adenylate cyclase may be mediated by G proteins, in particular G$_s$, which binds to the catalytic subunit of adenylate cyclase as a result of the interaction of VIP with its membrane receptor. The subsequent accumulation of cAMP causes the activation of a cAMP-dependent protein kinase which phosphorylates specific cellular proteins. The function of proteins phosphorylated as a result of VIP-receptor interaction has not yet been determined, although they may possibly be involved in VIP immunomodulatory effects.

Growth Hormone

Growth hormone (GH), also known as somatotropin, is a 191-amino acid hormone of the adenohypophysis [145] which has structural similarities to prolactin (PRL). Probably its best characterized activity is the promotion of growth of bone, cartilage, and soft tissues. Although GH secretion is maximal at puberty and declines after about 30 [146], detectable levels are found throughout the remainder of adulthood. This suggests that this hormone has other functions in addition to promotion of growth. In this respect, GH may be important for the maintenance of lean body mass. GH effects are mediated in part by insulin-like growth factor 1 (IGF-1) or somatomedin, which is induced by GH stimulation of hepatocytes.

Investigators have determined that the age-related changes in body composition of elderly men (61- to 81-year-old men) with low plasma IGF-1 concentration could be altered by the administration of recombinant biosynthetic human GH [147]. Treatment consisted of administering about 0.03 mg of GH/kg body weight subcutaneously 3 times a week. Plasma IGF-1 was used as an indirect measurement of GH secretion. The results of this study were that IGF-1 levels increased to a range similar to that of younger men. Physiologically, a significant increase in lean body mass (8.8%), average density of lumbar vertebra (1.6%), and sum of skin thickness (7.1%) was observed. In contrast, the adipose tissue mass decreased by 14.4%. It was concluded that diminished secretion of GH as indirectly measured by plasma IGF-1 levels is responsible, at least in part, for the changes associated with old age (lean body mass, adipose-tissue mass, and thinning of skin).

Given the likelihood that the decline of production of GH with age may play a role in the aging process, it is important to determine possible extrapituitary sources of GH. It is of particular interest that lymphocytes have been identified in the ectopic secretion of GH [148–150]. Nonstimulated rat lymphocytes secrete immunoreactive GH (irGH), which is similar in structure to pituitary-derived GH [148–150]. Lymphocyte-derived irGH is secreted under the control of GHRH.

Evidence has accumulated indicating that GH not only regulates growth of body tissues but can control important immune functions. One of the first lines of evidence to demonstrate how adenohypophyseal hormones are related to immunoregulation was that hypophysectomy caused thymic atrophy [151]. The functional significance of this finding has probably not been appreciated until recently. Studies have now shown that hypophysectomized rats were unable to exhibit an immune response [152]. Treatment with GH or PRL actually restored immunocompetence, whereas other pituitary hormones had no effect [153]. These observations are consistent with reports that lymphocytes express specific receptors for GH [151–156] and PRL [157, 158].

Thymic atrophy is seen in experimental hypophysectomy or advanced aging. Previously, investigators have tried to determine the deleterious consequences of aging on immune function by implanting GH and PRL secretory GH_3 pituitary adenomas cells into aging rats (18–24-months-old). Implantation here resulted in partial regeneration of thymic tissue and partial restoration of T-cell competence for proliferation [159]. The production of IL-2 was significantly increased in these rats. Since previous observations indicated that GH_3 implantation caused a dramatic rise in plasma GH and plasma PRL [160, 161], the authors surmised that these hormones may have been responsible for the restoration of T-cell responses seen in these animals. The findings do not exclude the possibility of other GH_3-derived hormones being important here. Further, treatment of these engrafted animals with GH- and/or PRL-specific antibodies could possibly provide information to clarify the role that GH and PRL play in the modulation of immunoregulation [162]. However, in support of these findings, exogenous GH injection of aging rats resulted in augmented spleen cell proliferation and NK cell activity [162]. Yet no morphologic alterations were seen in the thymus of the animals. However, thymopoietic activity of GH is suggested by the results of another study using DW/J dwarf mice [163]. These mice are GH-deficient and have hypoplastic thymi with losses of CD4/CD8 double-positive T cells. Treatment of these mice with GH resulted in normal distribution of T-cell progenitor cells in the thymus. Studies determining the combined effects of coadministration of exogenous GH and PRL on restoration of immune function would be of interest.

GH is also responsible for modulating other immunologic activities such as augmenting cytolytic activity of T cells, antibody synthesis, GM-CSF-dependent granulocyte differentiation, TNFα production, superoxide anion generation from peritoneal macrophages of hypophysectomized mice and NK activity [163].

The regulatory mechanisms governing immunoreactive GH (irGH) secretion and its effects on lymphocytes have recently been examined [164]. Administration of an antisense oligonucleotide of GH mRNA to lymphocytes inhibited T- and B-cell proliferation. Antisense, but not sense, oligonucleotides were able to significantly inhibit irGH production and [^{3}H]TdR incorporation in both resting and Con A-stimulated lymphocytes. These findings suggest that irGH is important for lymphocyte proliferation and that this activity may be facilitated through an 'autocrine/paracrine mechanism'. Importantly, lymphocyte-derived GH appears to be necessary for interleukin-induced lymphocyte growth, although it is not directly mitogenic.

Prolactin

PRL is a 170-amino acid long neuropeptide secreted from the adenohypophysis [145]. It has been demonstrated to participate in a multitude of physiologic activities [165]; however it is best known for its role in the initiation and maintenance of lactation [145]. Also, it is ubiquitous in nature in that it has been identified in all vertebrates [165]. Several lines of evidence have accumulated to suggest that PRL has important immunoregulatory activity. Factors that cause hypoprolactinemia are generally associated with inducing immunoincompetence [166, 167].

One of the first lines of evidence to suggest the importance of PRL as well as GH on immune function was the observation that hypophysectomy resulted in the regression of the thymus [151] and, more recently, has been shown to result in loss of immune competence [152]. Treatment with PRL restored immune competence [153]. In another study, chemically induced hypo-prolactinemia in mice using bromocriptine, a dopamine type 2 agonist, resulted in decreased macrophage-mediated tumoricidal activity, inhibition of mitogen-driven proliferation of splenic lymphocytes, and increased mortality from intraperitoneal challenge of the bacterial pathogen *Listeria monocytogenes* [166]. Coadministration of ovine PRL reversed these effects. Similarly, CQP 201–403, a more potent, longer-acting dopamine type 2 agonist, was used to suppress PRL levels in a rat cardiac allograft model [167]. Maximal dose administration caused a significant increase in graft survival as compared with controls. Concurrent administration of a low dose of cyclosporin resulted in a doubling of graft survival time compared to cyclosporin alone. Increased circulating levels of PRL have been seen in patients experiencing acute cardiac allograft rejection [168]. This may be due to the fact that cyclosporin, which was used to suppress graft rejection, can act as an antagonist to PRL binding to the PRL receptor on lymphocytes [157]. Hence, one mechanism of cyclosporin-induced immunosuppression may be to block the immunostimulatory effects of PRL on lymphocytes. As alluded to earlier, therapy that is directed at reducing circulating levels of PRL may facilitate the use of subtoxic and yet immunosuppressive doses of immunosuppressive drugs such as cyclosporin to prevent allograft rejection [167].

There is evidence that PRL may act as a lymphocyte growth factor [169–172]. Increased expression of growth-related genes, such as ornithine decarboxylase and c-myc, have been shown to occur in cells treated with PRL [169–171]. The mechanism of expression of the above genes appears to involve activation of protein kinase C by PRL, particularly activation at the level of the nuclear membrane [170].

It has been established that human PRL is normally secreted from the adenohypophysis, chorion or endometrium. Ectopic secretion of PRL is rarely seen with certain carcinomas [173]. Intracellular PRL has been detected in certain nonpituitary malignant cell lines; however secretion of PRL was not documented [174]. More recently, PRL has been shown to be secreted from a human B lymphoblastoid cell line variant designated as IM-9-P3 [175]. PRL synthesized by these cells was indistinguishable from human pituitary PRL, however the mRNA species expressed differed from that of pituitary origin in that it was approximately 150 bases longer than expected. The authors speculated that there was an elongation of the 5' and/or 3' untranslated regions of IM-9-P3 derived PRL mRNA. Further confirmation of the identity of this PRL is demonstrated by the fact that the immunoaffinity-purified lymphocyte PRL is of the same molecular weight as human pituitary PRL [175].

A 46-kD PRL-like molecule has been shown to be secreted by mitogen-driven rodent lymphocytes as compared to a 25-kD pituitary PRL [176]. One group has reported that a PRL-like mRNA from proliferating splenocytes is larger than other species of PRL-like mRNAs [150]. The size of mRNAs from PRL-like molecules from nonlymphoid tissues are generally in the range of 1 kb [177–179]. Thus, in addition to PRL, there are also PRL-like molecules from lymphocytes as well as nonlymphoid tissues.

The findings presented above suggest that PRL or PRL-like molecules play an important role in positive regulation of lymphocyte functions. Future studies should address the relationship of PRL activation of lymphocytes to that of interleukins such as IL-2.

Somatostatin

Somatostatin (SOM) is a 14-amino acid peptide found in the hypothalamus and central and peripheral nervous system. It is also located in the gastrointestinal tract and pancreatic islets. Its activities are pervasive in that it is responsible for inhibiting the secretion of GH, VIP, TSH, glucagon, insulin, secretin, gastrin, and cholecystokinin. Whereas GH and PRL have immunoenhancing capabilities, SOM has potent inhibitory effects on immune responses.

SOM has been shown to significantly inhibit Molt-4 lymphoblast proliferation and PHA stimulation of human T lymphocytes at $10^{-12}\,M$ [180]. Also, nanomolar concentrations were able to inhibit the proliferation of both spleen- and Peyer's-patches-derived lymphocytes [92]. Interestingly, intravenous infusion of SOM in patients to treat active duodenal ulcers caused a significant reduction in proliferative responses of mitogen-stimulated circulating lymphocytes [181]. Other immune responses, such as SEA-stimulated IFNγ secretion [182] (fig. 3), endotoxin-induced leukocytosis [183] and colony-stimulating activity release [184] are also inhibited by SOM. These functional data suggest that these responsive tissues express receptors for SOM.

Several studies have demonstrated that cells of the immune system express receptors for SOM [185, 186]. Recently, one group has described the existence of distinct subsets of SOM receptors on the Jurkat line of human leukemic T cells and U266 IgE-producing human myeloma cells [185]. They showed that these cells have both high and low affinity receptors with K_d values in the pM and nM range, respectively. The authors speculate that two subsets of receptors may account for the biphasic concentration-dependent nature of the effects of SOM in some systems [180, 187].

Thus, pituitary hormones such as GH and PRL have immunoenhancing effects on T cells, causing increased responses to mitogen stimulation and lymphokine production, while SOM, a potent hypothalamus-derived inhibitor of GH release, inhibits T-cell proliferation. An interesting loop involving positive and negative signals emerges concerning GH, PRL and SOM regulation of immune function.

Conclusions

There is a functional and structural relationship between the immune and neuroendocrine systems. As presented in this chapter, neuroendocrine hormones such as ACTH, endorphins, enkephalins, AVP, TSH, substance P, VIP, GH, PRL, and SOM can regulate a number of important immune functions. Some of these are: (a) enhancement and suppression of antibody production; (b) enhancement and suppression of lymphocyte cytotoxicity and proliferation; (c) modulation of lymphokine production and mediation of lymphokine function; (d) initiation of hypersensitivity events and possibly some immune complex diseases; (e) modulation of macrophage and neutrophil functions, and (f) enhancement of primary lymphoid organ functions such as thymic regeneration. The fact that lymphocytes can produce many of the neuroendocrine hormones that act on the immune system also makes these substances lymphokines by definition, and provides evidence that their regulation of immune functions may be part of the natural immunoregulatory repertoire.

Acknowledgments

This work was supported in part by National Institutes of Health grants AI25904 and CA38587. This paper is Florida Agriculture Experiment Station Journal Series R-05792.

References

1   Blalock JE: Peptide hormones shared by the neuroendocrine and immunologic systems. J Immunol 1985;135:858s–861s.
2   Smith EM, Galin S, LeBoeuf RD, Coppenhaver DH, Harbour DV, Blalock JE: Nucleotide and amino acid sequence of lymphocyte-derived corticotropin: Endotoxin induction of a truncated peptide. Proc Natl Acad Sci USA 1990;87:1057–1060.
3   Douglas J, Civelli O, Herbert E: Polyprotein gene expression: Generation of diversity of neuroendocrine peptides. Annu Rev Biochem 1984;53:665–715.
4   Blalock JE, Smith EM: Human leukocyte interferon: Structural and biological relatedness to adrenocorticotropic hormone and endorphins. Proc Natl Acad Sci USA 1981;77:5972–5974.
5   Smith EM, Blalock JE: Human lymphocyte production of cotricotropin- and endorphin-like substances: Association with leukocyte interferon. Proc Natl Acad Sci USA 1981;78:7530–7534.
6   Johnson HM, Smith EM, Torres BA, Blalock JE: Regulation of the in vitro antibody response by neuroendocrine hormones. Proc Natl Acad Sci USA 1982;79:4171–4174.
7   Mishell RI, Dutton RW: Immunization of dissociated spleen cell cultures from normal mice. J Exp Med 1976;126:423–442.
8   Mosier DE, Scher I, Paul WE: In vitro responses of CBA/N mice: Spleen cells of mice with an X-linked defect that precludes immune responses to several thymus-independent antigens can respond to TNP-lipopolysaccharide. J Immunol 1976;117:1363–1369.
9   Clarke BL, Bost KL: Differential expression of functional adrenocorticotropic hormone receptors by subpopulations of lymphocytes. J Immunol 1989;143:464–469.
10 Alvarez-Mon M, Kehrl JH, Fauci AS: A potential role for adrenocorticotropin in regulating B lymphocyte functions. J Immunol 1985;135:3823–3826.
11 Aebischer I, Stampfli MR, Miescher S, Horn M, Zurcher AW, Stadler BM: Neuropeptides accentuate interleukin 4-induced human immunoglobulin E synthesis in vitro. Exp Dermatol 1996;5:38–44.
12 Munn NA, Lum LG: Immunoregulatory effects of α-endorphin, β-endorphin, methionine-enkephalin, and adrenocorticotropic hormone on anti-tetanus toxoid antibody synthesis by human lymphocytes. Clin Immunol Immunopathol 1989;52:376–385.
13 Carr DJJ, Radulescu RT, DeCosta BR, Rice KC, Blalock JE: Differential effect of opioids on immunoglobulin production by lymphocytes isolated from Peyer's patches and spleen. Life Sci 1990;47:1059–1069.
14 Johnson HM, Torres BA, Smith EM, Dion LD, Blalock JE: Regulation of lymphokine (γ-interferon) production by corticotropin. J Immunol 1984;132:246–250.
15 Epstein LB, Cline MJ, Merigan TC: The interaction of human macrophages and lymphocytes in the phytohemmaglutinin-stimulated production of interferon. J Clin Invest 1971;50:744–753.
16 Torres BA, Farrar WL, Johnson HM: Interleukin-2 regulates immune interferon (IFNγ) production by normal and suppressor cell cultures. J Immunol 1982;128:2217–2219.
17 Torres BA, Yamamoto JK, Johnson HM: Cellular regulation of gamma interferon production: Lyt phenotype of the suppressor cell. Infect Immun 1982;35:770–776.
18 Wybran J, Appelboom T, Famaey J-P, Govaerts A: Suggestive evidence for receptors for morphine and methionine-enkephalin on normal human blood T lymphocytes. J Immunol 1979;123:1068–1070.
19 Hazum E, Chang K-J, Cuatrecasas P: Specific nonopiate receptors for β-endorphin. Science 1979;205:1033–1035.
20 Gilmore W, Weiner LP: β-Endorphin enhances interleukin 2 (IL 2) production in murine lymphocytes. J Neuroimmunol 1988;18:125–138.
21 Heijnen C, Bevers C, Kavelaars A, Ballieux RE: Effect of α-endorphin on the antigen-induced primary antibody response of human blood B cells in vitro. J Immunol 1986;136:213–216.
22 Hazum E, Chang K-J, Cuatrecasas P: Interaction of iodinated human [D-Ala₂]β-endorphin with opiate receptors. J Biol Chem 1979;221:309–323.
23 Udenfriend S, Kilpatrick DL: Biochemistry of the enkephalins and enkephalin-containing peptides. Archs Biochem Biophys 1983;221:309–323.
24 Morgan EL, McClurg MR, Janda JA: Suppression of human B lymphocyte activation by β-endorphin. J Neuroimmunol 1990;28:209–217.

25 Williamson SA, Knight RA, Lightman SL, Hobbs JR: Effects of beta-endorphin on specific immune responses in man. Immunology 1988;65:47–51.

26 Rowland RR, Tokuda S: Dual immunomodulation by met-enkephalin. Brain Behav Immun 1989; 3:171–174.

27 Morgan EL: Regulation of human B lymphocytes activation by opioid peptide hormones: Inhibition of IgG production by opioid receptor class (mu-, kappa-, and delta-) selective agonists. J Neuroimmunol 1996;65:21–30.

28 Sizemore RC, Dienglewicz RL, Pecunia E, Gottlieb AA: Modulation of concanavalin A-induced, antigen-nonspecific regulatory cell activity by leu-enkephalin and related peptides. Clin Immunol Immunopathol 1991;60:310–318.

29 Shavit Y, Lewis JW, Terman GW, Gale RP, Liebeskind JC: Opioid peptides mediate the suppressive effect of stress on natural killer cell cytotoxicity. Science 1984;223:188–190.

30 Flores CM, Hernandez MC, Hargreaves KM, Bayer BM: Restraint stress-induced elevation in plasma corticosterone and β-endorphin are not accompanied by alterations in immune function. J Neuroimmunol 1990;28:219–225.

31 Mathews PM, Froelich CJ, Sibbitt WL, Bankhurst AD: Enhancement of natural cytotoxicity by β-endorphin. J Immunol 1983;13:1658–1662.

32 Kay N, Morley JE, Allen JI: Interaction between endogenous opioid and IL-2 on PHA-stimulated human lymphocytes. Immunology 1990;70:485–491.

33 Faith RE, Liang HJ, Murgo AJ, Plotnikoff NP: Neuroimmunomodulation with enkephalins: Enhancement of human natural killer (NK) cell activity in vitro. Clin Immunol Immunopathol 1984;31:412–418.

34 Foster JS, Moore RN: Dynorphin and related opioid peptides enhance tumoricidal activity mediated by murine peritoneal macrophages. J Leukocyte Biol 1987;42:171–174.

35 Oleson DR, Johnson DR: Regulation of human natural cytotoxicity by enkephalins and selective opiate agonists. Brain Behav Immun 1988;2:171–186.

36 Carr DJJ, DeCosta BR, Jacobson AE, Rice KC, Blalock JE: Cotricotropin-releasing hormone augments natural killer cell activity through a naloxone-sensitive pathway. J Neuroimmunol 1990; 28:53–61.

37 Gilman SC, Schwartz JM, Milner RJ, Bloom FE, Feldman JD: β-Endorphin enhances lymphocyte proliferative responses. Proc Natl Acad Sci USA 1982;79:4226–4230.

38 McCain HW, Lamster IB, Bozzone JM, Grbic JT: β-Endorphin modulates human immunity via non-opiate receptor mechanisms. Life Sci 1982;31:1619–1624.

39 Glimore W, Moloney M, Bernstein T: The enhancement of polyclonal T cell proliferation by beta-endorphin. Brain Res Bull 1990;24:687–692.

40 Hemmick L, Bidlack JM: β-Endorphin stimulates rat T lymphocyte proliferation. J Neuroimmunol 1990;29:239–248.

41 Miller GC, Murgo AJ, Plotnikoff NP: Enhancement of active T-cell rosettes from lymphoma patients. Clin Immunol Immunopathol 1983;26:446–451.

42 Van Epps DE, Saland L: β-Endorphin and [Met]-enkephalin stimulate human peripheral blood mononuclear cell chemotaxis. J Immunol 1984;132:3046–3053.

43 Ruff M, Schiffmann E, Terranova V, Pert CB: Neuropeptides are chemoattractants for human tumor cells and monocytes: A possible mechanism for metastasis. Clin Immunol Immunopathol 1985;37:387–396.

44 Brown SL, Van Epps DE: Suppression of T lymphocyte chemotactic factor production by the opioid peptides β-endorphin and [Met]-enkephalin. J Immunol 1985;134:3384–3390.

45 Peterson PK, Sharp B, Gekker G, Brummitt C, Keane WF: Opioid-mediated suppression of interferon-γ production by cultured peripheral blood mononuclear cells. J Clin Invest 1987;80:824–831.

46 Morgano A, Setti M, Poerri I, Barabine A, Lotti G, Indiveri F: Expression of HLA-class II antigens and proliferative capacity in autologous mixed lymphocyte reactions of human T lymphocytes exposed in vitro to α-endorphin. Brain Behav Immun 1989;3:214–222.

47 Brownstein MJ, Russell JT, Gainer H: Synthesis, transport, and release of posterior pituitary hormones. Science 1980;207:373–378.

48 Sawyer WH: Neurohypophyseal hormones. Pharmacol Rev 1961;13:225–277.

49   Rossi NF, Schier RW: Role of arginine vasopressin in regulation of systemic arterial pressure. Annu Rev Med 1986;37:13–20.

50   Gibbs DM: Vasopressin and oxytocin: Hypothalamic modulations of the stress response: A review. Psychoneuroendocrinology 1986;11:131–140.

51   Doris PA: Vasopressin and central integrative processes. Neuroendocrinology 1984;38:75–85.

52   Clements JA, Funder JW: Arginine vasopressin (AVP) and AVP-like immune reactivity in peripheral tissues. Endocr Rev 1986;7:449–460.

53   Jessop DS, Murphy D, Larsen PJ: Thymic vasopressin (AVP) transgene expression in rats: A model for the study of thymic AVP hyper-expression in T cell differentiation. J Neuroimmunol 1995;62:85–90.

54   Jessop DS, Chowdrey HS, Lightman SL, Larsen PJ: Vasopressin is located within lymphocytes in the rat spleen. J Neuroimmunol 1995;56:219–223.

55   Geenen V, Benhida A, Kecha O, Achour I, Vandermissen E, Vanneste Y, Goxe B, Martens H: Development and evolutionary aspects of thymic T cell education to neuroendocrine self. Acta Haematol 1996;95:263–267.

56   Geenen V, Martens H, Vandermissen E, Kecha O, Benhida A, Cormann-Goffin N, Lefebvre PJ, Franchimont P: Thymic neuroendocrine self peptides and T cell selection. Adv Exp Med Biol 1994;355:21–26.

57   Robert FR, Martens H, Cormann N, Benhida A, Schoenen J, Geenen V: The recognition of hypothalamo-neurohypophyseal functions by developing T cell. Dev Immunol 1992;2:131–140.

58   Robert F, Geenen V: Thymic neuropeptides and T lymphocyte development. Ann NY Acad Sci 1992;650:99–104.

59   Johnson HM, Farrar WL, Torres BA: Vasopressin replacement of interleukin-2 requirement in gamma interferon production: Lymphokine activity of a neuroendocrine hormone. J Immunol 1982;129:963–986.

60   Johnson HM, Torres BA: Regulation of lymphokine production by arginine vasopressin and oxytocin: Modulation of lymphocyte function by neurohypophyseal hormones. J Immunol 1985;135:773s–775s.

61   Manning M, Olma A, Klis W, Kolodziejczyk A, Nawrocka E, Misicka A, Seto J, Sawyer WH: Carboxy terminus of vasopressin required for activity but not binding. Nature 1984;308:652–653.

62   Torres BA, Johnson HM: Arginine vasopressin (AVP) replacement of helper cell requirement in IFNγ production: Evidence for a novel AVP receptor on mouse lymphocytes. J Immunol 1988;140:2179–2183.

63   Bell J, Adler MW, Greenstein JI, Liu-Chen LY: Identification and characterization of [^{125}I]-arginine vasopressin binding sites on human peripheral blood mononuclear cells. Life Sci 1993;52:95–105.

64   Teppermann J, Teppermann HM: Metabolic and Endocrine Physiology, ed 5. Chicago, Year Book, 1987, p 131–132.

65   Contagliola S, Madec A-M, Benkirane MM, Orgiazzi J, Carayon P: Monoclonal antibody approach to the relationship between immunological structure and biological activity of thyrotropin. Mol Endocrinol 1988;2:613–618.

66   Pierpaoli W: Psychoneuroimmunology. New York, Academic Press, 1981, pp 575–606.

67   Smith EM, Phan M, Kruger TE, Coppenhaver D, Blalock JE: Human leukocyte production of immunoreactive thyrotropin. Proc Natl Acad Sci USA 1983;80:6010–6013.

68   Peele ME, Carr FE, Baker JR, Wartofsky L, Burman KD: TSH beta subunit gene expression in human lymphocytes. Am J Med Sci 1993;305:1–7.

69   Harbour DV, Kruger TE, Coppenhaver D, Smith EM, Meyer WJ: Differential expression and regulation of thyrotropin (TSH) in T cell lines. Mol Cell Endocrinol 1989;64:229–241.

70   Coutelier J-P, Kehrl JH, Bellur SS, Kohn LD, Notkins AL, Prabhaker BS: Binding and functional effects of thyroid stimulating hormone on human immune cells. J Clin Immunol 1990;10:204–210.

71   Francis T, Burch HB, Cai WY, Lukes Y, Peele M, Carr FE, Wartofsky L, Burman KD: Lymphocytes express thyrotropin receptor-specific mRNA as detected by the PCR technique. Thyroid 1991;1:223–228.

72   Blalock JE, Johnson HM, Smith EM, Torres BA: Enhancement of the in vitro antibody response by thyrotropin. Biochem Biophys Res Comm 1984;125:30–34.

73 Kruger TE, Blalock JE: Cellular requirements for thyrotropin enhancement of in vitro antibody production. J Immunol 1986;137:197–200.

74 Provinciali M, DiStefano G, Fabris N: Improvement in the proliferative capacity and natural killer cell activity of murine spleen lymphocytes by thyrotropin. Int J Immunopharmacol 1992;14: 865–870.

75 Harbour-McMenamin D, Smith EM, Blalock JE: Production of immunoreactive chorionic gonadotropin during mixe lymphocyte reactions: A possible mechanism for genetic diversity. Proc Natl Acad Soc JSA 1986;83:6834–6838.

76 Fuchs T, Hammarstrom L, Smith CI, Brundin J: Sex-dependent induction of human suppressor T cells by chorionic gonadotropin. J Reprod Immunol 1982;4:185–190.

77 Ricketts RM, Jones DB: Differential effect of human chorionic gonadotropin on lymphocyte proliferation induced by mitogens. J Reprod Immunol 1985;7:225–232.

78 Cooper JR, Bloom FE, Roth RH: The Biochemical Basis of Neuropharmacology, ed 5. New York, Oxford University Press, 1986, pp 352–393.

79 Pernow B: Substance P. Pharmacol Rev 1983;35:85–141.

80 Payan DG, Brewster DR, Goetzl EJ: Stereospecific receptors for substance P on cultured human IM-9 lymphoblasts. J Immunol 1984;133:3260–3265.

81 Payan DG, McGillis JP, Organist ML: Binding characteristics and affinity labeling of protein constituents of the human IM-9 lymphoblast receptor for substance P. J Biol Chem 1986;261: 14321–14329.

82 McGillis JP, Mitsuhashi M, Payan DG: Immunomodulation by tachykinin neuropeptides. Ann NY Acad Sci 1990;594:84–95.

83 Organist ML, Harvey J, McGillis JP, Mitsuhashi M, Melera P, Payan DG: Characterization of a monoclonal antibody against the lymphoblast substance P receptor. J Immunol 1987;139:1–5.

84 Foreman J, Jordan C: Histamine release and vascular changes induced by neuropeptides. Agents Actions 1983;13:105–116.

85 Kavelaars A, Jeurissen F, Heijnen CJ: Substance P receptors and signal transduction in leukocytes. Immunomethods 1994;5:41–48.

86 Goetzl EJ, Chernov T, Renold F, Payan DG: Neuropeptide regulation of the expression of immediate hypersensitivity. J Immunol 1985;135:802s–805s.

87 Marasco WA, Showell HJ, Becker EL: Substance P binds to the formylpeptide chemotaxis receptor on the rabbit neutrophil. Biochem Biophys Res Commun 1982;99:1065–1072.

88 Bar-Shavit Z, Goldman R, Stabinsky R, Gottlieb P, Fridkin M, Teichberg VI, Blumberg S: Enhancement of phagocytosis: A newly found activity of substance P in its N-terminal tetrapeptide sequence. Biochem Biophys Res Commun 1980;94:1445–1451.

89 Hartung H-P, Wolters K, Toyka KV: Substance P: Binding properties and studies on cellular responses in guinea pig macrophages. J Immunol 1986;136:3856–3863.

90 DeRose V, Robbins RA, Snider RM, Spurzem JR, Thiele GM, Rennard SI, Rubenstein I: Substance P increases neutrophil adhesion to bronchial epithelial cells. J Immunol 1994;152:1339–1346.

91 Payan DG, Brewster DR, Goetzl EJ: Specific stimulation of human T lymphocytes by substance P. J Immunol 1983;13:1613–1615.

92 Stanisz AM, Befus D, Bienenstock J: Differential effects of vasoactive intestinal peptide, substance P, and somatostatin on immunoglobulin synthesis and proliferation by lymphocytes from Peyer's patches, mesenteric lymph nodes, and spleen. J Immunol 1986;136:152–156.

93 Payan DG, Brewster DR, Missirian-Bastian A, Goetzl EJ: Substance P recognition by a subset of human T lymphocytes. J Clin Invest 1984;74:1532–1539.

94 Ruff MR, Wahl SM, Pert CB: Substance P receptor-mediated chemotaxis of human monocytes. Peptides 1985;2(suppl 6):10007–111.

95 Lotz M, Vaughn JH, Carson DA: Effects of neuropeptides on production of inflammatory cytokines by human monocytes. Science 1988;241:1218–1221.

96 Nair MP, Schwartz SA: Substance P induces tumor necrosis factor in an ex vivo model system. Cell Immunol 1995;166:286–290.

97 Lotz M, Carson DA, Vaughn JH: Substance P activation of rheumatoid synoviocytes: Neural pathways in pathogenesis of arthritis. Science 1987;235:893–895.

98   Yankner BA, Duffy LK, Kirschner DA: Neurotrophic and neurotoxic effects of amyloid β protein: Reversal by tachykinin neuropeptides. Science 1990;250:279–282.

99   Mitsuhashi M, Akitaya T, Turk CW, Payan DG: Amyloid β substituent peptides do not interact with the substance P receptor expressed in cultured cells. Mol Brain Res 1991;11:177–180.

100   Costa M, Furness JB: The origins, pathways, and terminations of neurons with VIP-like immunoreactivity in the guinea pig small intestine. Neuroscience 1983;8:665–676.

101   Morel G, Besson J, Rosselin G, Dubois PM: Ultrastructural evidence for endogenous vasoactive intestinal peptide-like immunoreactivity in the pituitary gland. Neuroendocrinology 1982;34:85–89.

102   Weithe E, Reinecke M: Peptidergic innervation of the mammalian sinus nodes: Vasoactive intestinal polypeptide, neurotensin, substance P. Neurosci Let 1981;26:283–288.

103   Barajas L, Sokolski DN, Lechago J: Vasoactive intestinal polypeptide-immunoreactive nerves in the kidney. Neurosci Lett 1983;43:263–269.

104   Bloom SR, Polak JM: Regulatory peptides and the skin. Clin Exp Dermatol 1983;8:3–18.

105   Felten DL, Felten SY, Carlson SL, Olschowska JA, Livnat S: Noradrenergic and peptidergic innervation of lymphoid tissue. J Immunol 1985;135:755s–765s.

106   Lundberg JM, Pernow AA, Hokfelt T: Neuropeptide Y-, substance P- and VIP-immunoreactive nerves in cat spleen in relation to autonomic vascular and volume control. Cell Tissue Res 1985; 239:9–18.

107   O'Dorisio MS, Wood CL, O'Dorisio TM: Vasoactive intestinal peptide and neuropeptide modulation of the immune response. J Immunol 1985;135:792s–799s.

108   Frawley LS, Neill JD: Stimulation of prolactin secretion in rhesus monkeys by vasoactive intestinal polypeptide. Neuroendocrinology 1981;33:79–83.

109   Feliu JE, Mojena M, Silvestre RA, Monge J, Marco J: Stimulatory effect of vasoactive intestinal peptide on glycogenolysis and gluconeogenesis in isolated rat hepatocytes: Antagonism by insulin. Endocrinology 1983;112:2120–2127.

110   Magisretti PJ, Morrison JH, Shoemaker WJ, Sapin V, Bloom FE: Vasoactive intestinal polypeptide induces glycogenolysis in mouse control of energy metabolism. Proc Natl Acad Sci USA 1981;78: 6535–6539.

111   Epelbaum J, Tapia-Aranciba L, Besson J, Rotszteyn WH, Kordon C: Vasoactive intestinal peptide inhibits release of somatostatin from hypothalamus in vitro. Eur J Pharmacol 1979;58:493–495.

112   Said SI, Geumi A, Hara N: Bronchodilator effect of VIP in vivo: Protection against bronchoconstriction induced by histamine or prostaglandin F_{2a}; in Said (ed): Vasoactive Intestinal Peptide. New York, Raven Press, 1982, pp 185–192.

113   Ottesen B, Gerstenberg T, Ulrichsen H, Manthrope T, Fahrenkrug J, Wagner G: Vasoactive intestinal polypeptide (VIP) increases vaginal blood flow and inhibits uterine smooth muscle activity in women. Eur J Clin Invest 1983;13:321–324.

114   O'Dorisio MS, O'Dorisio TM, Cataland S, Balcerzak SP: VIP as a biochemical marker for polymorphonuclear leukocytes. J Lab Clin Med 1980;96:666–672.

115   Cutz E, Chan W, Track NS, Goth A, Said S: Release of vasoactive intestinal polypeptide in mast cells by histamine liberatore. Nature 1978;275:661–662.

116   Leceta J, Martinez MC, Delgado M, Garrido E, Gomariz RP: Lymphoid cell populations containing vasoactive intestinal peptide in the rat. Peptides 1994;15:791–797.

117   Gomariz RP, Leceta J, Garrido E, Garrido T, Delgado M: Vasoactive intestinal peptide (VIP) mRNA expression in rat T and B lymphocytes. Regul Pept 1994;50:177–184.

118   Goetzl EJ, Sreedham SP, Turck CW: Structurally distinctive vasoactive intestinal peptides from rat basophilic leukemia cells. J Biol Chem 1988;263:9083–9086.

119   Ottaway CA, Greenburg GR: Interaction of vasoactive intestinal peptide with mouse lymphocytes: Specific binding and the modulation of mitogen responses. J Immunol 1984;132:417–423.

120   Ottaway CA, Bernaerts C, Chan B, Greenberg GR: Specific binding of VIP to human circulating mononuclear cells, Can J Physiol Pharmacol 1983;61:664–671.

121   Ottaway CA: Selective effects of vasoactive intestinal peptide on the mitogenic response of murine T cells. Immunology 1987;62:291–297.

122   Ganea D, Sun L: Vasoactive intestinal peptide downregulates the expression of IL 2 but not of IFN gamma from stimulated murine T lymphocytes. J Neuroimmunol 1993;47:147–158.

123 Sun L, Ganea D: Vasoactive intestinal peptide inhibits interleukin (IL)-2 and IL-4 production through different molecular mechanisms in T cells activated via the T cell receptor/CD3 complex. J Neuroimmunol 1993;48:59–69.

124 Wang HY, Xin Z, Tang H, Ganea D: Vasoactive intestinal peptide inhibits IL 4 production in myrine T cells by a post-transcriptional mechanism. J Immunol 1996;156:3243–3253.

125 Martinez C, Delgado M, Gomariz RP, Ganea D: Vasoactive intestinal peptide and pituitary adenylate cyclase-activating polypeptide-38 inhibit IL 10 production in murine T lymphocytes. J Immunol 1996;156:4128–4136.

126 Hassner A, Lau MS, Goetzl EJ, Adelman DC: Isotype-specific regulation of human lymphocyte production of immunoglobulins by sustained exposure to vasoactive intestinal peptide. J Allergy Clin Immunol 1993;92:891–901.

127 Elson CO, Heck JA, Strober W: T-cell regulation of murine IgA synthesis. J Exp Med 1979;149: 632–643.

128 Richman LK, Graeff AS, Yarchoan R, Strober W: Simultaneous induction of antigen-specific IgA helper T cell and IgG suppressor T cells in the murine Peyer's patch after protein feeding. J Immunol 1981;126:2079–2083.

129 Rola-Pleszcynski M, Bolduc D, St Pierre S: The effects of vasoactive intestinal peptide on human natural killer function. J Immunol 1985;135:2569–2573.

130 Sirianni MC, Annibale B, Tagliaferri F, Fais S, DeLuca S, Pallone F, DelleFave G, Aiuti F: Modulation of human natural killer activity by vasoactive intestinal peptide (VIP) family: VIP, glucagon, and GHRF specifically inhibit NK activity. Regul Pept 1992;38:79–87.

131 Holst JJ, Fahrenkrug J, Jensen SL, Nielsen OU: Peptidergic innervation of the pancreas; in Bloom SR, Polak JM (eds): Gut Hormones. Edinburgh, Churchill-Livingstone, 1981, pp 495–511.

132 Koff WC, Dunegan MA: Modulation of macrophage-mediated tumoricidal activity by neuropeptides and neurohormones. J Immunol 1985;135:350–354.

133 Yiangou Y, Serrano R, Bloom SR, Pena J, Festenstein H: Effects of preprovasoactive intestinal peptide-derived peptides on the murine immune response. J Neuroimmunol 1990;29:65–72.

134 Moore TC: Modification of lymphocyte traffic by vasoactive neurotransmitter substances. Immunology 1984;52:511–518.

135 Ottaway CA: In vitro alteration of receptors for vasoactive intestinal peptide changes in vivo localization of mouse T cells. J Exp Med 1984;160:1054–1069.

136 O'Dorisio MS, Hermina NS, O'Dorisio TM, Balcerzak SP: Vasoactive intestinal polypeptide modulation of lymphocyte adenylate cyclase. J Immunol 1981;127:2551–2554.

137 Gomariz RP, Garrido E, Leceta J, Martinez C, Abalo R, Delgado M: Gene expression of VIP receptor in rat lymphocytes. Biochem Biophys Res Commun 1994;203:1599–1604.

138 Beed EA, O'Dorsio MS, O'Dorsio TM, Gaginella TS: Demonstration of a functional receptor for vasoactive intestinal polypeptide on Molt-4B lymphoblasts. Regul Pept 1983;6:1–12.

139 Svoboda M, Tastenoy M, Van Rampelbergh J, Goosens JF, DeNeef P, Waelbroeck M, Robberecht P: Molecular cloning and functional characterization of a human VIP receptor from SUP-T1 lymphoblasts. Biochem Biophys Res Commun 1994;205:1617–1624.

140 Cheng PP, Sreedharan SP, Kishiyama JL, Goetzl EJ: The SKW6.4 line of human B lymphocytes specifically binds and responds to vasoactive intestinal peptide. Immunology 1993;79:64–68.

141 O'Dorsio MS: Biochemical characteristics of receptors for vasoactive intestinal polypeptide in nervous, endocrine, and immune systems. Fed Proc 1987;46:192–195.

142 Ottaway GA, Lay TE, Greenberg GR: High affinity specific binding of vasoactive intestinal peptide to human circulating T cells, B cells and large granular lymphocytes. J Neuroimmunol 1990;29: 149–155.

143 O'Dorisio MS, Wood CL, Wenger GD, Vassallo LM: Cyclic AMP-dependent protein kinase in Molt-4B lymphoblasts: Identification by photoaffinity labeling and activation in intact cells by the neuropeptides vasoactive intestinal polypeptide and peptide histidine isoleucine. J Immunol 1985; 134:4078–4086.

144 Gilman AG: G proteins and dual control of adenylate cyclase. Cell 1984;36:577–579.

145 Laycock JF, Wise PH: The hypothalamo-hypophyseal system; in Laycock JF: Essential Endocrinology, ed 2. New York, Oxford University Press, 1983, pp 29–76.

146 Rudman D: Growth hormone, body composition, and aging. J Am Geriatr Soc 1985;33:800–807.
147 Rudman D, Feller AG, Nagraj HS, Gergans GA, Lalitha PY, Goldberg AF, Schlenker RA, Cohn L, Rudman IW, Mattson DE: Effects of human growth hormone in men over 60 years old. N Engl J Med 1990;323:1–6.
148 Weigent DA, Baxter JB, Wear WE, Smith LR, Bost KL, Blalock JE: Production of immunoreactive growth hormone by mononuclear leukocytes. FASEB J 1988;2:2812–2818.
149 Hattori N, Shimatsu A, Sugita M, Kumagi S, Imura H: Immunoreactive growth hormone (GH) secretion by human lymphocytes: Augmented release by exogenous GH. Biochem Biophys Res Commun 1990;168:396–401.
150 Hiestand PC, Mekler P, Nordmann R, Grieder A, Permmongkol C: Prolactin as a modulator of lymphocyte responsiveness provides a possible mechanism of action for cyclosporine. Proc Natl Acad Sci USA 1986;83:2599–2603.
151 Smith PE: The effect of hypophysectomy upon the involution of the thymus in the rat. Anat Rec 1930;47:119–129.
152 Berczi I, Nagy E: A possible role of prolactin in adjuvant arthritis. Arthritis Rheum 1982;25:591–594.
153 Nagy E, Berczi I, Friesen HG: Regulation of immunity in rats by lactogenic and growth hormones. Acta Endocrinol (Copenh) 1983;102:351–357.
154 Arranbrecht S: Specific binding of growth hormone to thymocytes. Nature 1974;252:255–257.
155 Lesniak MA, Gordon P, Roth J, Gavin JR III: Binding of ^{125}I-human growth hormone to specific receptors in human cultured lymphocytes. J Biol Chem 1974;249:1661–1667.
156 Kiess W, Butenandt O: Specific growth hormone receptors on human peripheral mononuclear cells: Reexpression, identification, and characterization. J Clin Endocrinol Metab 1985;60:740–746.
157 Russell DH, Kibler R, Matrisian L, Larson DF, Poulos B, Magun BE: Prolactin receptors on human T and B lymphocytes: Antagonism of prolactin binding by cyclosporine. J Immunol 1985;134:3027–3031.
158 Russell DH, Matrisian L, Kibler R, Larson DF, Poulos B, Magun BD: Prolactin receptors on human lymphocytes and their modulation by cyclosporine. Biochem Biophys Res Commun 1984;121:899–906.
159 Kelley KW, Brief S, Westly HJ, Novakofski J, Bechtel PJ, Simon J, Walker EB: GH$_3$ pituitary adenoma cells can reverse thymic aging rats. Proc Natl Acad Sci USA 1986;83:5663–5667.
160 Prysor-Jones RA, Jenkins JS: Effect of excessive secretion of growth hormone on tissues of the rat, with particular reference to the heart and skeletal muscle. J Endocrinol 1980;85:75–82.
161 Seo H, Refetoff S, Fang VS: Induction of hypothyroidism and hypoprolactinemia by growth hormone producing rat pituitary tumors. Endocrinology 1977;100:216–226.
162 Davila DR, Brief S, Simon J, Hammer RE, Brinster RL, Kelley KW: Role of growth hormone in regulating T-dependent immune events in aged, nude, and transgenic rodents. J Neurosci Res 1987;18:108–116.
163 Kelley KW: The role of growth hormone in modulation of the immune response. Ann NY Acad Sci 1990;594:95–103.
164 Weigent DA, Blalock JE, LeBouef RD: An antisense oligodeoxynucleotide to growth hormone messenger ribonucleic acid inhibits proliferation. Endocrinology 1991;128:2053–2057.
165 Nicoll CS, Bern HA: On the actions of prolactin among the vertebrates: Is there a common denominator? In Wolstenholme GEW, Knight J (eds): Lactogenic Hormones. London, Churchill-Livingstone, 1972, pp 299–317.
166 Bernton EW, Meltzer MS, Holaday JW: Suppression of macrophage activation and T lymphocyte function in hypoprolactinemic mice. Science 1988;239:401–404.
167 Wilner ML, Ettenger RB, Koyle MA, Rosenthal JY: The effect of hypoprolactinemia alone and in combination with cyclosporine on allograft rejection. Transplantation 1990;49:264–267.
168 Carrier M, Russell DH, Wild JC, Emery RW, Copeland JG: Prolactin as a marker of rejection in human heart transplantation. J Heart Transplant 1987;6:290–292.
169 Berczi I, Nagy E, DeToledo SM, Matusik RJ, Friesen HG: Pituitary hormones regulate c-myc and DNA synthesis in lymphoid tissue. J Immunol 1991;146:2201–2206.

170 Russell DH: New aspects of prolactin and immunity: A lymphocyte-derived prolactin-like product and nuclear protein kinase C activation. Trends Pharmacol Sci 1989;10:40–44.

171 Tabor CW, Tabor H: Polyamines. Annu Rev Biochem 1984;53:749–790.

172 Clevenger CV, Russell DH, Appasamy PM, Prystowsky MB: Regulation in interleukin-2-driven T lymphocyte proliferation by prolactin. Proc Natl Acad Sci USA 1990;87:6460–6464.

173 Turkington RW: Ectopic production of prolactin. N Engl J Med 1971;285:1455–1458.

174 Rosen SW, Weintraub BD, Aaronson SA: Nonrandom ectopic protein production by malignant cells: Direct evidence in vitro. J Clin Endocrinol Metab 1980;50:834–841.

175 DiMattia GE, Gellersen B, Bohnet HG, Friesen HG: A human B lymphoblastoid cell line produces prolactin. Endocrinology 1988;122:2508–2517.

176 Montgomery DW, Zukoski CF, Shah GN, Buckley AR, Pacholczyk T, Russell DH: Concanavalin A-stimulated murine splenocytes produce a factor with prolactin-like bioactivity and immunoreactivity. Biochem Biophys Res Commun 1987;145:692–698.

177 Schuller LA, Hurley WL: Molecular cloning of a prolactin-related mRNA expressed in bovine placenta. Proc Natl Acad Sci USA 1987;84:5650–5654.

178 Duckworth ML, Kirk KL, Friesen HG: Isolation and identification of a cDNA clone of rat placental lactogen. J Biol Chem 1986;261:10871–10878.

179 Linzer DIH, Lee S-J, Ogren L, Talamantes F, Nathans D: Identification of proliferin mRNA and protein in mouse placenta. Proc Natl Acad Sci USA 1985;82:4356–4359.

180 Payan DG, Hess CA, Goetzl EJ: Inhibition by somatostatin of the proliferation of T lymphocytes and Molt-4 lymphoblasts. Cell Immunol 1984;84:433–438.

181 Malec P, Zeman K, Markiewicz K, Tchorzewski H, Nowak Z, Baj Z: Short-term somatostatin infusion affects T lymphocyte responsiveness in humans. Immunopharmacology 1989;17:45–49.

182 Muscettola M, Grasso G: Somatostatin and vasoactive intestinal peptide reduce interferon-gamma production by peripheral blood mononuclear cells. Immunobiology 1990;180:419–430.

183 Wagner M, Hengst K, Zierden E, Gerllach U: Investigations of the antiproliferative effect of somatostatin in man and rats. Metab Clin Exp 1979;27:1381–1386.

184 Hinterberger W, Cerny C, Kinast M, Pointer H, Trag KM: Somatostatin reduces the release of colony-stimulating activity (CSA) from PHA-activated mouse spleen lymphocytes. Experientia 1977;34:860–862.

185 Sreedharan SP, Kodama KT, Peterson KE, Goetzl EJ: Distinct subsets of somatostatin receptors on cultured human lymphocytes. J Biol Chem 1989;62:655–658.

186 Nakamura H, Koike T, Hiruma K, Sate T, Tomioka H, Yoshida S: Identification of lymphoid cell lines bearing receptors for somatostatin. Immunology 1987;62:655–658.

187 Pawlikowski M, Stepien M, Kunert-Radek J, Zelazowski P, Schally AV: Immunomodulatory action of somatostatin. Ann NY Acad Sci 1987;496:233–239.

Howard M. Johnson, PhD, University of Florida, Department of Microbiology and Cell Science, No Name and Museum Roads, Room 1019, Building 981, Gainesville, FL 32611 (USA)
Tel. (904) 846 0968, Fax (904) 392 5922

Blalock JE (ed): Neuroimmunoendocrinology, 3rd rev ed.
Chem Immunol. Basel, Karger, 1997, vol 69, pp 185–202

....
Hormonal Activities of Cytokines

Eric M. Smith

Departments of Psychiatry and Behavioral Sciences and Microbiology and
Immunology, University of Texas Medical Branch, Galveston, Tex., USA

Introduction

Systemic homeostatis is well known to be mediated by the nervous and
endocrine systems. Less understood is that the integrity of individual tissues
is maintained in a similar fashion by a third, perhaps more fundamental
mechanism [1]. This third mechanism is mediated through the production and
action of cytokines. These are a widely disparate group of molecules that are
similar to hormones in many respects. Like hormones, cytokines are generally
glycoproteins that are produced by one cell and act on others. In contrast to
hormones, cytokines are generally produced at very low levels or not at all
and their effects are therefore more localized. In cases where there is extreme
tissue trauma or chronic inflammation, cytokine levels rise to the level where
systemic effects may occur. Since all cells produce and respond to at least
some, and normally several, cytokines it is not surprising that many of their
effects are hormonal in nature. The aim of this chapter is to provide coverage
of the more significant advances concerning hormonal activities of cytokines
since the last update 4 years ago [2]. Many reports involving this topic have
appeared during this time. Due to space limitations and because of the neuro-
immunoendocrine focus of the book, the scope for this chapter has been
narrowed to those cytokines associated primarily with immunoregulatory roles
(i.e. as opposed to growth factors or neurotrophins). Also, discussion of cytokine effects on the nervous system is covered in detail elsewhere in this volume,
so in this chapter discussion of the neural effects will be restricted to their
impact on neuroendocrine mechanisms.

Table 1. Cytokine families

Families	Cytokines
Interleukins	IL-1α, IL-1β, IL-1ra, and IL-2–IL-17
Chemokines	C-X-C (IL-8), C-C (MCP-1), and C (lymphotactin)
Interferons	IFN-α, IFN-β, and IFN-γ
Tumor necrosis factors	TNFα, TNFβ$_1$, and TNFβ$_2$
Colony-stimulating factors	granulocyte, macrophage, and granulocyte-macrophage CSF
Growth factors	PDGF, FGF, EGF, FGF, IGF, and others
Transforming growth factors	TGFα, TGFβ (β1–5), and activins
Neurotrophic factors	NGF, BDNF, CNTF, NT
Others	erythropoietin, LIF, oncostatin M, angiogenin

Background

Although the first cytokines were described approximately 40 years ago, it is during the past decade that the field of cytokines has blossomed. In this period of time it has expanded from a few named interleukins (IL), to over 17 ILs and the realization that many otherwise named factors such as the interferons (IFN), tumor necrosis factors (TNF), and chemokines can be grouped under the domain of cytokines (table 1) [1, 3]. Paralleling the increasing number of recognized cytokines is an even greater increase in the activities attributed to each of these molecules. As can be seen in table 1 the cytokines can be subdivided into related families, based on general modes of activity. In many respects cytokines are hormones and would have probably been named so, had they been identified by endocrinologists. They are generally glycoproteins, are produced by one cell and active on another, sometimes distant cell. The primary difference is that the endogenous cytokine levels are very low or nonexistent and when induced are active at very low concentrations. Therefore, cytokine activities tend to be at a local level. The identification of common receptors, components and intracellular signal transduction pathways helps explain the pleiotropism of cytokine actions in the immune system. The similarities between the hematopoietic cytokines and other helix bundle peptides such as growth hormone (GH) and prolactin (PRL) clearly illustrate the molecular basis for the similarities in action of these particular molecules [4]. The chapter by Walter [this vol.] provides a detailed discussion of the structural biology of four helix bundle peptides and their receptors.

The cytokines receiving the most attention in the previous editions of this text were interferon-α (IFN-α) and interleukin 1 (IL-1) [2, 3]. Some of the earliest hormone-like activities were described for IFN [2, 3, 5]. IFN-α will increase the beat frequency of myocardial cells [6] and cause the release of corticosteroids from Y-1 adrenal tumor cells [7]. When injected intracerebroventricularly, IFN-α exhibits opioid effects, such analgesia and catatonia [8]. In vivo studies have shown IFN-α to attenuate a morphine-dependent withdrawal syndrome [9]. Further, human studies where large doses of IFN-α have been injected for antitumor therapy have borne out the predicted hormonal effects. Activation of the hypothalamic-pituitary-adrenal (HPA) axis, myocardial effects, plus CNS effects such as lethargy and malaise have been documented [5, 10].

About the same time, nervous and endocrine activities were described for a factor that was identified later as IL-1. Characterized initially as an endogenous pyrogen and lymphocyte activation factor, the use of purified IL-1 showed it caused activation of the HPA axis [11], plus the induction of sleep [12] as well as fever [13]. Now IL-1 is probably the best known and the most accepted mediator of neural-immune communication. A major focus of the previous two reviews concerned IL-1's activation of the HPA axis and whether the effect was by direct action on the pituitary or through the induction of corticotropin-releasing hormone (CRH) [2, 3]. Major questions then and yet to be answered, were whether significant quantities of cytokines could cross the blood-brain barrier. While specific transport mechanisms for IL-1 have been described [14], the finding that this cytokine is synthesized in the brain skirts this issue and probably has been the most convincing form of evidence leading to the acceptance of a neural/neuroendocrine role for cytokines.

While the field of cytokines has been expanding prodigiously, the rate of discovery of new hormonal activities for cytokines seems to have leveled off. The trend of the recent studies has been more to thoroughly characterize described hormonal actions than to identify new activities. This is not to say that the field has become stagnant, possibly just mature. But some relatively new cytokines such as IL-10 and GM-CSF now have hormonal activities attributed to them. Also, more cytokines are undergoing clinical trials for human therapy and the technology of transgenic animals has provided insights into the effects occurring with overproduction of certain cytokines.

New Hormonal Activities

IL-1
Since the first descriptions showed that bona fide IL-1 induced ACTH production by pituitary cells directly [15] and indirectly through the induction of corticotropin-releasing factor (CRF) [11, 16], the production of other hormones as well as cytokines by these cells have now been described. Especially

significant, is that IL-1 is found to be produced endogenously in anterior pituitary cells plus pituitary IL-1β protein and mRNA are increased following administration of bacterial lipopolysaccharide (LPS, endotoxin) [17–20].

The field has also moved beyond merely measuring hormone induction as an indicator of function, to characterizing the presence and pathways of specific receptors for IL-1 on neuroendocrine tissues. Elegant studies have shown binding activity [21–27], intracellular signal pathway activation [28–33], and mRNA expression for both types of IL-1 receptors (IL-1R) present on pituitary regions of brain slices and isolated cells [25, 26, 34]. On AtT-20 cells, CRF will increase the density of IL-1R without affecting the receptor's affinity [27]. Haour's group [23] in France has found high expression of IL-1R of a single affinity in murine hippocampus. The receptor's binding affinity did not change with LPS treatment whereas the pituitary binding density was increased by glucocorticoids. This shows an inverse relationship to the pituitary expression of IL-1β which is induced by LPS and inhibited by glucocorticoids [20, 21]. Using immunohistochemistry and RT-PCR techniques, Parnet et al. [25, 26] have shown that both the type I receptor seen by these previous groups and a type II receptor mRNA are expressed in murine brain and pituitary. The presence of at least two IL-1 receptor mechanisms is supported by a study that shows the pyrogenic and sickness behavior effects of centrally administered IL-1 are differentially mediated [35]. Since the type II receptor has a truncated cytoplasmic tail, the two receptors are likely to activate different intracellular signaling pathways which may expain some of IL-1's differential effects [25, 26].

IL-1 has been shown to induce pituitary cells to produce ACTH, endorphins, growth hormone (GH), luteinizing hormone (LH), and thyrotropin (TSH) [15, 28, 36–38]. The mechanisms for these multiple effects are just beginning to be determined. As mentioned above, two types of IL-1 receptors are expressed in the pituitary [26]. The truncated type II receptor has not been shown in the immune system to activate an intracellular signaling pathway, but it may be linked differently when expressed on pituitary cells. Fagarason et al. [29, 31] have shown that IL-1 induces c-*fos* and c-*jun* in AtT-20 cells, which form the AP-1 transcription factor and enhances proopiomelanocortin gene expression. In the immune sysem IL-1 is well known for inducing NF-κB transcription factor activity, which induces a number of cytokine genes, among them IL-6 [39]. NF-κB activity is expressed in AtT-20 cells [Cadet, Hughes, and Smith; unpubl. observation] and therefore may mediate IL-1's induction of pituitary IL-6 expression [40, 41].

There is a long-standing controversy over the role of IL-1 in induction of the HPA axis; particularly direct pituitary induction of ACTH [2, 3]. Indirect actions, possibly through the induction of IL-6 might be one factor in this regard. Another indirect mechanism might be related to the observation by Payne et al. [42] that CRF induces pituitary sensitivity to IL-1. Low levels of exogenous or endogenous CRF could sensitize the pituitary gland, enhancing the direct ACTH-releasing activity of IL-1. These indirect relationships extend to lymphocyte hormonal activities as well. We found that CRF would induce lymphocyte ACTH expression [43]. Kavelaars et al. [44] showed that CRF induced IL-1 expression which subsequently induced the POMC hormones. Schafer et al. [45, 46] have now shown this response in inflamed tissue and believe it may help account for stress-induced analgesia in inflammation. Likewise, Bhardwaj and Luger [47] have found that IL-1β stimulates cultured keratinocytes to synthesize POMC mRNA. Therefore IL-1's hormonal effects (CRF-like in this case) are not limited to the HPA axis, but may have important role(s) at peripheral sites.

Similarly, IL-1 elicits GH secretion by stimulating the release of hypothalamic GHRH. The inhibition of GH secretion after high doses of IL-1 was attributed to IL-1's induction of CRF [48]. Another factor that may mediate IL-1 actions on the pituitary is the IL-1 receptor antagonist (IL-1ra). Sauer et al. [49] have found IL-1ra mRNA expressed in cultures of all types of pituitary adenomas under basal conditions and following stimulation. In another study this group [50] found that IL-1ra would block IL-1 growth inhibition of cultured pituitary cells. Thus, besides indirect mechanisms of action there are also endogenous inhibitors of IL-1 in the pituitary.

Increasing evidence for a role of IL-1 in the pituitary-gonadal axis is being generated. Early studies indicated that IL-1 induced pituitary gonadotropin production [36]. Now, IL-1, IL-6 and TNF-α have been found to be produced in the mouse uterus during the estrous cycle and are induced by estrogen and progesterone [51]. Furthermore, gonadal steroids can modulate IL-1 and IL-6 production by peripheral blood mononuclear cells [52]. 17-β-Estradiol enhanced LPS-stimulated IL-1 and IL-6 secretion as well as the production of cell-associated IL-1. Whereas progesterone and testosterone at similar concentrations inhibited IL-1 secretion but had no significant effect on IL-6 secretion or on the production of cell-associated IL-1. These studies provide some specific mechanisms to explain the sexual dimorphism of the immune system [53].

Although it is a neurally mediated mechanism of action, recent studies suggest that peripheral IL-1 may induce its central activities through activating the subdiaphragmatic vagus. Disruption of the circuit by subdiaphragmatic vagotomy blocks IL-1-induced hyperthermia [54] and sickness behavior [55]. Goehler et al. [56] have found indications of IL-1 receptors on the vagus nerve. These studies demonstrate one means by which IL-1 can exert its effects across the blood-brain barrier, irrespective of having to physically cross the barrier. This may also be one means to induce endocrine effects as well.

IL-2

IL–2 was originally described as a T-lymphocyte growth factor and is a major regulatory factor for mediating T-cell activation and responses. Compared to the hormonal actions of IL-1, little is known of IL-2's hormonal actions. IL-2 has been shown previously to enhance POMC gene expression in pituitary cells [57] and to stimulate the HPA axis when administered in large doses intravenously [58]. IL-2 also can be involved with the pituitary under pathologic conditions. IL-2 and IL-2R expression have been detected in human corticotrophic adenoma and murine pituitary cells [59, 60]. The IL-2R is found on multiple pituitary cell lines including, corticotrophs and somatotrophs [61]. Phorbol myristic acetate could stimulate this expression. IL-2R has been shown co-localized with pituitary hormones in pituitary cells, but more so with PRL, ACTH, and GH, than TSH, FSH, or LH [50]. Recent studies have also suggested that IL-2 and IL-6 can be involved in anterior pituitary cell growth regulation [61]. Curiously, IL-2 and IL-6 stimulated GH3 pituitary tumor cell growth while inhibiting normal rat anterior pituitary cell growth. The authors suggest that regulation of pituitary cell growth by IL-2 and IL-6, together with their intrinsic pituitary production could be of importance in pituitary adenoma pathogenesis.

Clinical trails with IL-2 have demonstrated that IL-2 will activate the HPA axis, elevating ACTH, β-endorphin, and cortisol [58]. IL-2 also can be associated with thyroid function. Increased IL-2 levels have been observed during standard TRH testing in man [62]. Also, in cancer patients treated with IL-2 and LAK cells, there were significant decreases in serum T4, T3, and free thyroxine levels, but no change in TSH levels [63]. One patient developed compensated hypothyroidism (normal total T4, total T3, and free T4 but elevated TSH) and 4 patients had features of 'sick euthyroid syndrome'. Some of the changes could be associated with the clinical manipulations, but the authors concluded that some of the thyroid dysfunction may arise from direct hormonal effects of the IL-2.

The development of IL-2 transgenic mice has provided some interesting data regarding the role of IL-2 in the neuroimmune axis [64]. Surprisingly, the alterations associated with the overproduction of IL-2 were relatively minor for a cytokine with such major immune effects. Expression of human IL-2 and IL-2R light chain gene under control of the MHC class I promoter is accompanied by expression of the transgene in the thymus, spleen, bone marrow, lung, skin and muscles. The animals have gait disturbances and a loss of Purkinje cells in the cerebellum was noted when the MHC class I promoter was utilized. But use of a metallothionein promoter eliminated this change. Thus, in this model IL-2 seems to affect neural development rather than the HPA axis as might be expected from the studies described above.

IL-6

IL-6, a monokine, has many similarities to IL-1, both structurally and functionally. Identified independently by several laboratories, IL-6 has been variously named B-cell stimulatory factor, hepatocyte-stimulating factor, and IFN-β_2. We and others found that IL-6 (called hepatocyte-stimulating factor in our study) was a potent secretagogue for ACTH by AtT-20 cells [15, 37]. Recent studies have intensified the interest in IL-6, suggesting it may be very important in autocrine or paracrine actions within the pituitary.

Like IL-1, IL-6 is produced by many cell types, including pituitary and subject to several inducers of the HPA axis, like LPS and IL-1 [65–67]. Recent studies have shown folliculostellate cells to be a major source of IL-6 in the pituitary [68]. Using a folliculostellate cell line these authors found that a novel pituitary adenylate cyclase-activating peptide would induce IL-6 secretion along with cell proliferation. Several groups have reported the expression of IL-6 mRNA and protein in human pituitary adenomas [69]. These data combined with a study by Swada et al. [70] suggest that IL-6 may be a growth factor for pituitary cells.

Considering these activities attributed to IL-6, it is not surprising that the IL-6 expressing transgenic mice show gross alterations [71]. Overexpression of IL-6 in astrocytes of the CNS was induced under control of the GFAP (glial fibrillary acidic protein) promoter. Mice with abundant cerebral IL-6 expression are smaller than their nontransgenic littermates and died at the age of 3–10 weeks. The transgenic mice exhibited severe tremors, hind limb weakness, ataxia and seizures. Examination suggested that IL-6 may have participated in the induction of generalized neuronal toxicity. Expression in the CNS may not be the appropriate model for the HPA activities of IL-6. But, nonetheless, it shows that this is an important cytokine in the neuroimmune axis.

IL-10

Discovered in 1989, IL-10 was originally described as a cytokine synthesis inhibitory factor [72, 73]. IL-10 has been shown to be produced by Th2 lymphocytes, macrophages/monocytes and B lymphocytes and to act by inhibiting production of cytokines by activated Th1 cells, macrophages and NK cells. Numerous studies have shown that a plethora of both negative and positive immunoregulatory activities can be attributed to IL-10. In spite of this, little is know about its effects on neuroimmune functions.

IL-10 was found to be highly homologous to BCRF1 which corresponds to an open reading frame (ORF) coding for a protein expressed late in the replication cycle of EBV [74]. IL-10 and EBV-BCRF1/vIL-10 have been shown to have many properties in common. These findings coupled to the ability of

EBV to induce the production of ACTH [75], their similarities in inducers [72, 73] and the similarities of ACTH's and IL-10's effects on IFN-γ and B-lymphocyte responses [72, 73, 76], provided a strong rationale for us to study this cytokine in the immune and neuroendocrine axis.

Our studies were initially aimed at determining the effects of IL-10 in tissue of neuroendocrine origin. Due to the inherent difficulties of utilizing isolated pituitary cells, our initial approach was to determine the effects of IL-10 in vitro, employing AtT-20 mouse pituitary tumor cells. We treated AtT-20 cells with IL-10 at concentrations raging from 10 to 100 ng/ml. All concentrations of IL-10 induced ACTH, with induction occurring in a dose-dependent fashion [77]. The possibility that a sequence or structural similarity between IL-10 and CRF was also investigated. Computer-assisted amino acid sequence alignment and secondary structural comparisons (PC gene) revealed that this was not the case and indicated that a different mechanism of induction of ACTH was occurring, such as through specific IL-10 receptors.

Next, a recriprocal experiment was performed to determine if AtT-20 pituitary tumor cells produced IL-10. IL-10 was quantified by an indirect ELISA in which IL-10 standards or samples believed to contain IL-10 are first bound to the plate. Using this ELISA on supernatant fluids from untreated cells, we demonstrated a constitutive production of IL-10 from AtT-20 pituitary tumor cells. IL-10 was detected in both the supernatant fluids and the cellular lysates of these cells at levels of about 2–3 ng/ml. These levels corresponded to those at which IL-10 has been reported to be active in other systems [72, 73]. We next determined if as observed in AtT-20 cells IL-10 induced splenocytes to produce ACTH. IL-10, at 50 ng/ml, induced the production of ACTH from murine splenocytes as detected by radioimmunoassay.

To further determine if IL-10 is involved in the induction of ACTH, AtT-20 cells were treated with or without CRF for 3 and 6 h in the presence or absence of antibodies to IL-10 following which ACTH levels were measured by RIA. Our results indicated that ACTH levels are reduced in all samples treated with anti-IL10 [Cadet, Hughes, and Smith, unpubl. observation]. In the samples without anti-IL-10, ACTH levels increased in a time- and dose-dependent fashion. Authenticity of the pituitary-derived IL-10 was demonstrated by direct sequence analysis of cDNA fragments obtained from mouse splenocytes, AtT-20 pituitary tumor cells and freshly isolated mouse pituitaries (fig. 1) [77]. Starting with identical amounts of RNA from each tissue, we utilized reverse transcriptase (RT)-coupled polymerase chain reaction (PCR) with custom-designed primers. The amplification products corresponding to the expected molecular weight were then subjected to direct sequencing by using the consensus primers as sequencing primers. The RT-PCR amplification produced a major product at a molecular weight corresponding to 304 bp,

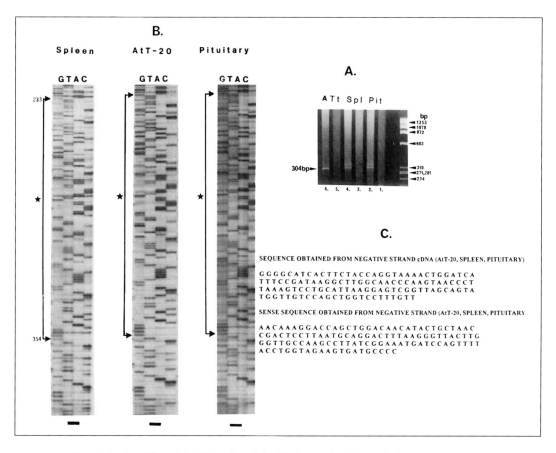

Fig. 1. Authenticity of AtT-20 cell and freshly isolated pituitary-derived IL-10. Total RNA isolated from the above tissues was subjected to RT-PCR for murine IL-10. *A* Ethidium bromide gel of RT-PCR. Expected molecular weight product was 304 bases. Lane 1 = Negative control; lane 2 = fragment amplified from mouse pituitary; lane 3 = negative control; lane 4 = fragment from splenocytes; lane 5 = negative control; lane 6 = fragment from AtT-20 cells. Molecular weight markers on side of gel. *B* Sequencing gel of the 304 molecular weight bands; bracketed areas indicate readable sequences and their respective location in IL-10 cDNA (nts 233–254). Both negative and positive strands sequenced, only negative strands shown. *C* Sequence from negative strand shown first then converted to sense orientation below. Reprinted with permission from Hughes et al. [77].

which was the expected size product. When these fragments were excised from the gel and submitted to sequence analysis, as shown in figure 1, 100% identity exists in sequences from all tissues tested. While this PCR is nonquantitative, identical amounts of RNA from each tissue were used in the amplification. Thus, the possibility that the 304-bp amplicon in lane 2 came solely from the small number of contaminating lymphocytes in the pituitary is unlikely, since similar amounts of amplification product were obtained from the lymphocyte-rich spleen preparations and lymphocyte-negative AtT-20 cell line [77].

We next determined whether a similar phenomenon could be demonstrated in humans [78]. Due to lack of human pituitary cells lines, we used pituitary and hypothalamus, poly(A^+) RNA (Clontech, Palo Alto, Calif., USA) derived from deceased human donors. The levels of cDNA derived from equivalent amounts of RNA for IFN-γ, a lymphocyte-specific product, and IL-10 were compared between the pituitary and the hypothalamus, with levels in peripheral blood leukocytes (PBLs) [78]. Furthermore, G3PDH levels were monitored to ensure that equal amounts of amplification had occurred in all tissues. A densitometric ratio of INF-γ or IL-10 to G3PDH (a 'housekeeping' gene present in all samples) was then determined. This ratio would provide information as to the relative amounts of PCR product that were contributed by each tissue. When the densitometric ratios of IL-10/G3PDH and (B) IFN-γ/G3PDH are compared between the tissues of (A/B), the ratio of the signals of IL-10 derived from the hypothalamus and the pituitary are about 124 and 8.5 times stronger, respectively, than that from the PBLs. Thus, while a component of the IL-10 RT-PCR product is derived from the lymphocytes in the vasculature, it appears that the majority is derived from the cells of the pituitary and hypothalamus.

Recently, the murine IL-10 receptor (mIL-10R) has been characterized. To further our contention that IL-10 acts in the neuroendocrine system, it was necessary to determine that the IL-10R was also present. Using specific oligonucleotides for mIL-10R, we determined if AtT-20 cells express IL-10R mRNA. The receptor appears to be expressed in AtT-20 cells and subject to negative regulation by IL-10. Furthermore, in our preliminary studies it appears that IL-10 mRNA is upregulated in AtT-20 cells treated with CRF.

IL-10 production has also been demonstrated in the CNS. It has been found in glioblastoma multiforme [79]. In particular, it was selectively expressed within invasive gliomas, possibly implying that the IL-10 inhibited host defenses or otherwise aided the invasion process. Also, IL-10 and IL-10R mRNA has been detected in microglia and astrocytes [80]. The expression of IL-10 mRNA and protein was enhanced by stimulation of the mouse glial cells with LPS. Furthermore, IL-10 is active at the CNS level. Intracerebroventricular injection of IL-10 alters cortical EEGs and decreases slow wave sleep, the opposite effect of IL-1 [81]. IL-10 knockout mice have been developed and show severe effects [82]. In these gene knockout mice the lymphocyte and antibody development appears normal, but most animals are growth retarded, anemic and suffer from chronic enterocolitis. No neuroendocrine or CNS effects have been reported to date.

The synthesis and action of IL-10 in the neuroendocrine and central nervous systems opens many possibilities for paracrine and autocrine regulation. In particular, it will be interesting to determine if IL-10 can function to inhibit Th1 type cytokine production in the HPA axis as it does in the immune system and brain [83]. It may serve as an endogenous regulator of those proinflammatory cytokines in the pituitary.

Tumor Necrosis Factor

TNF-α is another proinflammatory cytokine, like IL-1 in many of its actions, including activity on the pituitary [38, 84]. A potent cytokine originally identified as a product of activated macrophages, TNF is now known to be produced by many cell types and has been implicated in regulation of normal tissue homeostasis as well as in cellular differentiation. Recent studies have shown that like IL-1, TNF-α is also synthesized by pituitary cells. LPS administration induces TNF-α expression in the pituitary along with IL-1β and IL-6 [18]. IL-1β and TNF-α mRNA expression peaked at 1 h post induction in spleen, pituitary, hippocampus, and hypothalamic tissues. IL-6 expression lagged, however, peaking at 2 h in all these tissues, possibly secondary to IL-1β and TNF-α expression.

TNF-α may also have a role in the reproductive system. In humans and some rodents TNF is expressed in ovaries, oviducts, uteri, placentas and embryos [85]. The data indicate that TNF expression is regulated either directly or indirectly by ovarian and/or placental hormones. Estrogen and progesterone induce TNF-α along with IL-1 and IL-6 in the mouse uterus during the estrous cycle [51]. Interestingly, either hormone alone would induce IL-1, but both were needed for TNF and IL-6 expression. Furthermore, TNF-α decreases the in vitro synthesis of progesterone and increases estradiol and human chorionic gonadatropin by JEG-3 choriocarcinoma cells [86]. These findings have led some to speculate that TNF is involved in gamete development, cyclic changes in the uterus, cancers of the female reproductive tract, placental maturation, and embryonic development [85].

Various Cytokines

Numerous other cytokines have been implicated as having hormonal activities. CSF-1 and GM-CSF stimulate human cytotrophoblast differentiation into large multinucleated structures composed of extensive patches of syncytium interspersed with mononuclear cells [87]. Concomitantly with the morphological differentiation was upregulation of placental lactogen and chorionic gonadotropin. Also, TNF-α and IL-1 controlled the production of GM-CSF and CSF-1 by placental fibroblasts.

The novel production of leukemia inhibitory factor (ILF) has been described in fetal pituitary issue [88]. Messenger RNA transcripts, protein immunocytochemistry, and immuno-electron microscopy showed LIF expression in fetal pituitaries as young as 14 weeks plus adult tissues as well. LIF-binding sites are present on isolated pituitary and AtT-20 cells. Thirty-five percent of human pituitary fetal cells were immunoreactive for LIF receptor and ACTH or 33% positive for LIF and ACTH. Lower percentages for GH, TSH PRL, FSH, and LH double positive for either LIF or its receptor were also observed. LIF was active on AtT-20 cells, inducing ACTH secretion.

Clinical Studies and Implications

IFN was the first purified cytokine to be administered to humans in large-scale trials [89]. It turned out that the severe side effects associated with high doses of IFN were one of the major limiting factors for its use as an anti-tumor agent. Interesting then and now explainable, many of the side effects were neural or hormonal in nature [5]. Now IFN-α is approved by the FDA for treatment of viral hepatitis, hairy cell leukemia, condeloma acuminatum, plus Kaposi's sarcoma; and IFN-γ is approved for the treatment of chronic granulomatous disease [89]. This more common usage and with more highly purified, recombinant forms of the IFNs has proved that the neural and hormonal side effects are inherent activities of the IFNs. Clinically efficacious doses are usually associated with a 'flu-like' syndrome characterized by fever, chills, headache, lethargy, arthalgias and myalgias [89]. Very high doses may induce cardiocirculatory and neurologic toxicities [90].

Although not utilized to the extent of the IFNs, other cytokines are also being given to human subjects. A study by Nolten et al. [91] examined the effects of IFN-β, IFN-γ, and TNF-α given to cancer patients on the pituitary-adrenal axis. Injections of 90–450 million units of one of the IFNs or 125–275 μg/m^2 of TNF were given for a period of 15 days on alternating days. One to 2 h after injection of IFN-β, the median levels of cortisol, ACTH, PRL, and GH rose twofold. IFN-γ caused a comparable rise in plasma cortisol, whereas TNF induced a 2- to 4-fold rise in ACTH and cortisol. The hormonal response induced by the cytokines was unrelated to their pyrogenic effect, undiminished with repetitive treatment, and not dose-dependent above a threshold level.

As described above, treatment of cancer patients with IL-2 and lympho-kine-activated killer cells altered thyroid functions [63]. Lissoni et al. [92] treated cancer patients with recombinant IL-3. In contrast to the other effects of cytokines on the HPA axis, IL-3 did not significantly alter cortisol, β-endorphin, PRL, FSH, LH, TSH or melatonin levels. However, 6 h after IL-3 administration GH levels were 5-fold higher than with saline.

Table 2. Direct hormonal actions of cytokines

Tissue	Affected hormone	Cytokine
Adrenal	corticosteroids	IFN-α, IL-1
Gonadal	gonadal steroids	IL-1, IL-6, TNF-α
Pituitary	ACTH (POMC)	IL-1, IL-2, IL-6, IL-10, TNF-α, IFN-α, IFN-γ, LIF
	FSH	IL-1
	GH	IL-1, IFN-γ
	PRL	IL-1, IFN-γ
	TSH	IL-1
	IL-6	IL-1
Thyroid	T3, T4	IL-2

IL-10 has been administered i.v. as a single bolus injection (1–25 µg/kg) to humans in a controlled phase 1 trial [93]. It was effective at inhibiting inflammatory cytokine production, seemingly through alterations in cell populations and numbers. Unfortunately, no HPA axis hormone levels were reported and it was stated that there were no adverse symptoms or signs following IL-10 administration. It will be interesting to measure these hormones. Especially in phase II trials, with larger doses of IL-10 to see if it retains its in vitro, CRF-like activity.

Although the field has matured in many aspects, there are still no unifying conclusions one can make other than the observation that many if not most cytokines exert hormonal activities (table 2). Considering that only a few, of possibly hundreds of cytokines have been examined for hormonal functions, there is a lot of leeway for speculation about the physiological role(s) of these interactions. Are they merely redundant regulatory pathways? Or as suggested by Hopkins and Rothwell [1] do they maintain tissue homeostasis in the neuroendocrine and nervous systems as they do in the immune tissues? The presence of stimulatory (IL-1, IL-6) and inhibitory (IL-10) cytokines strengthens arguments for such autocrine and paracrine regulation. The scope and conservation through evolution [94] of the interactions points to their fundamental nature.

What will be the future directions of the field? Certainly, the discovery of new factors and development of newly purified cytokines as reagents will provide continued impetus for this line of study. In this regard, the chemokines represent a large group of cytokines that have only recently started to gain attention and appear to be potential signal molecules in neuroimmune regulation. New understandings of the intracellular signaling pathways may help decipher how activation of these hormone and cytokine receptors are integrated. Finally, further studies and clinical trials of genetically manipulated animals are sure to continue and provide new insights into the cytokines' many activities.

Acknowledgments

I would like to express my gratitude to my colleagues Drs. T.K. Hughes, M.R. Opp, P. Rady, G.B. Stefano and P. Cadet for helpful discussions and our collaborations described in this chapter. The author's studies discussed in this chapter were supported in part by the Office of Naval Research (N00014–89–J–1095), the National Institutes of Health (DK41034), and the National Institute of Drug Abuse (DA 08354).

References

1   Hopkines SJ, Rothwell NJ: Cytokines and the nervous system. I. Expression and recognition. Trends Neurosci 1995;18:83–88.
2   Smith EM: Hormonal activities of cytokines. Chem Immunol 1992;52:154–169.
3   Smith EM: Hormonal activities of lymphokines, monokines, and other cytokines. Prog Allergy 1988;43:121–139.
4   Horseman ND, Yu-Lee LY: Transcriptional regulation by the helix bundle peptide hormones: Growth hormone, prolactin, and hematopoietic cytokines. Endocr Rev 1994;15:627–649.
5   Smith EM, Blalock JE: The hormonal nature of the interferon system. Tex Rep Biol Med 1981; 41:350–358.
6   Blalock JE, Stanton JD: Common pathways of interferon and hormonal action. Nature 1980;283: 406–408.
7   Blalock JE, Harp C: Interferon and adrenocorticotropic hormone induction of steroidogenesis, melanogenesis and antiviral activity. Arch Virol 1981;67:45–49.
8   Blalock JE, Smith EM: Human leukocyte interferon (HuIFN-alpha): Potent endorphin-like opioid activity. Biochem Biophys Res Commun 1981;101:472–478.
9   Dafny N: Interferon as an endocoids candidate preventing and attenuating opiate addiction; in Lal H, LaBella F, Lane J (eds): Endocoids. New York, Liss, 1985, vol 192, pp 269–276.
10 Roosth J, Pollard RB, Brown SL, Meyer WJ 3d: Cortisol stimulation by recombinant interferon-alpha 2. J Neuroimmunol 1986;12:311–316.
11 Besedovsky H, del Rey A, Sorkin E, Dinarello CA: Immunoregulatory feedback between interleukin-1 and glucocorticoid hormones. Science 1986;233:652–654.
12 Krueger JM, Takahashi S, Kapas L, Bredow S, Roky RX, Fang J, Floyd R, Renegar KB, Guha-Thakurta N, Novitsky S: Cytokines in sleep regulation. Adv Neuroimmunol 1995;5:171–188.
13 Klir JJ, McClellan JL, Kluger MJ: Interleukin-1 beta causes the increase in anterior hypothalamic interleukin-6 during LPS-induced fever in rats. Am J Physiol 1994;266:RI845–1848.
14 Maness LM, Banks WA, Zadina JE, Kastin AJ: Selective transport of blood-borne interleukin-1 alpha into the posterior division of the spectrum of the mouse brain. Brain Res Dev Brain Res 1995;700:83–88.
15 Woloski BM, Smith EM, Meyer WJ 3d, Fuller GM, Blalock JE: Corticotropin-releasing activity of monokines. Science 1985;230:1035–1037.
16 Berkenbosch F, van Oers J, del Rey A, Tilders FX, Besedovsky H: Corticotropin-releasing factor-producing neurons in the rat activated by interleukin-1. Science 1987;238:524–526.

17 Koenig JI, Snow K, Clark BD, Toni R, Cannon JG, Shaw AR, Dinarello CA, Reichlin S, Lee SL: Intrinsic pituitary interleukin-1 beta is induced by bacterial lipopolysaccharide (published erratum appears in Endocrinology 1990;127:657). Endocrinology 1990;126:3053–3058.

18 Laye S, Parnet P, Goujon E, Dantzer R: Peripheral administration of lipopolysaccharide induces the expression of cytokine transcripts in the brain and pituitary of mice. Brain Res Dev Brain Res 1994; Mol Brain Res:157–162.

19 Takao T, Nakata H, Tojo C, Kurokawa H, Nishioka T, Hashimoto K, de Souza EB: Regulation of interleukin-1 receptors and hypothalamic-pituitary-adrenal axis by lipopolysaccharide treatment in the mouse. Brain Res Dev Brain Res 1994;649:265–270.

20 Takao T, Culp SG, De Souza EB: Reciprocal modulation of interleukin-1 beta (IL-1 beta) and IL-1 receptors by lipopolysaccharide (endotoxin) treatment in the mouse brain-endocrine-immune axis. Endocrinology 1993;132:1497–1504.

21 Ban E, Marquette C, Sarrieau A, Fitzpatrick F, Fillion G, Milon GX, Rostene W, Haour F: Regulation of interleukin-1 receptor expression in mouse brain and pituitary by lipopolysaccharide and glucocorticoids. Neuroendocrinology 1993;58:581–587.

22 Ban E, Milon G, Prudhomme N, Fillion G, Haour F: Receptors for interleukin-1 (alpha and beta) in mouse brain: Mapping and neuronal localization in hippocampus. Neuroscience 1991;43:21–30.

23 Haour F, Marquette C, Ban E, Crumeyrolle-Arias MX, Rostene W, Tsiang H, Fillion G: Receptors for interleukin-1 in the central nervous and neuroendocrine systems: Role in infection and stress. Ann Endocrinol (Paris) 1995;56:173–179.

24 Haour F, Marquette C, Tsiang H, Ban E, Crumeyrolle-Arias M, Rostene W, Fillion G: Interleukin-1 receptors in brain and pituitary: Characterization and modulation during infection and stress. Ann NY Acad Sci 1994;741:324–337.

25 Parnet P, Amindari S, Wu C, Brunke-Reese D, Goujon E, Weyhenmeyer JAX, Dantzer R, Kelley KW: Expression of type I and type II interleukin-1 receptors in mouse brain. Brain Res Dev Brain Res 1994; Mol Brain Res:63–70.

26 Parnet P, Brunke DL, Goujon E, Mainard JD, Biragyn A, Arkins SX, Dantzer R, Kelley KW: Molecular identification of two types of interleukin–1 receptors in the murine pituitary gland. J Neuroendocrinol 1993;4:213–219.

27 Webster EL, Tracey DE, De Souza EB: Upregulation of interleukin-1 receptors in mouse AtT-20 pituitary tumor cells following treatment with corticotropin-releasing factor. Endocrinology 1991; 129:2796–2798.

28 Fagarasan MO, Arora PK, Axelrod J: Interleukin-1 potentiation of beta-endorphin secretion and the dynamics of interleukin-1 internalization in pituitary cells. Prog Neuro-Psychopharmacol Biol Psychiatry 1991;15:551–560.

29 Fagarasan MO, Aiello F, Muegge K, Durum S, Axelrod J: Interleukin 1 induces beta-endorphin secretion via Fos and Jun in AtT-20 pituitary cells. Proc Natl Acad Sci USA 1990;87:7871–7874.

30 Fagarasan MO, Bishop JF, Rinaudo MS, Axelrod J: Interleukin 1 induces early protein phosphorylation and requires only a short exposure for late induced secretion of beta-endorphin in a mouse pituitary cell line. Proc Natl Acad Sci USA 1990;87:2555–2559.

31 Fagarasan MO, Axelrod J: Interleukin-1 amplifies the action of pituitary secretagogues via protein kinases. Int J Neurosci 1990;51:311–313.

32 Fagarasan MO, Axelrod J, Catt KJ: Interleukin 1 potentiates agonist-induced secretion of beta-endorphin in anterior pituitary cells. Biochem Biophys Res Commun 1990;173:988–993.

33 Fagarasan MO, Eskay R, Axelrod J: Interleukin 1 potentiates the secretion of beta-endorphin induced by secretagogues in a mouse pituitary cell line (AtT-20). Proc Natl Acad Sci USA 1989; 86:2070–2073.

34 Ban E, Haour F, Lenstra R: Brain interleukin 1 gene expression induced by peripheral lipopolysaccharide administration. Cytokine 1992;4:48–54.

35 Kent S, Bluthe RM, Dantzer R, Hardwick AJ, Kelley KWX, Rothwell NJ, Vannice JL: Different receptor mechanisms mediate the pyrogenic and behavioral effects of interleukin 1. Proc Natl Acad Sci USA 1992;89:9117–9120.

36 Bernton EW, Beach JE, Holaday JW, Smallridge RC, Fein HG: Release of multiple hormones by a direct action of interleukin-1 on pituitary cells. Science 1987;238:519–521.

37 Fukata J, Usui T, Naitoh Y, Nakai Y, Imura H: Effects of recombinant human interleukin-1 alpha, -1 beta, 2 and 6 on ACTH synthesis and release in the mouse pituitary tumor cell line AtT-20. J Endocrinol 1989;122:33–39.

38 McCann SM, Lyson K, Karanth S, Gimeno M, Belova NX, Kamat A, Rettori V: Mechanism of action of cytokines to induce the pattern of pituitary hormone secretion in infection (review). Ann NY Acad Sci 1995;771:386–395.

39 Baldwin SJ: The NF-kB and I-k B proteins: New discoveries and insights; in Paul WE, Fathman CG, Metzger H (eds): Annual Review of Immunology. Palo Alto, Annual Reviews Inc, 1996, vol 14, pp 649–683.

40 Spangelo BL, Judd AM, Isakson PC, MacLeod RM: Interleukin-1 stimulates interleukin-6 release from rat anterior pituitary cells in vitro. Endocrinology 1991;128:2685–2692.

41 Vankelecom H, Carmeliet P, Van Damme J, Billiau A, Denef C: Production of interleukin-6 by folliculo-stellate cells of the anterior pituitary gland in a histiotypic cell aggregate culture system. Neuroendocrinology 1989;49:102–106.

42 Payne LC, Weigent DA, Blalock JE: Induction of pituitary sensitivity to interleukin-1: A new function for coricotropin-releasing hormone. Biochem Biophys Res Commun 1994;198:480–484.

43 Smith EM, Morrill AC, Meyer WJ III, Blalock JE: Corticotropin releasing factor induction of leukocyte-derived immunoreactive ACTH and endorphins. Nature 1986;322:881–882.

44 Kavelaars A, Ballieux RE, Heijnen CJ: The role of IL-1 in the corticotropin-releasing factor and arginine-vasopressin-induced secretion of immunoreactive beta-endorphin by human peripheral blood mononuclear cells. J Immunol 1989;142:2338–2342.

45 Schafer M, Mousa SA, Zhang Q, Carter L, Stein C: Expression of corticotropin-releasing factor in inflamed tissue is required for intrinsic peripheral opioid analgesia. Proc Natl Acad Sci USA 1996;93:6096–6100.

46 Schafer M, Carter L, Stein C: Interleukin 1 beta and corticotropin-releasing factor inhibit pain by releasing opioids from immune cells in inflamed tissue. Proc Natl Acad Sci USA 1994;91:4219–4223.

47 Bhardwaj RS, Luger TA: Proopiomelanocortin production by epidermal cells: Evidence for an immune neuroendocrine network in the epidermis. Arch Dermatol Res 1994;287:85–90.

48 Payne LC, Krueger JM: Interactions of cytokines with the hypothalamus-pituitary axis. J Immunother 1992;12:171–173.

49 Sauer J, Stalla GK, Muller OA, Arzt E: Inhibition of interleukin-2-mediated lymphocyte activation in patients with Cushing's syndrome: A comparison with hypocortisolemic patients. Neuroendocrinology 1994;59:144–151.

50 Renner U, Newton CJ, Pagotto U, Sauer J, Arzt E, Stalla GK: Involvement of interleukin-1 and interleukin-1 receptor antagonist in rat pituitary cell growth regulation. Endocrinology 1995;136: 3186–3193.

51 De M, Sanford TR, Wood GW: Interleukin-1, interleukin-6, and tumor necrosis factor alpha are produced in the mouse uterus during the estrous cycle and are induced by estrogen and progesterone. Dev Biol 1992;151:297–305.

52 Li ZG, Danis VA, Brooks PM: Effect of gonadal steroids on the production of IL-1 and IL-6 by blood mononuclear cells in vitro. Clin Exp Rheumatol 1993;11:157–162.

53 Smith EM, Ebaugh MJ: Neuroimmunoendocrinology and sexual dimorphism of the immune response; in Bronson RA, Alexander NJ, Anderson D, Branch DW, Kutteh WH (eds): Reproductive Immunology. Cambridge, Blackwell Science, 1996, pp 103–126.

54 Watkins LR, Goehler LE, Relton JK, Tartaglia N, Silbert L, Martin D, Maier SF: Blockade of interleukin-1 induced hyperthermia by subdiaphragmatic vagotomy: Evidence for vagal mediation of immune-brain communication. Neurosci Lett 1995;183:27–31.

55 Bluthe RM, Pawlowski M, Suarez S, Parnet P, Pittman Q, Kelley KWX, Dantzer R: Synergy between tumor necrosis factor alpha and interleukin-1 in the induction of sickness behavior in mice. Psychoneuroendocrinology 1994;19:197–207.

56 Goehler LE, Relton J, Maier SF, Watkins LR: Biotinylated interleukin-1 receptor antagonist (IL-1ra) labels paraganglia in the rat liver hilus and hepatic vagus. Proc Soc Neurosci 1994;220: in press.

57 Brown SL, Smith LR, Blalock JE: Interleukin 1 and interleukin 2 enhance proopiomelanocortin gene expression in pituitary cells. J Immunol 1987;139:3181–3183.

58   Denicoff KD, Durkin TM, Lotze MT, Quinlan PE, Davis CLX, Listwak SJ, Rosenberg SA, Rubinow DR: The neuroendocrine effects of interleukin-2 treatment. J Clin Endocrinol Metab 1989;69: 402–410.

59   Arzt E, Stelzer G, Renner U, Lange M, Muller OA, Stalla GK: Interleukin-2 and interleukin-2 receptor expression in human corticotrophic adenoma and murine pituitary cell cultures. J Clin Invest 1992;90:1944–1951.

60   Smith LR, Brown SL, Blalock JE: Interleukin-2 induction of ACTH secretion: Presence of an interleukin-2 receptor alpha-chain-like molecule on pituitary cells. J Neuroimmunol 1989;21:249– 254.

61   Arzt E, Buric R, Stelzer G, Stalla J, Sauer J, Renner U, Stalla GK: Interleukin involvement in anterior pituitary cell growth regulation: Effects of IL-2 and IL-6. Endocrinology 1993;132:459–467.

62   Komorowski J, Stepien H, Pawlikowski M: Increased interleukin-2 levels during standard TRH test in man. Neuropeptides 1994;27:151–156.

63   Kung AW, Lai CL, Wong KL, Tam CF: Thyroid functions in patients treated with interleukin-2 and lymphokine-activated killer cells. Q J Med 1992;82:33–42.

64   Geiger K, Sarvetnick N: The influence of cytokines on the central nervous system of transgenic mice. Curr Top Microbiol Immunol 1996;206:101–117.

65   Lafortune L, Nalbantoglu J, Antel JP: Expression of tumor necrosis factor alpha (TNF alpha) and interleukin 6 (IL-6) mRNA in adult human astrocytes: Comparison with adult microglia and fetal astrocytes. J Neuropathol Exp Neurol 1996;55:515–521.

66   Liao J, Keiser JA, Scales WE, Kunkel SL, Kluger MJ: Role of epinephrine in TNF and IL-6 production from isolated perfused rat liver. Am J Physiol 1995;268:R896–901.

67   Norris JG, Tang LP, Sparacio SM, Benveniste EN: Signal transduction pathways mediating astrocyte IL-6 induction by IL-1 beta and tumor necrosis factor-alpha. J Immunol 1994;152:841–850.

68   Matsumoto H, Koyama C, Sawada T, Koike K, Hirota KX, Miyake A, Arimura A, Inoue K: Pituitary folliculo-stellate-like cell line (TtT/GF) responds to novel hypophysiotropic peptide (pituitary adenylate cyclase-activating peptide), showing increased adenosine 3′,5′-monophosphate and interleukin-6 secretion and cell proliferation. Endocrinology 1993;133:2150–2155.

69   Jones TH, Daniels M, James RA, Justice SK, McCorkle RX, Price A, Kendall-Taylor P, Weetman AP: Production of bioactive and immunoreactive interleukin-6 (IL-6) and expression of IL-6 messenger ribonucleic acid by human pituitary adenomas. J Clin Endocrinol Metab 1994;78:180–187.

70   Sawada T, Koike K, Kanda Y, Ikegami H, Jikihara H, Maeda T, Osako Y, Hirota K, Miyake A: Interleukin-6 stimulates cell proliferation of rat pituitary clonal cell lines in vitro. J Endocrinol Invest 1995;18:83–90.

71   Campbell IL: Neuropathogenic actions of cytokines assessed in transgenic mice. Int J Dev Neurosci 1995;13:275–284.

72   Moore KW, O'Garra A, de Waal Malefyt R, Vieira PX, Mosmann TR: Interleukin-10. Ann Rev Immunol 1993;11:165–190.

73   Mosmann TR: Properties and functions of interleukin-10. Adv Immunol 1994;56:1–26.

74   Vieira P, de Waal-Malefyt R, Dang MN, Johnson KEX, Kastelein R, Fiorentino DF, deVries JE, Roncarolo MG, Mosmann TR, Moore KW: Isolation and expression of human cytokine synthesis inhibitory factor cDNA clones: Homology to Epstein-Barr virus open reading frame BCRFI. Proc Natl Acad Sci USA 1991;88:1172–1176.

75   Oates EL, Allaway GP, Armstrong GR, Boyajian RA, Kehrl JH, Prabhakar BS: Human lymphocytes produce pro-opiomelanocortin gene-related transcripts: Effects of lymphotropic viruses. J Biol Chem 1988;263:10041–10044.

76   Johnson HM, Torres BA, Smith EM, Dion LD, Blalock JE: Regulation of lymphokine (gamma-interferon) production by corticotropin. J Immunol 1984;132:246–250.

77   Hughes TK, Cadet P, Rady PL, Tyring SK, Chin R, Smith EM: Evidence for the production and action of interleukin-10 pituitary cells. Cell Mol Neurobiol 1994;14:59–69.

78   Rady PL, Smith EM, Cadet P, Opp MR, Tyring SK, Hughes TK Jr: Presence of interleukin-10 transcripts in human pituitary and hypothalamus. Cell Mol Neurobiol 1995;15:289–296.

79   Nitta T, Hishii M, Sato K, Okumura K: Selective expression of interleukin-10 gene within glioblastoma multiforme. Brain Res Dev Brain Res 1994;649:122–128.

80   Mizuno T, Sawada M, Suzumura A, Marunouchi T: Expression of cytokines during glial differentiation. Brain Res Dev Brain Res 1994;656:141–146.
81   Opp MR, Smith EM, Hughes TK Jr: Interleukin-10 (cytokine synthesis inhibitory factor) acts in the central nervous system of rats to reduce sleep. J Neuroimmunol 1995;60:165–168.
82   Kuhn R, Lohler J, Rennick D, Rajewsky K, Muller W: Interleukin-10-deficient mice develop chronic enterocolitis. Cell 1993;75:263–274.
83   Di Santo E, Sironi M, Pozzi P, Gnocchi P, Isetta AMX, Delvaux A, Goldman M, Marchant A, Ghezzi P: Interleukin-10 inhibits lipopolysaccharide-induced tumor necrosis factor and interleukin-1 beta production in the brain without affecting the activation the hypothalamus-pituitary-adrenal axis. Neuroimmunomodulation 1995;2:149–154.
84   Sharp BM, Matta SG, Peterson PK, Newton R, Chao CX, Mcallen K: Tumor necrosis factor-alpha is a potent ACTH secretagogue: Comparison to interleukin-1 beta. Endocrinology 1989;124: 3131–3133.
85   Hunt JS: Expression and regulation of the tumor necrosis factor-alpha gene in the female reproductive tract. Reprod Fertil Dev 1993;5:141–153.
86   Pedersen AM, Fulton SK, Porter L, Francis GL: Tumor necrosis factor-alpha affects in vitro hormone production by JEG-3 choriocarcinoma cell cultures. J Reprod Immunol 1995;29:69–80.
87   Garcia-Lloret MI, Morrish DW, Wegmannn TG, Honore L, Turner AR, Guilbert LJ: Demonstration of functional cytokine-placental interactions: CSF-1 and GM-CSF stimulate human cytotrophoblast differentiation and peptide hormone secretion. Exp Cell Res 1994;214:46–54.
88   Akita S, Webster J, Ren SG, Takino H, Said J, Zand O, Melmed S: Human and murine pituitary expression of leukemia inhibitory factor: Novel intrapituitary regulation of adrenocorticotropin hormone synthesis and secretion. J Clin Invest 1995;95:1288–1298.
89   Tyring SK: Introduction to clinical uses of interferons; in Baron S (ed): Interterons: Principles and Medical Applications. Galveston, UTMB, 1992, pp 399–407.
90   Quesada JR: Toxicity and side effects of interferons; in Baron S (ed): Interferon: Principles and Medical Applications. Galveston, UTMB, 1992, pp 427–432.
91   Nolten WE, Goldstein D, Lindstrom M, McKenna MV, Carlson IH, Trump DL, Schiller J, Borden EC, Ehrlich EN: Effects of cytokines on the pituitary-adrenal axis in cancer patients. J Interferon Res 1993;13:349–357.
92   Lissoni P, Rovelli F, Tisi E, Ardizzoia A, Perlangeli V, Barni S, Tancini G: Endocrine effects of human recombinant interleukin-3 in cancer patients. Int J Biol Markers 1992;7:230–233.
93   Chernoff AE, Granowitz EV, Shapiro L, Vannier EX, Lonnemann G, Angel JB, Kennedy JS, Rabson AR, Wolff SM, Dinarello CA: A randomized, controlled trial of IL-10 in humans. Inhibition of inflammatory cytokine production and immune responses. J Immunol 1995;154:5492–5499.
94   Smith EM: Corticotropin and immunoregulation; in Scharrer B, Smith EM, Stefano GB (eds): Neuropeptides and Immunoregulation. Berlin, Springer, 1994, pp 28–45.

Eric M Smith, PhD, University of Texas Medical Branch, Department of Psychiatry,
Galveston, TX 77555-0428 (USA)
Tel (409) 772 6747, Fax (409) 772 3511

Blalock JE (ed): Neuroimmunoendocrinology, 3rd rev ed.
Chem Immunol. Basel, Karger, 1997, vol 69, pp 203–222

···················

Interactive Signaling Pathways of the Neuroendocrine-Immune Network

Thomas L. Roszman, William H. Brooks

Department of Microbiology and Immunology, University of Kentucky Medical
Center, Lexington, Ky., USA

Introduction

Evidence continues to accumulate indicating that interaction between the
neuroendocrine and immune systsems has potential biological significance.
Similar to the well-described hormonal loops within the endocrine system,
neuroendocrine-immune interactions would be anticipated to involve feedback
and feedforward loops thus maintaining homeostasis. These bidirectional
loops occur as a consequence of neurohormones (NH) acting on cells of the
immune system while cytokines or antibodies secreted by lymphocytes and
macrophages in turn influence neuroendocrine function. It is important to
note that such interactions are not only inhibitory but facilitory as well,
fulfilling important teleologic considerations. Furthermore, examination of
data related to neuroendocrine-immune interactions reveals that under physiologic conditions alterations occurring in either system generally are small both
in magnitude and duration, thereby suggesting the existence of a homeostatic
relationship between these two systems. The ability of one system to dominate
the other would lead to chaos. Similar to all biological regulatory systems this
interaction should exhibit the ability to generate an amplified response to low
levels of stimuli as well as manifest the ability to adapt to prolonged high levels
of stimuli further underscoring the function of these systems as maintaining
homeostasis within the host.

The focus of this review is to amplify these concepts and pose questions concerning the relationship between the neuroendocrine and immune systems with
emphasis on possible mechanisms of how NH modulate lymphocyte function.

Supported in part by NIH grant AI-38568 and a Research Scientist Award K05
MH01069 to Thomas L. Roszman.

Can the Pituitary Gland Modulate the Immune System?

It is reasonable to hypothesize that if the pituitary gland can influence the immune system, then its absence or removal should result in detectable alterations in immunity. Indeed, there are a number of reports using different approaches which support this contention. Two ways this problem have been approached is to examine the immune potential of either hypophysectomized animals or through the use of hypopituitary mice. The majority of these studies but not all [1–4], show that hypophysectomized animals exhibited impaired humoral [5–8] and cell-mediated immunity [7–11]. A number of similar immunologic studies have been done with hypopituitary Snell-Bagg mice. These mice generally exhibit a decrease in the number of lymphocytes in the thymus, bone marrow and peripheral lymphoid with accompanying impairment in both humoral and cell-mediated immune responses [12–18], although there are reports indicating that the immune system of these animals is normal [19, 20].

Recently, we examined the immunologic characteristics and responsiveness of the Snell-Bagg dwarf mice [21]. The results show that the immunologic competency of these animals is entirely dependent on when the animals are weaned and the age at which they are examined immunologically. Thus, dwarf mice weaned at 21 days of age and sacrificed at that time or 7 days later have decreased numbers of splenocytes and thymocytes as well as impaired responsiveness to concanavalin A as compared to heterozygous littermates. However, splenocytes obtained from these dwarf mice responded normally to lipopolysaccharide. If the dwarf mice weaned on day 21 of age are analyzed at 32 days of age or weaned at day 30 of age and analyzed 7 days later, their ability to respond to mitogen stimulation does not differ from control animals. No anomaly was noted in the percentage of CD4+/CD8+ thymocytes as well as CD4+ or CD8+ thymocytes in dwarf mice weaned at 30 days of age and sacrificed 7 days later. Of considerable interest is the observation that dwarf mice weaned at 30 days of age and sacrificed 7 days later had a normal V-β T-cell receptor repertoire. Moreover, the dwarf mice responded normally to primary immunization with sheep red blood. Collectively, these data indicate that hypopituitary dwarf mice are immunologically normal.

In general, there have been few if any, attempts to examine at the mechanistic level the effects of hypophysectomy on immune function. However, it is clear that a hypophysectomized animal can be immunologically reconstituted by a number of relatively straightforward maneuvers including the administration of either growth hormone or prolactin, as well as ectopic pituitary grafts [22–24]. The immunomodulatory role of these hormones is further substantiated by the observation that implantation of GH_3 pituitary tumor cells into aged syngeneic rats results in cellular and functional restoration of the thymus to levels comparable to that of 3-month-old animals [25]. Although direct proof is lacking, the presumption is that this restoration results from the production of prolactin and growth hormone by the GH_3 tumor cells. We have demonstrated that normal C57BL/6 mice given pituitary grafts under the kidney capsule, which have a 2- to 3-fold sustained increase in prolactin, have markedly greater primary antibody responses to sheep red blood cells as compared to normal values [26]. Interestingly, placement of pituitary grafts under the kidney capsule of 24-month-old mice does not result in cellular or functional restoration of the thymus to comparable levels observed in young animals, suggesting that prolactin may not have a role in this process [27].

There is other evidence sugesting that the pituitary gland has a key role in modulating immune function. We initiated a series of experiments directed at confirming earlier reports that anterior hypothalamic ablation is associated with diminished immune reactivity [28]. In these studies we demonstrated that electrolytic lesioning of the anterior hypothalamic areas of rats induces a decrease in the numbers of nucleated spleen cells and thymocytes as compared to control lesioned and normal animals [29]. This modulation extends also to mitogen [29] and antigen-driven lymphocyte proliferation (30) as well as natural killer cell function [11]. The observed diminished immune reactivity was short-lived, returning to normal within 14 days. Exploration of other areas of the brain indicated that in addition to areas that are associated with down-regulation of immunity, there are specific areas (hippocampus and amygdaloid complex) that facilitate lymphocyte reactivity with a markedly enhanced proliferative response [31]. These effects also disappeared by 14 days after lesioning. The acuteness of the effects is attributed to the remarkable plasticity of the central nervous system (CNS) and the subsequent re-establishment of dendritic-axonal networks [32].

From these experiments demonstrating that changes in the CNS function can be correlated with alterations in immune reactivity, we began the search for the functional link between the CNS and mediators of immunity. We have shown that modulation of immunity by neural lesions is not related to changes in corticosterone [29]; yet certain pituitary-derived hormones are influenced by anterior hypothalamic lesions and these are capable of impairing cellular activation. To test this hypothesis, neurally induced changes in lymphocyte responsiveness were assessed before and after hypophysectomy [33]. The results of these investigations suggest that the CNS is capable of modulating splenocyte blastogenesis and number via the endocrine system because pituitary removal abrogates both the inhibitory as well as the facilitory immunologic effects induced by neural lesions. In a similar system [34], we have also examined the effects of 'chemical' neural lesions produced by the cisterna magna injection of 6-hydroxydopamine (6-OHDA). Treatment of animals with 6-OHDA 48 h prior to immunization results in a profound suppression of the primary IgM and IgG antibody response which is not the result of increased levels of corticosterone. However, if 6-OHDA is injected into hypophysectomized mice 48 h prior to immunization, the primary antibody response is not impaired compared to the response of noncatecholamine-depleted hypophysectomized mice [35]. These results strongly suggest that modulation of the immune response as a consequence of central catecholamine depletion is emanating from the pituitary gland.

Collectively, these data indicate that the pituitary gland via the hormones it elaborates has a decided modulatory effect on immune function. Precisely how these hormones can modulate immunity remains to be determined. In fact there are few, if any, experiments which probe the mechanism of action of hypophysectomy on immune function. For example, does hypophysectomy influence immune function by inducing alterations in the balance between helper-suppressor circuits, TH1 vs. TH2 responses, lymphocyte maturation or cell trafficking? It is clear that the immunosuppressive effects of hypophysec-tomy can be overcome by either growth hormone or prolactin [22, 24] thus possibly providing an important clue as to the mechanisms responsible for this effect. While hypophysectomy does establish the importance of neurohor-mones in modulating immune function, it may be difficult to use this approach to decipher the precise mechanism. Removal of the pituitary gland causes a compounding number of changes in the normal physiology of the animal thereby making it difficult to determine precisely what factor or combination of factors are responsible for the observed alterations in immune function.

Are There Receptors for Neurohormones (NH) Present on Cells of the Immune System?

Data implicating the pituitary gland in modulating antigen independent and dependent maturation of the immune system suggest that NH have a vital role in this process. A pivotal concept in neuroendocrine-lymphocyte interactions is the presence of receptors in or on cells of the immune system. Therefore, if NH are to modulate immune function there must be external and/or internal receptors for these peptides in order for the cells of the immune system to receive and subsequently interpret the putative signal and, there is evidence for such receptors on these cells. Because the results of these studies have been reviewed often and recently [23, 36–47] only salient features required to illustrate certain points will be highlighted. Some of the better characterized receptors for pituitary-derived hormones reported to be detectable on

Table 1. Receptors for pituitary hormones on cells of the immune system

Hormone	Source of cells	References
Prolactin	human T cells, B cells, monocytes or thymocytes	50–53, 57
	rat splenocytes, bone marrow, lymph node and peripheral blood lymphocytes	54
	murine splenocytes, lymph node or peripheral blood lymphocytes	55, 56
Growth hormone	human lymphocyte cell line IM-9	61, 60
	human peripheral blood T cells, B cells and monocytes	62, 64
	murine lymphoid cells	63
	calf and mouse thymocytes	65
β-Endorphin	cultured human lymphocytes	66
	human peripheral blood lymphocytes	67, 68
	mouse thymocytes	69
	monkey thymocytes	70
ACTH	mouse splenic mononuclear cells	71
	human mononuclear lymphocytes	72
	rat T and B cells	73
Thyrotropin	human monocytes and polymorphonuclear leukocytes	74
	human monocytes, natural killer cells, and activated B cells	75

lymphoid and myeloid cells are listed in table 1. Although these data provide presumptive evidence for the presence of neurohormone receptors, there is clearly a need for confirmatory studies using antibodies and molecular probes. Recently, these data have been forthcoming for the presence of prolactin, growth hormone or opioid receptors on lymphocytes. The availability of a panel of monoclonal antibodies (mAb) to the prolactin receptor [48, 49] has revealed that these receptors are found on thymocytes and peripheral T and B cells [53–57]. Between 80 and 90% of thymocytes from either rats or mice are prolactin receptor positive [54, 56] while about 75% human peripheral blood T cells and thymocytes are stained with antiprolactin receptor mAb [57]. Additionally, using reverse transcription with the polymerase chain reaction the expression of the prolactin receptor gene has been shown in human T cells, B cells and monocytes [53] and in murine thymocytes and splenocytes [58]. The expression of mRNA for both the long and short form of the prolactin receptor is detected in rat peripheral blood lymphocytes [59]. The presence of growth hormone receptors were first detected on IM-9 lymphocytes using ^{125}I-growth hormone [60, 61]. More recently, these receptors have been detected on lymphocyte subsets using fluorochrome-labeled growth hormone [62, 63] or a mAb to the receptor [64]. The presence of opioid receptors on lymphocytes is less well-established. The opioid family of peptides can bind to three classes of membrane receptors termed μ, δ and κ. There are numerous reports using a variety of techniques indicating the presence of these receptors on lymphocytes [66–70]. Recently, the identification of κ transcripts were detected in human peripheral blood lymphocytes and monocytes [68] and δ transcripts in monkey lymphocytes [70]. The presence of κ receptors were detected on mouse thymocytes using a high-affinity fluorescein-conjugated opioid ligand [69]. These results correlate with the observation that κ receptors can be detected on human peripheral blood lymphocytes using a κ receptor mAb [Morgan, pers. commun.]. In addition, receptors for ACTH [71–73] and thyrotropin [74, 75] have been detected on lymphocytes as well as monocytes. These studies illustrate a number of important corollaries concerning the presence of neurohormone receptors on lymphocytes. For example, these receptors may be differentially expressed on certain subsets of T cells; not all lymphocytes may possess neurohormone receptors and hence would be refractory to hormonal modulation. Moreover, expression of neurohormone receptors may be autoregulated during activation of the lymphocyte; an increase in receptor expression might amplify the effects of neurohormones on cellular function whereas a diminution or loss of receptors would be expected to have an opposing effect. Finally, although the utility of employing cloned T-cell lines or lymphoblastoid cells have obvious advantages, it is important to realize that the presence of neurohormone receptors on these 'transformed' cells does not guarantee their presence on normal lymphocytes.

Can NH Influence the Immune System?

The biological significance of the presence of neurohormone receptors on the cells of the immune system is supported by the in vitro and in vivo evidence attesting to the ability of NH to modify cellular behavior. Because there are a number of comprehensive recent reviews regarding the effects of NH on immune function [22–24, 38–40, 43–46, 76–82], we will restrict our comments to a general overview of the phenomenology revealed by these studies. One readily apparent observation drawn from these studies is that NH have broad immunomodulatory effects on various types of cells involved in the immune response. For example, β-endorphin alters the function of lymphocytes, natural killer cells, macrophages, polymorphonuclear cells and mast cells [43]. Moreover, the effects of a specific NH on cell function can either be facilitory or inhibitory [43, 45, 76, 79]. This appears to be a general pattern for most NH. Overall, these data imply that the various and diverse cells encompassing the immune system have receptors for NH and that the biochemical and molecular signals elicited in these cells as a consequence of ligand-receptor interactions are differentially encoded and interpreted. Unfortunately, there is currently a paucity of data to substantiate this hypothesis; more research is required to clarify these interesting but confounding observations. This will not be a trivial undertaking considering the complexity of the immune system and its cells, compounded by the fact that many NH exert only modest alterations in immune function.

How Do NH Modulate T-Cell Function?

During the last 10 years, evidence has accrued to establish that lymphocytes have high affinity receptors for NH. The challenge remains to elucidate how NH modulate immune function. Because we believe this to be a propitious time for initiation of these types of investigations, it is reasonable to conceptualize potential approaches to explicate these mechanisms. Although neural-immune interactions are bidirectional this presentation is concerned solely with a unidirectional approach in which considerations are limited to discussion of the potential mechanistic effects of NH on acquired immunity. Specific features of this interaction are crucial to a functional understanding of the features neuroimmunomodulation. Chief among these is the fact that the immune response displays specificity, diversity, memory; is self-regulating and can discriminate self from non-self. These collectively support the concept that the immune response is for the most part autonomous and self-regulatory. That NH can influence the outcome of immune responsiveness has been demonstrated, yet the question remains unanswered as to the extent and exactly how this is accomplished. In accordance with the experimental evidence the immunomodulatory potentialities of NH are limited to 'fine tuning' and/or 'setting of the gain' of immune potential and functional. The assertion of more or a higher degree of modulatory effects on immune function by NH would theoretically promote immunologic chaos for which experimental data are lacking and moreover would be deleterious to the host.

In this discussion of the potential mechanisms responsible for this form of neuroimmunomodulation, we will restrict our comments to acquired immunity involving CD4+ T cells. These T-cell subpopulations are central to many cellular events required for acquired immunity including the activation and function of B cells and CD8+ T cells. It must be emphasized that it is not implied that natural immunity is refractory to modulation by NH. Indeed, growth hormone has a facilitory effect on phorbol ester-induced superoxide production by polymorphonuclear cells [83]. Although a teleological argument or the existence of NH modulation of natural immunity may be presented, further evidence is required. Similarly, the effects of NH on T-cell and B-cell development and lymphocyte trafficking remain in an embryonic stage of investigation. These nonetheless are fertile and interesting areas for future study.

The CD4 + T-cell subpopulation is a complex mixture of phenotypic and functional lymphocytes which occupy a central position in cell-mediated and humoral immunity. Influences of immune responsiveness contingent on the interaction of pituitary-derived hormones with these pivotal T-cell subpopulations provide the infrastructure for those investigators exploring the mechanisms of neuroimmunomodulation. The initiation of an antigenic specific response; transition from the acquisition of competency to generation of appropriate signaling required for progression and proliferation; and, differentiation of abilities of CD4 + T-cell subsets to promote specific types of immune responses (cellular vs. humoral) are sensitive avenues of the immune pathway that may be open to the modulatory effects of NH.

Naive CD4 + T cells require two signals (two signal model) for the induction of proliferation and differentiation into effector cells [84]. The initial signal is delivered to the T-cell receptor (TCR) complex which recognizes antigenic peptide fragments bound to the major histocompatibility complex II (MHC). The second signal which is neither specific nor interacts with the TCR is termed the costimulatory signal. One of the most important of these costimulatory signals results from the ligation of CD28 on CD4 + T cells with either B7 or B7.2 present on antigen presenting cells. A naive CD4 + T cell that receives only the first signal (one signal model) undergoes apoptosis or becomes anergic [85]. Subsequent to receiving appropriate signals from antigen and costimulators, the CD4 + T cell begins to progress from the Go phase of the cell cycle. As CD4 + T cells move into the cell cycle they must pass through an important restriction point at the G1/S interface. At this juncture, antigen stimulated T cells must synthesis and secrete interleukin 2 (IL-2) and upregulate the high-affinity IL-2 receptor (IL-2R). The binding of IL-2 to its receptor allows the CD4 + T cell to pass through the G1/S restriction point into the cell cycle. Interestingly, the cellular receptors for growth hormone and prolactin belong to the type I cytokine receptor family (hematopoietic receptors) which also includes the IL-2R. This is discussed in detail in the chapter by Walter [this vol.]. After the naive CD4 + T cell undergoes activation and differentiation, it may return to a resting state where it is referred to as a memory or activated T cell. These activated/memory CD4 + T cells differ both phenotypically and functionally from naive CD4 + T cells. One phenotypic difference between the two types is that activated T cells are CD45RO + while naive cells remain with a CD45RA + marker. Additionally, activated T cell also express more lymphocyte function antigen-1. Importantly, these memory T cells can become activated upon binding antigen-MHC on the surface of an antigen-presenting cell in the absence of costimulatory signals. The CD4+ T cells can be induced to differentiate into TH1 or TH2 subsets which have different functions. The TH2-type helper cell is responsible for promoting B-cell proliferation and differentiation into antibody producing cells during the humoral immune response while TH1 cells secrete macrophage activating cytokines thus supporting the acquisition of cell-mediated immunity. Because there are no known phenotypic markers to differentiate between these two T-cell subsets, TH1- and TH2-type activity currently is distinguished via cytokine secretion profiles. The molecular events associated with differentiation of naive CD4 T cells into TH1- and TH2-type helper function remains to be determined although cytokines, costimulatory molecules and antigen concentration all seemingly are important [86]. The differentiation of CD4+ T cells in accordance with their abilities to promote specific types of immune response, e.g. cellular or humoral, is one area where pituitary-derived hormones may modulate immune readiness.

Thus, immune responsiveness, cellular and humoral, is dependent on the activation and differentiation of CD4+ T cells within a microenvironment of antigen, costimulatory molecules and cytokines. These interactions ultimately lead to a variety of outcomes for the CD4+ T cell including effector cell function, anergy and/or apoptosis. Each developmental stage of this process provides a focal point for the interdiction of pituitary-derived hormones to modulate the ensuing response. The ability of a NH to productively interact with its specific receptor on CD4+ T cells and subsequently exert a perceivable effect on immune function is dependent on a number of variables. These include: (i) the sensitivity of the CD4+ T cells to NH-derived signals which in part is dependent on the quantitative and qualitative nature of neurohormone receptor; (ii) the physiologic state of the CD4+ T cell at the time of interaction with NH which would be reflected in alterations in the normal biochemical and molecular cascades on which lymphocyte function is contingent, and (iii) derivation of the teleologic and/or homeostatic advantages of NH-lymphocyte interaction. When considered as a mediating influence within the processes of the development of immunity these variables would be expected to be operant in a biologic milieu (noise) influencing the potential sensitivity and magnitude amplification of CD4+ T-cell function and finally modulate the amplitude of the subsequent response.

Neurohormone-CD4 T-Cell Interactions: Signaling Models

There is a substantial wealth of information describing the effects of pituitary hormones on a variety of immune parameters [81, 82]. The majority of these studies are phenomenologic in nature but nonetheless contribute in important ways to describe and define the limits of the immunomodulatory potential of NH. Therefore, the question no longer turns on whether this form of neuroimmunomodulation exists, but rather on how it is effected mechanistically. In considering possible approaches to unraveling the mechanisms of neuroendocrine-immune modulation we have found it useful to develop models which may serve as a template for subsequent inquiry. We have modified previously described models by casting them in terms of the one and two immune signal model of antigen activation of CD4+ T cells. It is within the context of this model of immunological activation that NH must act in order to be capable of influencing T-cell function. Furthermore, these models represent an extension of the tenets of neurohormone-CD4+ T-cell interaction as discussed previously and are based on the integrated biologic systems of signal amplification and the cascade of biochemical and molecular events which result in modulation of function and adaptability.

The binding of a NH to its receptor on CD4+ T cells results in the generation of a biochemical and molecular wave of intracellular events through the cell. This is dependent on the local concentration of NH as well as the number and affinity of the specific neurohormone receptor on the exposed T cell. Thus, a rise in the concentration of NH above normal steady state levels is anticipated to induce a magnitude amplification of intracellular biochemical cascades dependent on the number of molecules of NH bound to its receptor found on the CD4+ T cells. For example, 500 molecules of NH binding to their specific receptor could, for example, elicit 10^4 molecules of a specific second messenger. If this sould occur in a resting CD4+ T cell concurrently receiving no immune signaling, the biochemical cascade of activity should have no persisting biologic effect on lymphocyte function. Although interactions of the NH with the CD4+ T cell may result in a number of diverse biochemical and molecular alterations within the cell, the signal is insufficient and inappropriate to activate the cell thereby promoting immune signaling and/or reactivity. This may in part be explained by the ability of the CD4+ T cell to process this biochemical information in such a manner as to abrogate any physiological effect otherwise expected after neurohormone receptor ligation. The interaction of ACTH with T cells serves as a useful illustration. As a consequence of physiological stress the concentration of circulating ACTH is increased which enhances the potential of T cells to bind this peptide [71–73] thereby eliciting the second messenger cAMP [73]. During this brief time, a resting T cell receiving no other inputs, i.e. immune signals, represents an example of the one-signal model of neuroendocrine-immune modulation. Biochemical and molecular changes occur within the cell as a result of its interaction with ACTH yet no physiological changes are observed in these resting T cells. This adaption to non-immune signals occurs through a number of well-known mechanisms including receptor desensitization downregulation, uncoupling of adenylyl cyclase and increasing cAMP phosphodiesterase. Concurrent with the return of ACTH to baseline levels, the T cell completes its biochemical adaptation and again becomes receptive to this peptide. This is precisely how the CD4+ T cell must respond to NH signaling. To do otherwise would not be homeostatic or teleologically viable and result in an unprovoked chaotic nonantigenic induced and unregulated immune response. There is no evidence that a NH can 'activate' a resting CD4+ T cell to acquire immune effector function.

A CD4+ T cell interacting with antigen-MHC class II on antigen presenting cells (immune signal 1) in the absence of costimulatory signals (immune signal 2) becomes anergized or apoptotic. Thus, a CD4+ T cell stimulated with antigen alone will not proliferate and secrete IL-2 when later restimulated with antigen and costimulatory signals (immune signal 2). However, proliferation is induced if exogenous IL-2 is provided to these anergized CD4 T cells. Although the exact biochemical and molecular details responsible for the induction of these cellular states remain to be determined [87], it is useful in explicating models of neuroimmunomodulation to speculate as to where NH may be effective in modulating CD4+ T cells which have received only the initial signal (immune signal 1) required for immune responsiveness. Because growth hormone and prolactin belong to the hematopoietic receptor superfamily which includes receptors for IL-2 through 7, it is interesting to hypothesize that either of these NH can functionally substitute for IL-2. This speculation is further strengthened by the observation that prolactin can activate RAF-1 [88] and JAK-2 [89] similar to that observed when IL-2 binds to its high affinity receptor. The availability of NH which can functionally mimic IL-2 thus activating anergic T cells would have major implications, implying a deleterious potential for growth hormone or prolactin to participate and facilitate autoimmune diseases. Indeed, there is evidence implicating these neurohormones in autoimmune disease processes [90–95], but a discussion of this is beyond the scope of this review.

Although there is no evidence that a NH can competitively inhibit the binding of either antigen or costimulatory molecules to their respective receptors on CD4 T cells, the potential interaction of NH with CD4+ T cells receiving both immune signals, antigen and costimulator, presents a number of complex and fundamentally important possibilities relating to neuroendocrine modulation of immunity. A NH potentially may bind to its respective receptors (assuming availability) on an antigen activated T cell at any time during the differentiative and proliferative process. When all three signals (immune signal 1, 2 and NH-linked) are delivered simultaneously, the CD4+ T cell is required to integrate the second messengers elicited by the NH with those emanating from stimulation of the TCR and the CD28 molecule. Those second messengers linked to the neurohormone receptor are decoded and potentially available to associate with, substitute for, or abrogate intracellular transduction events within CD4+ T cells evoked via immune signals 1 and 2. The immune responsiveness of these cells may be facilitated or inhibited depending on the cross talk, e.g. phosphorylation-dephosphorylation of molecules required for CD4+ T-cell activation and proliferation, among NH and immune-linked second messengers. Hence, attenuation or amplification of the effects of the various kinases, phosphatases and/or proteases on which an antigen driven CD4+ T-cell response is contingent would be manifest as the ability of a specific NH to modulate immunity. Indeed, evidence exists that such interactions occur among second messengers in many cells including T cells [96, 97]. For example, increasing the concentration of cAMP generally results in a decrease in the proliferative capacity of appropriately stimulated T cells. Similar observations occur when stimulated T cells are exposed to ACTH [73]. However, the interaction of NH with lymphocytes does not always result in downregulation of function. For example, prolactin can enhance in vitro and in vivo lymphocyte function and immune responsiveness [81]. Thus, altering the magnitude and kinetics of transmembrane signals linked to TCR and costimulatory ligands by second messengers and activated via the neurohormone may result in either facilitation or attenuation of CD4+ T-cell function.

The limitation of this particular model resides in the temporal frame during which NH, antigen and costimulatory ligands simultaneously bind to their respective receptors on CD4+ T cells. It is unlikely that this would occur with high frequency in vivo. Moreover, this model ignores the dynamics and autonomous regulatory complexity of the neuroendocrine and immune systems. For example, circulatory levels of NH normally vary and have a short functional half-life. Concurrently, a given number of CD4+ T cells constantly are undergoing activation. Paramount to any model of neuroimmunomodulation is consideration that most likely these signals will temporally occur asynchronously. An antigen-stimulated CD4+ T cell may receive a signal generated by NH at any time throughout the cell cycle. This interaction with NH can influence lymphocyte responsiveness in an additive or synergistic manner; the magnitude of modulation being governed by the strength of the NH-linked signals. Additionally, NH-derived signaling may alter the differentiation of CD4+ T cells into TH1 or TH2 subsets as well as influencing the secretion of cytokines specifically attributed to these subsets. Subtle abrogations of lymphocyte function would be consistent with the hypothesis that the potential exists for these hormones to incrementally modify the immune response.

Although the reality of in vitro studies indicating the potential of NH to alter lymphocyte responsiveness may be more apparent than real, this experimental approach has provided useful and important information that afford an opportunity to develop investigative models of neuroendocrine-immune interactions. For example, growth hormone and prolactin synergistically enhance the mitogen-induced responsiveness of T cells [81]. Thus, the cellular proliferative response elicited after stimulation with both NH and immune signals are significantly greater than the sum of activation induced by either NH or immune signals alone. Alternatively, ACTH can synergize with immune signals to inhibit T-cell proliferation [73]. Although these observations indicate that these signals can cross-talk at the biochemical and molecular levels, the mechanism(s) responsible for synergy remains to be established. It is possible that a particular NH binds and modulates all CD4+ T cells or that only a subset of these T cells are involved, e.g. TH1 or TH2. Furthermore, different types of signal amplification can occur during the interaction of NH with CD4+ T cells. One form of signal amplification, termed magnitude amplification, is characterized by a small concentration of stimulus eliciting a large number of effector molecules [98]. For example, a small concentration of ACTH generates a large number of cAMP molecules in the lymphocytes. The other form of signal amplification, sensitivity amplification, is characterized by a greater than expected increase in the response than that anticipated from the percentage change (increase) in the stimulus. Sensitivity amplification appears to be operant in the three signal model of neuroimmunomodulation in which a synergistic effect on the lymphocyte function is observed. Utilizing this model, it is hypothesized that the binding of a NH and immune stimulus to their respective receptors on T cells results in a far greater generation of second messengers than anticipated from a given concentration of either stimulus alone. Thus, the binding of ACTH to its receptor on a lymphocyte results in an increase in the concentration of cAMP within the cell, yet the concentration of cAMP is synergistically enhanced in lymphocytes concurrently stimulated via an immune signal and identical concentrations of ACTH. This form of signal amplification has enormous significance for neuroendocrine-immune interactions. It would suggest that large increases in circulating levels of a NH are not absolutely required to effect a change in a particular lymphocyte function. Thus, a slight increase in NH above normal homeostatic levels results in a synergistic increase in those second messengers elicited via neurohormone receptor activation in the presence of immune signaling. This synergistically enhanced cellular signaling provides a greater probability for physiological levels of NH to modulate immune responsiveness. We have initiated experiments to explore this hypothesis using resting human T cells stimulated with isoproterenol to activate the β-adrenergic receptor and phytohemagglutinin (PHA) or anti-CD3 mAb to provide the 'immune' stimulus. Stimulation of T cells with increasing concentrations of isoproterenol results in a progressive increase in cAMP with maximal values obtained at 10^{-5} M isoproterenol. Neither PHA nor anti-CD3 mAb elicits cAMP to any appreciable level but rather activate PLCγ1 which results in the turnover of phosphatidylinositol (PI) and generation of increased $[Ca^{2+}]_i$ and activation of PKC [99]. When T cells are exposed to both isoproterenol and PHA or anti-CD3 mAb there is a synergistic rise in cAMP and a reduced proliferative response when compared to that observed with PHA stimulation alone [96, 97]. These results support the hypothesis that the operant interactions of immune with NH linked signals are best described as the induction of a form of sensitivity amplification resulting in otherwise unpredicted significant increases in biochemical and molecular signals capable of modulating lymphocyte reactiveness.

Additional investigations have indicated that a more complex form of sensitivity amplification may occur in vivo. Addition of physiologic concentrations of the synthetic glucocorticoid dexamethasone and prostaglandin E_2 to anti-CD3 mAb stimulated human T cells or CD4 + T cells results in synergistic inhibition of T-cell proliferation [100, 101]. Interestingly, the proliferative response of CD4 + T cells are more susceptible to suppression than unseparated T cells. Although the mechanism(s) responsible for this phenomenon remain to be established, the findings reveal yet another level of complexity that may operate during neuroendocrine-immune interactions. It suggests that not only can combinations of neurally-derived substances simultaneously bind to T cells but that at physiologic concentrations can impair T-cell function. Moreover, this form of neuroimmunomodulation primarily affects a subset of T cells, i.e. CD4 + cells.

Collectively, these data would suggest that if sensitivity amplifiction is operating in these models, small increases in the concentration of neurally derived substances above physiologic levels results in large alterations in lymphocyte function. Thus, this form of amplification has the potential to provide an enormous advantage to neural-immune interactions and correlates well with the role of these interactions in immune homeostasis. It will be interesting to determine if a similar phenomenon occurs with neurohormones and an immune stimulus.

NH Modulation of Immune Function – Future Directions

The evidence is overwhelming that NH can modulate immune function both in vivo and in vitro. What is not clear is how this is effected. In this section we will define some of the questions which are amenable to analysis and whose answers thereto will help establish the biological significance of this particular form of neural-immune regulation.

It would seem reasonable that if NH are to interact effectively with and modulate lymphocyte or macrophage function, these cells should have high-affinity receptors for the various peptides. As previously discussed, membrane receptors for a number of these peptides have been demonstrated on lympho-cytes; however, confirmation of some of these receptors is still lacking. Additionally, there is a paucity of information on the cellular distribution of these receptors although this data is rapidly forthcoming for prolactin and growth hormone receptors (table 1). These data will greatly aid in deciding what types of functional assays should be performed. Moreover, it is equally important to gain an understanding of factors involved in the expression and modulation of these receptors. For example, is the density or affinity of these receptors altered when lymphocytes are activated? Another important missing piece of information is whether the molecular structure of the receptor present on lymphocytes is identical to that found on the target cells for the hormone. The advent of antibodies to these receptors will provide a valuable tool for determining the number of receptor-positive cells as well as the temporal expression of the receptors in relationship to lymphocyte activation.

With the rigorous establishment of membrane receptors for NH on lymphoid cells, attention can then be focused on their mode of action. As previously discussed, there are ample data describing the phenomenologic events which occur when various NH are added to cultures of lymphoid cells. What is lacking for the most part is an in-depth analysis of the biologic, biochemical and molecular events which transpire in the context of the signaling models presented.

Conclusions

In this review we have presented a chain of evidence establishing motive, opportunity and means for interaction between the neuroendocrine and immune systems (table 2). The motive is to enable neurohormones to exert homeostatic control over immune function. This can take the form of either

Table 2. Chain of evidence for neuroendocrine-immune interactions

Motive	immune homeostasis
Opportunity	availability of neurohormones and presence of neurohormone receptors on cells of the immune system
Means	modulates biochemical and molecular events involved in lymphocyte function

facilitatory or inhibitory modulations in immunity. Under normal physiologic conditions the magnitude and duration of this immunomodulation will be limited because the immune system has developed finely-tuned networks and circuits which provide for efficient control. Thus, NH will not have a major influence on immune function but rather an associative and governing role. The opportunity for this form of neuroimmunomodulation to occur is provided by the availability of NH to encounter cells of the immune system in concentrations sufficient to bind to functional receptors on these cells. Because lymphoid and myeloid cells reside in a number of different anatomical sites, their availability to NH will differ. Finally, the means for neurohormonal modulation of immunity occurs as a consequence of NH binding to their receptors on lymphoid and myeloid cells and subsequent induction of biochemical and molecular events which alter cellular function. We have various signaling models which can as first approximations be employed to explore these receptor-ligand interactions. It is important to stress that there is no conclusive evidence indicating that a NH binding to its receptor on a resting lymphocyte (one-signal model) will induce this cell to proliferate or differentiate. This is consistent with the observations indicating that a lymphocyte must receive a number of immune-derived signals to achieve full function.

References

1   Kalden JR, Evans MM, Irvin WJ: The effect of hypophysectomy on the immune response. Immunology 1970;18:671–679.
2   Thrasher SG, Bernardis LL, Cohen S: The immune response in hypothalamic-lesioned and hypophysectomized rats. Int Arch Allergy Appl Immunol 1971;41:813–820.
3   Tyrey L, Nalbandov AV: Influence of anterior hypothalamic lesions on circulating antibody titres in the rat. Am J Physiol 1972;22:179–185.
4   Dann JA, Wachtel SS, Rubin AL: Possible involvement of the central nervous system in graft rejection. Transplantation 1979;27:223–226.
5   Lundin PM: Action of hypophysectomy on antibody formation in the rat. Acta Pathol Microbiol Scand 1960;48:351–357.
6   Gisler RH, Schenkel-Hullinger L: Hormonal regulation of the immune response. II. Influence of pituitary and adrenal activity on immune responsiveness in vitro. Cell Immunol 1971;2:646–657.
7   Comsa J, Leonhardt H, Schwartz JA: Influence of the thymus-corticotropin-growth hormone interaction on the rejection of skin allografts in the rat. Ann NY Acad Sci 1975;249:387–401.
8   Nagy E, Berczi I: Immunodeficiency in hypophysectomized rats. Acta Endocrinol 1978;89:530–537.
9   Prentice ED, Lipscomb H, Metcalf WK, Sharp JG: Effects of hypophysectomy on DNCB-induced contact sensitivity in rats. Scand J Immunol 1976;5:955–961.
10 Saxena QB, Saxena RK, Adler WH: Regulation of natural killer activity in vivo. III. Effect of hypophysectomy and growth hormone treatment on the natural killer activity of the mouse spleen cell population. Int Arch Allergy Appl Immunol 1982;67:169–174.
11 Cross RJ, Markesbery WR, Brooks WH, Roszman TL: Hypothalamic-immune interactions. Neuromodulation of natural killer activity by lesioning of the anterior hypothalamus. Immunology 1984; 51:399–405.

12   Baroni CD, Fabris N, Bertoli G: Effects of hormones on development and function of lymphoid tissues: Synergistic action of thyroxin and somatropic hormone in pituitary dwarf mice. Immunology 1969;17:303–313.

13   Baroni CD, Pesando PC, Bertoli G: Effects of hormones on development and function of lymphoid tissue. II. Delayed development of immunological capacity in pituitary dwarf mice. Immunology 1971;21:455–461.

14   Duquesnoy RJ, Kalpaktsoglou PK, Good RA: Immunological studies on the Snell-Bagg pituitary dwarf mouse. Proc Soc Exp Biol Med 1970;133:201–206.

15   Fabris N, Pierpaoli W, Sorkin E: Hormones and the immunological capacity. III. The immunodeficiency disease of the hypopituitary Snell-Bagg dwarf mouse. Clin Exp Immunol 1971;9:209–225.

16   Fabris N, Pierpaoli W, Sorkin E: Hormones and the immunological capacity. IV. Restorative effective of developmental hormones of lymphocytes on the immunodeficiency syndrome of the dwarf mouse. Clin Exp Immunol 1971;9:227–240.

17   Okouchi E: Thymus, peripheral tissue and immunological responsiveness of the pituitary dwarf mouse. J Physiol Soc Jpn 1976;38:325–335.

18   Murphy WJ, Durum SK, Anver MR, Longo DL: Immunologic and hematologic effects of neuro-endocrine hormones: Studies on DW/J dwarf mice. J Immunol 1992;148:3799–3805.

19   Dumont F, Robert F, Bischoff P: T and B lymphocytes in pituitary dwarf Snell-Bagg mice. Immunology 1979;38:23–31.

20   Schneider GB: Immunological competence in Snell-Bagg pituitary dwarf mice: Response to the contract-sensitizing agent oxazolone. Am J Anat 1976;145:371–380.

21   Cross RJ, Bryson JS, Roszman TL: Immunologic disparity in the hypopituitary dwarf mouse. J Immunol 1992;148:1347–1352.

22   Berczi I: The effects of growth hormone and related hormones on the immune system; in Berczi I (ed): Pituitary Function and Immunity. Boca Raton, CRC Press, 1986, pp 134–159.

23   Berczi I: Immunoregulation by pituitary hormones; in Berczi I (ed): Pituitary Function and Immunity. Boca Raton, CRC Press, 1986, pp 227–240.

24   Berczi I, Nagy E: Prolactin and other lactogenic hormones; in Berczi (ed): Pituitary Function and Immunity. Boca Raton, CRC Press, 1986, pp 162–183.

25   Kelley KW, Brief S, Westly HJ, Novakofski J, Bechtel PJ, Simon J, Walker EB: GH_3 pituitary adenoma cells can reverse thymic aging in rats. Proc Natl Acad Sci USA 1986;83:5663–5667.

26   Cross RJ, Campbell J, Roszman TL: Potentiation of antibody responsiveness after the transplantation of a syngeneic pituitary gland. J Neuroimmunol 1989;25:29–35.

27   Cross RJ, Brooks WH, Roszman TL, Markesbery WR: Transplantation of syngeneic pituitary graft fails to restore T-cell function and thymus morphology in aged mice. Mech Aging Dev 1990;56:11–22.

28   Stein M, Schiavi RC, Camerino M: Influene of brain and behavior on the immune system. Science 1976;191:435–440.

29   Cross RJ, Markesbery WR, Brooks WH, Roszman TL: Hypothalamic-immune interactions. I. The acute effect of anterior hypothalamic lesions on the immune response. Brain Res 1980;196:79–87.

30   Roszman TL, Cross RJ, Brooks WH, Markesbery WR: Neuroimmunomodulation: Effects of neural lesions on cellular immunity; in Guillemin R, Cohn M, Melnechuk T (eds): Neural Modulation of Immunity. New York, Raven Press, 1985, pp 95–109.

31   Brooks WH, Cross RJ, Roszman TL, Markesbery WR: Neuroimmunomodulation: Neural anatomical basis for impairment and facilitiation. Ann Neurol 1982;12:56–61.

32   Goldowitz D, Scheff S, Cotman C: The specificity of reactive synaptogenesis: Comparative study in the adult rat hippocampal formation. Brain Res 1979;170:427–441.

33   Cross RJ, Brooks WH, Roszman TL, Markesbery WR: Hypothalamic-immune interactions. Effects of hypophysectomy on neuroimmunomodulation. J NeuroSci 1982;53:557–566.

34   Cross RJ, Jackson JC, Brooks WH, Sparks DL, Markesbery WR, Roszman TL: Neuroimmunomodulation: Impairment of humoral immune responsiveness by 6-hydroxydopamine treatment. Immunology 1986;57:145–152.

35   Cross RJ, Brooks WH, Roszman TL: Modulation of T-suppressor cell activity by central nervous system catecholamine depletion. J Neurosci Res 1987;18:75–81.

36 Besedovsky HD, Sorkin E: Immunologic-neuroendocrine circuits: Physiological approaches; in Ader R (ed): Psychoneuroimmunology. New York, Academic Press, 1981, pp 545–574.
37 MacLean D, Reichlin S: Neuroendocrinology and the immune process; in Ader R (ed): Psychoneuroimmunology. New York, Academic Press, 1981, pp 405–428.
38 Blalock JE: The immune system as a sensory organ. J Immunol 1984;132:1067–1070.
39 Blalock JE, Smith EM: A complete regulatory loop between the immune and neuroendocrine systems. Fed Proc 1985;44:108–111.
40 Blalock JE, Smith EM, Meyer WJ: The pituitary-adrenocortical axis and the immune system. Clin Endocrinol Metab 1985;14:1021–1038.
41 Payan DG, McGillis JP, Goetzl E: Neuroimmunology. Adv Immunol 1986;39:299–323.
42 Plaut M: Lymphocyte hormone receptors. Annu Rev Immunol 1987;5:621–669.
43 Sibinga NES, Goldstein A: Opioid peptides and opioid receptors in cells of the immune system. Annu Rev Immunol 1988;6:219–249.
44 Bost KL: Hormone and neuropeptide receptors on mononuclear leukocytes. Prog Allergy 1988;43: 68–83.
45 Kelley KW: Growth hormone, lymphocytes and macrophages. Biochem Pharmacol 1989;38:705–713.
46 Carr DJJ, Blalock JE: Neuropeptide hormones and receptors common to the immune and neuroendocrine systems: Bidirectional pathway of intersystem communication; in Ader R, Felten D, Cohen N (eds): Psychoneuroimmunology. San Diego, Academic Press, 1991, pp 573–588.
47 Auernhammer CJ, Strasburger CJ: Effects of growth hormone and insulin-like growth factor I on the immune system. Eur J Endocrinol 1995;133:635–645.
48 Katoh M, Raguet S, Zachwieja J, Dijane J, Kelly PA: Hepatic prolactin receptors in the rat: Characterization using monoclonal antireceptor antibodies. Endocrinology 1987;120:739–749.
49 Okamura H, Zachwieja J, Raguet S, Kelly PA: Characterization and applications of monoclonal antibodies to the prolactin receptor. Endocrinology 1989;124:2499–2508.
50 Russell DH, Matrisian L, Kibler R, Larson DF, Poulos B, Magun BE: Prolactin receptors on human lymphocytes and their modulation by cyclosporine. Biochem Biophys Res Commun 1984; 121:899–906.
51 Russell DH, Kibler R, Matrisian L, Larson D, Poulos B, Magun BE: Prolactin receptors on human T and B lymphocytes: Antagonism of prolactin bindidng by cyclosporine. J Immunol 1985;134: 3027–3031.
52 Bellussi G, Mucciioli G, Ghe C, DiCarlo R: Prolactin binding sites in human erythrocytes and lymphocytes. Life Sci 1987;41:951–959.
53 Pellegrini I, Lebrun JJ, Ali S, Kelly PA: Expression of prolactin and its receptor in human lymphoid cells. Mol Endocrinol 1992;6:1023–1031.
54 Yoh CY, Phillips JT: Prolactin rreceptor exxpression by lymphoid tissues in normal and immunized rats. Mol Cell Endocrinol 1993;92:R21–R25.
55 Gala RR, Shevach EM: Identification by analytical flow cytometry of prolactin receptors on immunocompetent cell populations in the mouse. Endocrinology 1993;133:1617–1623.
56 Gagnrault M-C, Touraine P, Savino W, Kelly PA, Dardenne M: Expression of prolactin receptors in murine lymphoid cells in normal and autoimmune situations. J Immunol 1993;150:5673–5681.
57 Dardenne M, do Carmo M, De Moraes L, Kelly PA, Gagnerault M-C: Prolactin receptor expression in human hematopoietic tissues analyzed by flow cytometry. Endocrinology 1994;134:2108–2114.
58 O'Neal KD, Schwarz LA, Yu-Lee LY: Prolactin receptor gene expression in lymphoid cells. Mol Cell Endocrinol 1991;82:127–135.
59 Di Carlo R, Bole-Feysot C, Gualillo O, Meli R, Nagano M, Kelly PA: Regulation of prolactin receptor mRNA expression in peripheral lymphocytes in rats in response to changes in serum concentrations of prolactin. Endocrinology 1995;136:4713–4716.
60 Lesniak MA, Roth J, Gorden P, Gavin JR: Human growth hormone radioreceptor assay using cultured human lymphocytes. Nature 1973;241:20–22.
61 Lesniak MA, Gorden P, Roth J, Gavin JR: Binding of ^{125}I-human growth hormone to specific receptors in human cultured lymphocytes. J Biol Chem 1974;249:1661–1667.

62   Rapaport R, Sills IN, Green L, Barrett P, Labus J, Skuza KA, Chartoff A, Goode L, Stene M, Peterson BH: Detection of human growth hormone receptors on IM-9 cells and peripheral blood mononuclear cell subsets by flow cytometry: Correlation with growth hormone-binding protein levels. J Clin Endocrinol Metabolism 1995;80:2612–2619.

63   Gagnerault M-C, Postel-Vinay M-C, Dardenne M: Expression of growth hormone receptors in murine lymphoid cells analyzed by flow cytofluorometry. Endocrinology 1996;137:1719–1726.

64   Badolato R, Bond HM, Valerio G, Petrella A, Morrone G, Waters MJ, Venuta S, Tenore A: Differential surface expression of growth hormone receptor on human peripheral blood lymphocytes detected by dual fluorochrome flow cytometry. J Clin Endocrinol Metab 1994;79:984–990.

65   Arrenbrecht S: Specific binding of growth hormone to thymocytes. Nature 1974;242:255–257.

66   Hazum E, Chang K, Cuatrecassas P: Specific nonopiate receptors for beta-endorphin. Science 1979; 205:1033–1035.

67   Mehriski JN, Mills IH: Opiate receptors on lymphocytes and platelets. Clin Immunol Immunopathol 1983;27:240–249.

68   Gaveriaux C, Peluso J, Simonin F, Laforet J, Kieffer B: Identification of κ- and δ-opioid receptor transcripts in immune cells. FEBS Lett 1995;369:272–276.

69   Lawrence DMP, El-Hamouly W, Archer S, Leary JF, Bidlack JM: Identification of κ opioid receptors in the immune system by indirect immunofluorescence. Proc Natl Acad Sci USA 1995;92:1062–1066.

70   Chuang LF, Chuang TK, Killam KF Jr, Chuang AJ, Kung H-F, Yu L, Chuang RY: Delta opioid receptor gene expression in lymphocytes. Biochem Biophys Res Commun 1994;202:1291–1299.

71   Johnson HM, Smith EM, Torres BA, Blalock JE: Neuroendocrine hormone regulation of in vitro antibody production. Proc Natl Acad Sci USA 1982;79:4171–4174.

72   Smith EM, Brosan P, Meyer WJ, Blalock JE: A corticotropin (ACTH) receptor on human mononuclear lymphocytes: Correlation with adrenal ACTH receptor activity. N Engl J Med 1987;317: 1266–1269.

73   Clarke BL, Bost KL: Differential expression of functional adenocorticotropic hormone receptors by subpopulation of lymphocytes. J Immunol 1989;143:464–469.

74   Chabaud O, Lissitzky S: Thyrotropin-specific binding to human peripheral blood monocytes and polymorphonuclear leukocytes. Mol Cell Endocrinol 1977;7:79–87.

75   Coutelier JP, Kehrl JH, Bellur SS, Kohn LD, Nokins AL, Prabhakar BS: Binding and functional effects of thyroid-stimulating hormone on human immune cells. J Clin Immunol 1990;10:204–210.

76   Bernton EW: prolactin and immune host defenses. Prog Neuroendocrinimmunol 1989;2:21–29.

77   Besedovsky H, Del Ray A, Sorkin E: Regulatory immune-neuro-endocrine feedback loops; in Berczi I (ed): Pituitary Function and Immunity. Boca Raton, CRC Press, 1986, pp 241–249.

78   Roszman TL, Carlson SL: Neural-immune interactions: Circuits and networks. Prog Neuroendocrinimmunol 1991;4:69–78.

79   Cross RJ, Roszman TL: Neuroendocrine modulation of immune function: The role of prolactin. Prog Neuroendocrinimmunol 1989;2:17–20.

80   Johnson HM, Torres BA: Immunoregulatory properties of neuroendocrine peptide hormones. Prog Allergy, Basel, Karger, 1988, vol 43, pp 37–67.

81   Murphy WJ, Rui H, Longo DL: Effects of growth hormone and prolactin immune development and function. Life Sci 1995;57:1–14.

82   Besedovsky HO, Del Ray A: Immune-neuro-endocrine interactions: Facts and hypotheses. Endocr Rev 1996;17:64–102.

83   Fu YK, Arkins S, Wang BS, Kelley KW: A novel role of growth hormone and insulin-like growth factor-1: Priming neutrophils for superoxide anion secretion. J Immunol 1991;146:1602–1608.

84   Janeway CA, Bottomly K: Signals and signs for lymphocyte responses. Cell 1994;76:275–285.

85   Jenkins MK, Ashwell JD, Schwartz RH: Allogeneic non-T helper cells restore the responsiveness of normal T-cell clones stimulated with antigen and chemically modified antigen-presenting cells. J Immunol 1988;140:3324–3330.

86   Paul WE, Seder RA: Lymphocyte responses and cytokines. Cell 1994;76:241–251.

87   Schwartz RH: Models of T-cell anergy: Is there a common molecular mechanism. J Exp Med 1996; 184:1–8.

88 Clevenger CV, Torigoe T, Reed JC: Prolactin induces rapid phosphorylation and activation of prolactin receptor-associated RAF-1 kinase in a T-cell line. J Biol Chem 1994;269:5559–5565.

89 Dusanter-Fourt I, Muller O, Ziemiecki A, Mayeux P, Drucker B, Kjiane J, Wilks A, Harpur AG, Fischer S, Gisselbrecht S: Identification of JAK protein tyrosine kinases as signaling molecules for prolactin: Functional analysis of prolactin receptor and prolactin-erythropoietin receptor chimera expressed in lymphoid cells. EMBO J 1994;13:2583–2591.

90 Palestine AG, Muellenberg-Coulombre CG, Kim MK, Gelato MC, Nussenblatt RB: Bromocriptine and low dose cyclosporine in the treatment of experimental autoimmune uveitis in the rat. J Clin Invest 1987;79:1078–1081.

91 Buskila D, Sukenik S, Shoenfeld Y: The possible role of prolactin in autoimmunity. Am J Reprod Immunol 1991;26:118–123.

92 McMurray R, Keisler D, Kanuckel K, Izui S, Walker SE: Prolactin influences autoimmune disease activity in the female B/W mouse. J Immunol 1991;147:3780–3787.

93 Riskind PN, Massacesi L, Doolittle TH, Hauser SL: The role of prolactin in autoimmune demye-lination: Suppression of experimental allergic encephalomyelitis by bromocriptine. Ann Neurol 1991;29:542–547.

94 Jara LJ, Lavalle C, Fraga A, Gomez-Sanchez C, Silveria LH, Martinez-Osuna P, Germain BF, Espinoza LR: Prolactin, immunoregulation, and autoimmune diseases. Semin Arthritis Rheum 1991;20:273–284.

95 Hawkins TA, Gala RR, Dunbar JC: Prolactin modulates the incidence of diabetes in male and female NOD mice. FASEB J 1993;7:A20.

96 Carlson SL, Brooks WH, Roszman TL: Neurotransmitter-lymphocyte interactions: Dual receptor modulation of lymphocyte proliferation and cAMP production. J Neuroimmunol 1989;24:155–162.

97 Carlson SL, Trauth K, Brooks WH, Roszman TL: Enhancement and adaptation of beta-adrenergic-induced cAMP accumulation in T-cells. J Cell Physiol 1994;161:39–48.

98 Koshland DE, Goldbeter A, Stock JB: Amplification and adaptation in regulatory and sensory systems. Science 1982;217:220–225.

99 Altman A, Coggeshell KM, Mustelin T: Molecular events mediating T-cell activation. Adv Immunol 1990;48:227–360.

100 Elliott LH, Brooks WH, Roszman TL: Inhibition of anti-CD3 monoclonal antibody induced T-cell proliferation by dexamethosone, isproterenol or prostaglandin E_2 either alone or in combination. Cell Mol Neurobiol 1992;14:1–7.

101 Elliott LH, Levay AK, Sparks B, Miller M, Roszman TL: Dexamethosone and prostaglandin E_2 modulate T-cell receptor signaling through a cAMP-independent mechanism. Cell Immunol 1996; 169:117–124.

Thomas L. Roszman, PhD, University of Kentucky College of Medicine,
Department of Microbiology and Immunology, Lexington, KY 40536-0084 (USA)
Tel. (606) 323 5913, Fax (606) 257 8994

Author Index

Subject Index

Cytokine, *see also* specific cytokines
  central nervous system feedback 120, 121
  classification 186
  common properties 42, 43
  four-helix bundle motif 81–84
  glial cell response 48–61
  hormonal activities 185–198
Cytokine receptor, *see also* specific cytokines
  crystal structures 77, 79, 80
  domains 79, 80
  oligomerization 84
  signal transduction 77, 78
  structural comparison of classes 80, 81
  superfamily classes 77

Dopamine receptor
  lymphocyte expression 137, 138
  subtypes 137

Endorphin
  functions in immune system 21, 22,
    158–161, 208
  induction and properties in immune
    system 10, 11
  processing 16, 158
  receptor expression in immune cells 138,
    139, 207
Enkephalin
  functions in immune system 160, 161
  induction and properties in immune
    system 3, 4
Experimental autoimmune encephalitis
  cytokine expression 42
  glial cell function abnormalities 39,
    41, 42
  inflammatory infiltrate composition
    31, 32

Follicle-stimulating hormone, induction and
  properties in immune system 6

Glial cell, *see also* Astrocyte, Microglia,
  Oligodendrocyte
  abnormal function in neurological disease
    39, 41, 42
  classification and functions 32–35, 37–39
  cytokine response 48–61

Granulocyte-macrophage colony
  stimulating factor
  hormonal activities 195
  microglia response 54, 55
Growth hormone
  age-related changes in expression 172
  cell types in immune system
    production 17
  crystal structure of complex with receptor
    86–89
  epitopes 89
  functions in immune system 20, 21, 172,
    173, 204, 205, 209
  induction and properties in immune
    system 6, 14
  receptor 84, 85, 207
  structure 85
Growth hormone-releasing hormone,
  induction and properties in immune
  system 7, 8, 14

Inflammatory infiltrate, cellular
  composition in central nervous system
    disease 31, 32
Insulin-like growth factor-I
  functions in immune system 20, 21
  induction and properties in immune
    system 9
  receptor expression in immune cells
    146
Interferon-α
  clinical applications 196
  hormonal activities overview 187, 188
Interferon-γ
  astrocyte effects 49–52
  clinical applications 196
  immune cell secretion 46
  induction by arginine vasopressin
    161–163
  microglia response 56
  oligodendrocyte effects 58, 60
  receptor
    components 46, 91
    crystal structure of ligand complex
      92–94
    signal transduction 46, 91, 94, 95
  structure 91, 92